Nursing Evidence-Based Practice

Karen Holland and **Colin Rees**

Series Editor **Karen Holland**

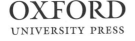

OXFORD

UNIVERSITY PRESS

Great Clarendon Street, Oxford ox2 6DP

Oxford University Press is a department of the University of Oxford.
It furthers the University's objective of excellence in research, scholarship,
and education by publishing worldwide in

Oxford New York

Auckland Cape Town Dar es Salaam Hong Kong Karachi
Kuala Lumpur Madrid Melbourne Mexico City Nairobi
New Delhi Shanghai Taipei Toronto

With offices in

Argentina Austria Brazil Chile Czech Republic France Greece
Guatemala Hungary Italy Japan Poland Portugal Singapore
South Korea Switzerland Thailand Turkey Ukraine Vietnam

Oxford is a registered trade mark of Oxford University Press
in the UK and in certain other countries

Published in the United States
by Oxford University Press Inc., New York

British Library Cataloguing in Publication Data

Data available

Library of Congress Cataloging in Publication Data

Data available

Typeset by MPS Limited, A Macmillan Company
Printed in Great Britain on acid-free paper by
Ashford Colour Press Limited, Gosport, Hampshire

ISBN 978–0–19–956310–4

1 3 5 7 9 10 8 6 4 2

Foreword

This book reflects a significant moment in time for the nursing profession. Over the next few years the majority of newly qualified nurses will graduate with an expectation that they have been prepared to fulfil pivotal clinical leadership roles. An ageing population will bring an unprecedented increase in demand for nursing care. The numbers of individuals living with long-term and often multiple conditions will grow exponentially, resulting in more patients living with a range of health problems such as pain, anxiety, fatigue, or reduced mobility. The management of all of these problems lies at the heart of nursing practice and the quality of life of patients and their families will be heavily influenced by the effectiveness of the clinical decisions made by nurses

In future, the registered nurse will be responsible and accountable for the provision of compassionate, expert and **evidence-based** interventions across all domains of nursing care. There will also be growing pressures on nurses to assess the impact of these clinical decisions on patient outcomes using a range of measures or metrics. The key to meeting these agendas resides in clear articulation and implementation of evidence-based nursing care. Student nurses and their educators must therefore embrace this concept and demonstrate a robust understanding of research principles as well as the skills to identify and critique existing research which can inform best practice. This excellent new text by Karen Holland and Colin Rees is ideally placed to support the next generation of nurses in embedding evidence-based care in practice.

Of course evidence-based nursing is not new, indeed Florence Nightingale's success in achieving radical changes to hygiene practices was realized by the use of rigorously analysed epidemiological data when arguing with politicians! Since then growing numbers of nurses have led research and every nurse is expected to be research aware. All pre-registration courses now include evidence-based nursing modules and numerous textbooks have been written to support this learning. However, few texts have addressed the translation of an understanding of research methods into taking responsibility for applying evidence to nursing practice. Instead, research has largely been seen as an 'add on' extra. This new book has been designed to fill that vacuum by clearly articulating the meaning of evidence-based nursing practice. This includes embedding an understanding of research and evidence into all aspects of care, taking responsibility for ensuring that nursing decisions are based on up-to-date evidence, recognizing evidence gaps and making the case for more research effort in these areas. Karen and Colin have produced a book which will give student nurses a firm foundation for building professional confidence as evidence base practitioners. They use straightforward language and well-chosen scenarios to bring the concepts of evidence-based practice to life. They cover a range of research methods and clearly identify the types of evidence each method will generate. Their approach will help nurses make informed decisions about managing nursing care.

This text makes an invaluable contribution to the evidence-based nursing agenda. Giving students a clear steer from the beginning of their course, it will set them on the right path to becoming confident, accountable, evidence-based professionals. This new generation will be able to think critically on all aspects of nursing care, be accountable for their clinical decisions, and for assessing the outcomes. In turn means they will deliver the highest quality nursing care and have the greatest possible impact on the health of patients and their families.

Professor Dame Jill Macloed Clark

To my son Gareth who qualified as a mental health nurse in 2009, for his contribution to my understanding of the student nurse experience and to the online material for the book. I am proud of his achievement, dedication, and commitment to nursing practice.

Karen Holland

To my mum Enid and granddaughter Nia: one left this world and the other entered it during work on this book. With heartfelt appreciation and love to my wife Brenda, who supported me and shared both events.

Colin Rees

Series editor preface

A message from the Series Editor

Learning to be a nurse requires students to develop a set of skills and a knowledge base which will enable them to make the transition from learner to qualified nurse. As with any transition this can often seem at times to be a daunting prospect, and one where the student may ask 'how am I *ever* going to learn all that I need to know to get through this course and become a qualified nurse?'.

For student nurses this experience entails learning in 'two worlds', that of the university and that of the clinical environment. Although there is a physical distinction between the two, it is important that the learning that takes place in one is integrated with the learning in the other. This series of books has set out to do just that.

These 'two worlds' require that students learn two sets of skills in order to qualify as a nurse and be ready to take on further sets of skills in whatever nursing environment they are employed in. The skills which will be a core part of this series are numerous, and central to them is that of 'coping with the unknown'. This being in relation to facing a new environment each time they start a new clinical placement, communicating with patients and a large number of health and social care professionals, dealing with difficult and often complex situations, and sometimes stressful clinical experiences. In the university there are also situations which may be unknown, such as learning new study skills, working with others, searching and finding information, and managing workloads. It is every student's goal to complete their course with the required foundation for the future and it is the essential goal of this series to enable the student to develop skills for a successful learning and nursing experience.

The central ethos to all the books therefore is to facilitate and enhance the student learning experience and develop their skills, through engaging with a variety of reflective accounts, exercises, and web-based resources. We hope that you as the reader and learner enjoy reading these books and that the guidance within them supports your goal of successfully completing your course of study.

Karen Holland
Series Editor

Preface and acknowledgements

Learning to become a qualified nurse involves not only engaging with theoretical learning experiences but most importantly engaging with patients in clinical practice. Ensuring that their care is based on the best possible and appropriate evidence is an essential part of the role of the nurse, and learning the skills and knowledge to enable you to do this is the essential reason for why we chose to write this book. Our overall aim therefore is to enable you to have a learning resource which will support your ability to link the theory of research and evidence-based practice with the actual reality of your learning experiences, both in the classroom and in clinical practice.

Our approach to setting out the content in the book, is based on many years of engaging with both student and qualified nurses and learning from them what relevant skills and knowledge they require to be able to progress in their careers. Our approach has been whenever possible, to place ourselves in that student experience.

This is not a book that will tell you absolutely everything you need to know about research and evidence-based practice. It will give you a foundation on which to build more advanced knowledge and skills in the future or that stimulates your interest to learn more. We have structured the book in such a way that will enable you to do this, each chapter introduces a key element of evidence-based practice and together they should be viewed as making up the whole picture of what is required to implement evidence based nursing practice.

Acknowledgements

We wish to acknowledge the support given to us by Geraldine Jeffers, who inspired us to write this book as well as her enthusiasm and commitment to the student experience. Our thanks also to the excellent reviewers for their constructive feedback which we have used to shape the development of the chapters and acknowledge their contribution to some of the ideas we have introduced to facilitate student learning. Thanks also to the many students we have both taught over our careers, who have shaped our thinking and enabled us to gain an insight into their learning needs to write this book.

Karen Holland and Colin Rees

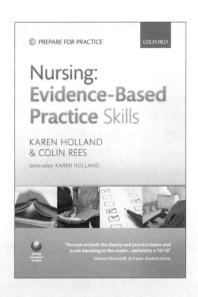
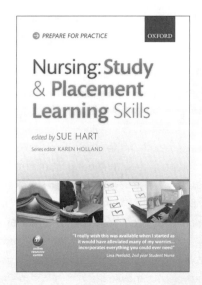

Contents

Detailed table of contents

About the authors

Karen Holland

Karen Holland is Editor of *Nurse Education in Practice* an international nurse education journal. She is author of two published books which are widely used by student nurses, as well as published articles focusing on their experiences. She has had an extensive career in both nursing practice and education, with her main area of work focusing on teaching research and evidence-based practice, undertaking small and large research projects as well as developing the skills and knowledge of practitioners to understand and use research and evidence in practice. Her main area of interest and ongoing project activity at the University of Salford is in enhancing the student learning experience through ensuring their programmes of learning are evidence-based. She is an advocate of students learning to write for publication and to dissemination of their learning.

Colin Rees

Colin Rees is a lecturer at Cardiff University where he has taught research methods on a variety of courses for many years. He is author of *An Introduction to Research for Midwives*, now about to appear in its third edition and has published frequently on a variety of health topics. Unusually, he is not a health professional but a sociologist by training. However, through his teaching of health professionals from a variety of disciplines, he is able to apply research principles to health care issues. He sees his main role as enabling health professionals to become confident users of research, and to help them see research as part of professional and clinical practice within the context of evidence-based practice. Colin teaches research internationally to nurses and others in Wales, the Caribbean, Germany, and Oman.

Walk through preface

Nursing: Evidence-Based Practice Skills explains what nursing research is and outlines the skills of evidence based practice required to be a nurse. This brief tour of the book shows readers how to get the most out of this textbook and web package.

It's all new to me!

Find what you need fast!

The detailed list of contents in the front of the book and the chapter aims at the start of each chapter will help you find what you need quickly.

What does that mean?

Nursing research has a language of its own but it's easy to understand! Each new term is highlighted in colour in the text and explained in the glossary at the back of the book – you can also revise these online.

Click search and you will get a more recent search. For each neath the reference for options such as 'cited by' followed by will give you more recent articles that have cited this article is an example of 'Forward chaining', described later. There 'Related Articles' and clicking this will allow you to find other search.

Helping you to develop your skills

EBP in action

These activities provide guidance on key aspects of the research process and are intended to help you to acquire the practical skills that are required for your academic assignments and your evidence-based nursing practice.

+ ⋯⋯⋯⋯⋯⋯⋯⋯⋯⋯⋯⋯⋯⋯⋯⋯⋯⋯

EBP in action

Imagine you are receiving treatment for a chronic health pro an outpatient basis every 6 months or so. At one visit you are ment trial about to start and you are asked if you would like questions that you might like answered before you make a de or not.

Key points

Essential facts, advice, and tips are highlighted to help you understand particular issues and to avoid common mistakes.

! **Key points**

Before undertaking an interview you need to prepare, pre should have a thoroughly prepared set of questions, with involved. The participants need to be invited with plenty o bring an extra set of batteries for your digital recorder!

Thinking about

Issues relating to research and evidence-based practice can be complex – these boxes encourage readers to develop an awareness of key concepts and practices, and build their knowledge beyond an introductory level.

> **? Thinking about**
>
> How far would you support the view that learning the skill d important a professional skill as learning a clinical techniqu one's health be disadvantaged or life put in danger becaus the literature?

Research examples

It is often said that the most important features to look for when buying a house are location, location, location! A parallel for learning about nursing research is examples, examples, examples! Real examples of seminal and contemporary nursing research provide a context for the concepts and skills which are discussed in the chapter text.

> **The Unpopular Patient by Felicity Stockwell**
>
> A study which utilized non-participant observation a today is that of the Unpopular Patient undertaken b 33) (see Chapter 1 for access to this report on the RC 'observations of incidents, conversations and comment study' and had told the staff only 'that the researcher relationships on the ward'. Her observations were sel different focus to her observations during her observat above) obtain a copy of her study and decide whethe from your experience in clinical practice. In other words about still valid in relation to patients you have come int such as this undertaken over 35 years ago may still be val replicated to determine for definite. You may also wish of an assignment (see Chapter 9).

Nursing case studies

It can be difficult to integrate research theory and evidence-based skills into real practice at first, so these case studies highlight how evidence can be utilized in care delivery.

> **+ Case study** Emma:
>
> Emma, a 6 year old child has undergone a tonsillectomy (rem are trying to get her to eat and drink post-operatively withou know she can do this before they send her home. Her mothe was unsure whether she should. She felt however that she her do things.
> What does the research evidence tell us about this scenari

Summary and further information

Every chapter ends with a list of the most important points for readers to take note of and to aid easy review and revision. Readers are then prompted to visit the online resource centre (where they will find useful tools including online references for essay writing). The authors have also identified helpful books and websites which are highly useful for study, assignments, and practice.

> ■ **Online resource centre**
>
> To learn more about searching the literature, please ne
> www.oxfordtextbooks.co.uk/orc/holland/ to find mor
>
> ■ **References**
>
> Beecroft, C., Rees, A. & Booth, A. (2006) Finding the evidenc *The Research Process in Nursing* (5th edn). Oxford Blackwell.
> Bryman, A. (2008) *Social Research Methods* (3rd edn.) Oxfor
> Burns, N., & Grove, S. (2009) *The Practice of Nursing R Generation of Evidence* (6th ed.) St. Louis: Saunders.
> Cronin, P., Ryan, F., & Coughlin, M. (2008) Undertaking a literat

Online resource centre

Nursing students need to use a variety of online nursing materials throughout their course to find information, research, and develop their 'literature searching' skills – this book has a dedicated website to help you get started! Just save the url in your 'favourites' in your web browser and go there when instructed to in the book:

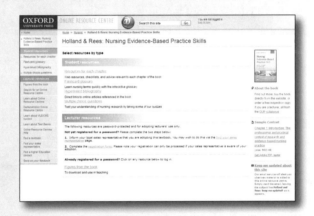

www.oxfordtextbooks.co.uk/orc/holland/

Students can:

- Learn nursing terms quickly with the interactive glossary
- Download practical checklists for placements
- Save time by using the hyper links to the references in the book which will take you straight to the journal articles
- Get ahead with 'insider' sources of further information and guidelines
- Look at examples of evidence-based resources and packages to help you with project work
- Test your understanding of nursing research by taking some of our quizzes

For lecturers:

- You can download the figures for the book and use the resources in your classes

Introduction

The professional and practical context of research and evidence-based nursing practice

Karen Holland and Colin Rees

The aims of this chapter are:

➤ To outline the structure and rationale for the book.

➤ To show how research and evidence-based practice skills will help you to meet some of the standards and competencies required of a student and registered nurse.

➤ To show the importance of research and evidence-based practice in relation to nursing and health care.

Introduction

The first idea about why you might find this book of interest or of value to you as a student nurse is in the title: *Nursing: evidence-based practice skills*. You may have seen in your course handbook that there is a module you have to undertake with a similar title, or you may have been introduced to the term evidence in relation to undertaking your first assignment. So what is 'research', 'evidence', and 'evidence-based practice' (EBP) and why are they important topics for inclusion in your course? These topics can at first seem very daunting and you may wonder 'what have they to do with what I need to learn to be a nurse–I am not here to learn to be a researcher!'

We believe that they are essential not only because they ultimately have an impact on patient care, but also because through learning about them you will also develop a set of skills that can be transferred into other areas of your learning experience as a student nurse, such as problem solving, critical thinking, and analysis and how to use the nursing process: assessing, planning, implementing, and evaluating care.

This book is aimed at helping you to understand the relevance of research and EBP to you as a student nurse and when you achieve registration to practise as a qualified nurse. It must be made clear at the outset that this book cannot give you all the information about research and EBP—both subjects are enormous and library shelves are filled with volumes of books on the subject. We believe that as a student nurse you need an introduction to the key concepts together with practical tips on how to use research and evidence in your nursing practice as well as in your academic work. For those who wish to study research in more depth (for final year projects or post qualified courses), supplementary reading of traditional research textbooks will be necessary and you will be directed to other texts for supplementary reading when relevant.

One manuscript reviewer challenged us to consider what was so different about this book to all the others on the book shelves. We believe it is different in that it actually links the subject to the student learning experience, i.e. what knowledge you *need* to know and how to develop skills to *use* that knowledge as a nurse. Too many books just describe the research process or only tell you how to implement evidence in practice, they rarely do both or do both well. Instead we have focused on both the fundamental theory of research and on the practical use of research and evidence that you require as a student nurse so that on registration as a qualified nurse you have the skill set you need.

Throughout the chapters you will find short 'EBP in action' boxes with exercises which help to guide you to a better understanding of some of the issues being addressed and also illustrations of how others have experienced either doing research or utilizing evidence in practice. You may choose not to do these of course, but we have based them on our own experiences of supporting students to understand both the topics themselves and how they can be used to achieve your learning goals in university assignments, classroom work but most importantly in your clinical practice.

The book sets out to 'talk to you' as a student nurse, and possibly someone with very little knowledge of research and experience of EBP. From our experience students are often daunted by the words research and EBP, yet become less so if they are explained clearly and in a language which they can relate to from their own personal experience. We have tried to do so in this book and much of the content is based on our teaching and related practice experience, including feedback from students.

Each chapter focuses on topics that will help you to both understand the principles of EBP and demonstrate their usefulness and relevance to your learning in university and practice. They can be read and used as individual chapters but also viewed as a whole approach to learning about different aspects of research and evidence, their utilization in practice and in your academic work.

Overview of the book's content

Chapter 1 (this chapter) focuses on the rationale for the book and the key concepts as they relate to nursing and health care.

Chapter 2 focuses on the basic principles of EBP. It also focuses on the hierarchy of evidence because it is important for the student nurse to appreciate different kinds of evidence and gain an understanding of how this is evident in the literature.

Chapter 3 seeks to demystify research and relate it to a similar process you might meet in practice: the nursing process. It will also help you to understand the different components of a research proposal and will establish the background to some of the chapters which explore some of components in more depth.

Chapter 4 will give an explanation of qualitative research design, including different methodologies such as ethnography and phenomenology and associated methods such as non-participant observation, focus group interviews and interviews. The ethical issues related to qualitative research will also be explored as will various approaches to analysis of data.

Chapter 5 will focus on quantitative research design, including methodological approaches such as survey, experiments, and randomized control trials. Ethical issues associated with quantitative research will be discussed.

Chapter 6 is a critical chapter in the book, in that it focuses on how evidence can be found and in particular offers a systematic way of doing so.

Chapter 7 will focus on how the knowledge and understanding gained in Chapters 2–6 can be used in evaluating and appraising evidence in a constructive and critical way. These earlier chapters are essential in helping you understand terminology found in research articles, why the different methodologies have been used and most importantly enable you to appraise the quality of the study in relation to different aspects of the research process and overall design.

Patient care needs to be delivered and supported by the best and most appropriate evidence. Chapter 8 will facilitate your understanding of the importance of EBP and in particular how it can be implemented in nursing and health care. It offers examples of how you the student can link learning and developing skills in research and EBP in such areas as developing a care plan in practice or how to search for evidence to undertake feedback to a group when undertaking a problem/enquiry-based learning scenario related to a practice experience.

During your programme of study from student to registered nurse there will be many assignments to complete, including for some a dissertation or extended study. Chapter 9 will help you to develop the skills in relation to using different kinds of evidence and to make best use of it within your written work.

There will also be occasions during your programme of study when a presentation of work undertaken will be required. This could either be on your own or as a group.

You may also be required to provide written work as part of this activity. Chapter 10 will focus on how to make the best use of evidence for this kind of activity, and also how to disseminate and publish some of your course work or other writing.

The language of 'research' and 'evidence' can be daunting and to help you there is also a Glossary of terms included which gives you easy access to key words, which can be referred to as a memory aid in those situations where you might just need a quick reference. It could be to check for example on a word or term you have found in an article but couldn't quite remember what it meant.

Although in the main this book is aimed at student nurses in the United Kingdom, there are many similarities to the student experience in other countries. The issue of what research skills and knowledge are required to register as a qualified nurse and enable the implementation of EBP is a global one. We will refer to this issue in the book.

Before we look at the professional and practice context of evidence-based nursing, it is important to introduce what some of the key terms of 'research' and 'evidence' mean. Many of these will also be found in the Glossary of terms for easy access and you will find them indicated in **bold and in colour** throughout the text.

What is research?

It appears that there are many different definitions of research, but for the purpose of this book, which focuses on nursing research, the following definition by Parahoo (1997: 7) remains a useful one:

> 66 Nursing research is an umbrella term for all research into nursing practice and issues related to it. It can be defined as the systematic and rigorous collection of data on the organisation, delivery, uses and outcomes of nursing care for the purpose of enhancing clients' health. It is not only about what nurses do, but also about clients' behaviour, knowledge, beliefs, attitudes, perceptions and other factors influencing how they make use of, and experience, care and treatment. 99

Parahoo does however state (2006: 9) that:

> 66 definitions of nursing research are difficult to find mainly because of the lack of consensus in the definition of nursing and because nurses' roles are constantly evolving and expanding in order to meet new demands. 99

Students in their final year of a nursing course may have already seen changes since they began on the course in how their mentors, as qualified nurses, deliver care.

> **?** **Thinking about it**
>
> Consider this explanation and examine your own view of what nursing is. Do you think that nursing is difficult to define and in particular if nurses' roles are changing, is the breadth of nursing practice now changing?

As we write this book even pre-registration nursing education itself is being evaluated (NMC 2008) and what students of the future need to be able to undertake on qualifying is being determined—see the online resource centre for updates on this post publication.

You will also come across research that has been undertaken to enhance your learning experience (there are several journals on the subject of nurse education) and so the above definition of research could be applied just as effectively to nurse education instead of nursing care, nurse educators not nurses, students not clients and teaching and learning not care and treatment.

We also need to consider how nurses now work within multi-disciplinary teams to deliver care, so that previous areas of practice may now need to be considered differently when planning research. However in many situations, delivery of care is still the domain of nurses, but as Professor Dame Jill Macleod Clark alluded to at the Royal College of Nursing (RCN) Research Conference in 2009, it would appear that, from her analysis of the research presented in conference papers and other evidence, nurses are no longer researching nursing interventions (the care we deliver to patients) and cannot therefore determine the nursing impact on patient care and its improvement (Macleod Clark 2009) (see **http://www.rcn.org.uk/development/ researchanddevelopment/rs/research2009/keynotes/**: accessed December 2009).

Some of you may consider at some point in the future becoming involved in such research and may already have skills and knowledge which go beyond the scope of this book. Consider these chapters as a point of reference for applying these in the context of your course of study and the application to a clinical nursing context. As Macleod Clark (2009) alluded to it is essential for the future of patient care that we not only pursue the research questions in relation to the art of nursing but also not lose sight of those which require a different scientific approach which could impact on how we deliver nursing care and which also allows the outcome to be measured in some way. These are both essential for ensuring that EBP has a rigorous foundation.

Another definition by Thompson et al. (2002: 85) highlights that it is more than just the gathering of data or information on a topic:

> 66 Research is a rigorous process of inquiry designed to provide answers to questions about phenomena of concern in an academic discipline or profession. 99

Hockey (1984: 4) also linked research to a process activity and most importantly to the acquiring of a 'body of knowledge':

> 66 ... an attempt to increase the sum of what is known, usually referred to as a 'body of knowledge' by the discovery of new facts or relationships through a process of systematic scientific enquiry, the research process. 99

Undertaking research involves gathering information to provide answers to questions and how this occurs will depend very much on the nature of the questions themselves and what kind of information is required to answer them. This will in turn require the researcher to approach it in different ways and has led to what can sometimes be a misleading division between what has become to be commonly expressed as 'quantitative research' and 'qualitative research'. The former being research which seeks to measure something and the latter which is more focused on the experience of people.

You may even have been asked to participate in and have experienced this research process by being a part of someone else's research. This will have given you an insight into issues such as questionnaires, interviews, focus groups and informed consent, all of which are discussed in later chapters.

Some of you may have also undertaken a small research project yourself as part of your course of study but this is not a requirement for student nurses in most UK universities. Using research findings and other forms of evidence however is an essential part of being a student nurse in both clinical practice and university contexts. As a qualified nurse you will also be involved in developments linked to research, which Gerrish & McMahon (2006: 5) state:

> 66 involves the systematic use of knowledge obtained through research and/ or practical experience for the purpose of producing new or improved products, processes, systems or services. 99

and which for nurses very much links to practice development. They cite the definition for this by Garbett & McCormack (2002) as:

> 66 Practice development encompasses a broad range of innovations that are initiated to improve practice and the services in which that practice takes place. It involves a continuous process of improvement towards increased effectiveness in patient-centred care. This is brought about by helping health care teams to develop their knowledge and skills and to transform the culture and context of care. 99

Another term often used alongside research and EBP is that of *effectiveness of care* (see above definition) and the term clinical effectiveness is often used in this context. This is a term that you will meet when reading about EBP in particular and it is worth noting some definitions:

> ❝ The extent to which specific clinical interventions when deployed in the field for a particular patient or population do what they are intended to do i.e. maintain and improve health and secure the greatest possible health gain from available resources. ❞

> (NHS Executive 1996)

The Royal College of Nursing (1996) simplified this by stating that:

> ❝ Clinical effectiveness ... is about doing the right thing in the right way for the right person at the right time. This involves getting evidence of what works into everyday clinical practice and evaluating its effect on patient care. ❞

We know however that what was the right evidence to underpin practice 20 years ago may no longer be the best evidence for care in today's nursing and health care. This will be explored further in Chapter 8.

What is evidence-based practice?

Given that research is about gathering evidence through different methods of inquiry then EBP is about **using** this research as evidence. Given that the main focus of this book relates to nursing, we will re-phrase this as evidence-based **nursing** practice.

One of the most well-known definition of EBP is that by Sackett *et al.* (1997: 2):

> ❝ The conscientious, explicit and judicious use of current best evidence about the care of individual patients. ❞

It is important to remember however that the drive for EBP came from the discipline of medicine, and that as Parahoo (2006) cautions, given that nursing practice is so varied and also person-centred we need to ensure that nursing develops its own way rather than 'adopt[ing] the medical definition of evidence-based practice, with its heavy emphasis on systematic reviews and RCT's' (p. 460). His challenge for nursing is:

> " … to take what it finds useful from it, while developing its own body of knowledge using a range of approaches. The strength of nursing research resides in its openness to different research and development methodologies. To impose a medical model of practice development on nursing will be a retrograde step. "
>
> (Parahoo 2006: 460)

However, in order to ensure that the patient receives the best possible care it is important to work collaboratively with other care professions, and that whilst it is important for nursing to develop its unique evidence base, a combined body of knowledge on aspects of care and therefore evidence has a great deal more to offer in terms of effective outcomes for the patient than a uni-professional one. We will be returning to this challenge throughout the book, as we help you develop the skills and knowledge to be a part of evidence-based nursing practice developments.

Of course there are many different types of evidence, which will be explained later in this book, but in the main we shall refer to research evidence when discussing evidence-based (nursing) practice. Other types of evidence will be discussed in Chapter 2.

Newell & Burnard (2006: 203) note that, like research,

> " evidence-based practice is also a process which consists of five stages, which can be aimed at meeting the health needs of an individual or group. "

These are:

1. Asking answerable questions.
2. Finding the best available evidence.
3. Appraising the evidence for its validity and applicability.
4. Applying the results of this appraisal in clinical practice.
5. Evaluating the performance of EBP.

All these stages will be explored throughout the following chapters in the context of nursing and health care practice.

The Joanna Briggs Institute in Australia (which is a Centre for EBP) offers a number of linked definitions focusing on an 'evidence base' to nursing and health care practice: (www.joannabriggs.edu.au/about/eb_nursing.php/)

> 66 *Evidence-based **health care** relates to all the health professions—medicine, nursing and allied health—as well as health policy makers, planners and executives. Simply defined, evidence-based **practice** is the melding of individual clinical judgement and expertise with the best available external evidence to generate the kind of practice that is most likely to lead to a positive outcome for a client or patient.*
>
> *Evidence-based **nursing** is nursing practice that is characterized by these attributes. Evidence-based **clinical practice** takes into account the context within which care takes place; the preferences of the client; and the clinical judgement of the health professional, as well as the best available evidence.* 99

We can see that there is a need for a combination of evidence to be considered, including that of the expert clinical judgement of the practitioner. As a student nurse you will learn to develop this ability to make clinical judgements alongside the skills and knowledge to implement EBP. The latter will depend on your ability to understand and determine the quality and value of research evidence, together with consideration of the patient's situation and preference for care. You will however be doing this under the supervision of a qualified nurse.

EBP in action

During a recent clinical placement experience you will have met many clients/patients and possibly their families and carers. What kind of decisions did the nurses make about their care? Could you determine whether this was based on research based evidence or was the decision very often made on the previous experience and possible 'expert' knowledge of the nurse? Consider how you could meet the following NMC Standard:

- Identify relevant changes in practice or new information and disseminate to colleagues (NMC 2004)

You may choose to search for evidence via the university databases (see Chapter 6) together with talking to specialist nurses, social care workers, and community nurses about the evidence they use to make decisions. Talking to the patient/client and gaining an insight into their personal experience may be another form of evidence. You need to ensure that they give permission to share this knowledge with others and for you to use this as part of their planned care. Gathering this information can be one of your learning goals for that placement. Disseminating it to other students during that placement can be another goal. The information and evidence you have gathered could then be kept in that placement to enable it to be used by the team. Discuss this with your mentor and personal tutor.

Whatever your plan, the decisions made by qualified nurses in practice are not always based on a research evidence base, and at times it may be difficult to discern how they made that decision. It is hoped however that whenever possible that decisions about care will involve the patient. However, this may not always be possible; for example, when a nurse chooses an appropriate wound care treatment this must be based on clinical evidence rather than on patient preference, but if a nurse is considering a different approach to helping a patient to give up smoking this would be a shared decision between nurse and patient.

Why do student nurses need research skills and be able to implement evidence-based practice?

Understanding research, gaining knowledge of how to undertake research and being able to determine what is the best research, together with being able to use research evidence and implement it in practice are key to becoming a qualified nurse. The vast majority of student nurses around the world need to prove they are skilled in this area before they can register. For example, in the United Kingdom the **Nursing and Midwifery Council** (NMC 2004) include specific Standards of Proficiency that all student nurses are expected to achieve as part of their learning to be a registered nurse. Standard 7 relates to education, and Box 1.1 outlines what proficiencies for EBP it includes.

> **Box 1.1** Proficiencies for EBP
>
> Standards of proficiency: Care Delivery (Entry to Branch Outcomes)
>
> Demonstrate evidence of a developing knowledge base which underpins safe and effective practice:
>
> * Access and discuss research and other evidence in nursing and related disciplines.
> * Identify examples of the use of evidence in planned nursing interventions.
>
> Standards of proficiency: Care Delivery (Entry to Register)
>
> * Ensure that current research findings and other evidence are incorporated into practice.
> * Identify relevant changes in practice or new information and disseminate to colleagues.
> * Engage with and evaluate the evidence base that underpins safe nursing practice.
>
> Standards of proficiency: Personal and professional Development (Entry to Branch Outcomes)
>
> * Begin to engage with and interpret the evidence base which underpins nursing practice.

You can see from the above how important it is for you to develop skills and gain a certain level of knowledge to achieve these outcomes, all of which are included in either your assessments in practice or your academic assessments which are more theoretical in focus but still require you to make links to nursing practice. We will be returning to this issue of assessment and assignments in more detail in Chapter 9, but please consider the following in order for you to begin to make connections to your learning:

+ . . . .

EBP in action

Consider your career pathway as a nurse, that is, are you undertaking children's nursing, adult nursing, mental health nursing or learning disability nursing. What evidence did you obtain in order for you to determine which of these pathways you were going to follow and what made you decide whether that evidence was useful to you?

. . . .

In responding to this question you will already be thinking about the fact that you may have obtained both verbal and non-verbal types of information and that its usefulness depended on how that was presented to you or who gave it to you. Choosing nursing as a career would require obtaining information in itself and this would have been a major career choice without the added choice of also deciding which pathway to take, requiring extra information! Obtaining the right information as well as it being the best information available would have been essential to your choice. This is not unlike research and EBP, which is also dependent on:

- understanding how to obtain information
- understanding what approach to take
- deciding on what is the best evidence and then using it to make an informed decision.

Once you have made your choice of career in nursing, you are then faced with a number of further decisions. Where to undertake a course of study would be an important decision as would everything that went with it, such as: do you have the right qualifications, where is the university and can you travel to it easily, are the clinical placements associated with it within easy travelling distance of where you live, will I get a bursary, and so on. Making decisions become an important part of being a student nurse, not only as these questions relating to your course of study demonstrate but also those related to what you will actually be doing in clinical practice or what is often called clinical placement.

Asking questions in order to access information (data) and evidence as described above is exactly the kind of skill we would like to encourage. This is a transferable skill which can not only help you with being a student nurse but also, if undertaken in the appropriate manner, will be invaluable in obtaining important data from the patients and clients in your care and as a consequence being able to use this to assess their health

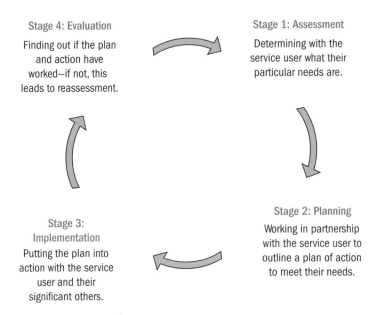

Stage 4: Evaluation
Finding out if the plan
and action have
worked—if not, this
leads to reassessment.

Stage 1: Assessment
Determining with the
service user what their
particular needs are.

Stage 3:
Implementation
Putting the plan into
action with the service
user and their
significant others.

Stage 2: Planning
Working in partnership
with the service user to
outline a plan of action
to meet their needs.

Figure 1.1 The Nursing Process: a problem-solving cycle

needs and plan and evaluate their nursing care. This is often called the nursing process (Haberman & Uys 2005) and has similar stages to that of the research process,
which is explained in Chapter 3. These are: assess, plan, implement, and evaluate
(see Fig. 1.1).

How to link evidence-based practice and care planning will be included in Chapter 8.

The importance of research and evidence-based practice in nursing and health care

We have seen from the NMC standards the importance of student nurses achieving
skills and knowledge of research and EBP. This is built into the requirements of their
future profession and also into their programme of learning to become a nurse. The
student therefore has to both gain the relevant knowledge and skills to be able to understand research and EBP but also then gain experience in being able to implement this
in practice. To achieve these key competencies, students need to gain skills in finding
and appraising evidence and we will explore how to do this throughout this book. First,
however we need to consider the much wider nursing and health care context for EBP.
Cullum (2007) points out that:

> 66 *Policy and professional developments over the last 15 years have placed increas-ing pressure on nurses to be more accountable for their actions. At the same time, research into nurses decision-making and research information use by nurses has also increased. The advent of National Service Frameworks, The Commission for Health Improvement (CHI) and the National Institute for Clinical Excellence (NICE) mean that evidence-based approaches to nursing practice have become firmly established in research, professional and policy agendas.* 99

Her study examined the use of research information in clinical decision-making of nurses, and, as we have seen, this will involve making clinical judgements about the patient. Of significance to you as a student nurse are the findings related to 'barriers to using research based information in clinical decisions'. In order to achieve the NMC Standards of proficiency there is an expectation that your mentor will be able to support and guide you to know the best possible evidence to underpin care practices. Many of the nurses in Callum's study felt they had a limited ability in 'working with research products' in particular because of the perceived 'lack of research appreciation skills and confidence'.

+...

EBP in action

Consider the following example from a recent study by Lauder *et al.* (2008), where a student believed that not having up to date evidence-based knowledge, as she had experienced it, affected the student–mentor relationship:

> 66 *There's an instance that happened recently giving an injection … this is just an example (re: the student knowing more than the mentor) … that you do not expel the air bubble be-cause the air bubble is at the bottom so the patient gets the full dose but I was with the nurse who expelled the bubble and when we went back to the trolley I said to her "I hope you don't mind me asking but can you tell me why you did that" …. (her reply…) "We've always done it like that"…. But I said to her "that's actually not what you do, you actually leave the bubble in" … (her reply) … "Who says?"' (student nurse).* 99

1. What is your understanding of this scenario from an evidence base?
2. What is the evidence base to this example regarding injection technique?
3. What have you been taught to do on your course and on what evidence is this based?
4. Is the student correct in her assessment or is there a variety of issues to be considered?
5. We will explore this briefly but you may find it helpful to discuss this in more detail with your mentor or personal tutor.

....

Some of you may have experienced similar situations and as a student you may have expected that all qualified nurses use evidence to underpin and inform their practice. From the research it is clear that this is not the case and that just as student nurses are often mystified by aspects of how to read research papers or understand their meaning, so are many qualified practitioners. Using the evidence then becomes much harder and requires a set of skills and knowledge to do so.

Managing situations whereby the student nurse knows more than her mentor or other nurses is clearly an individual one. However wherever care is compromised in some way due to inappropriate practice, the student needs to ensure that no harm comes to the patient and has a duty of care to report this to a senior person in the placement and discuss it with her personal tutor. Situations like this are discussed in Sue Hart's (2010) book *Nursing: Study and Placement Learning Skills*.

With regards to the student's quote, it would appear that there are different opinions on the issue of evidence in relation to the giving of injections. A paper by Roger & King (2000) reviewing the practice of drawing up and administering intramuscular (IM) injections concluded that the 'air bubble technique' in IM injections was contentious. However on accessing the National Rheumatoid Arthritis Society website (2007) it was noted that in the new Metoject Methotrexate (sub cutaneous) injection in which the mixture is already prepared, included an air bubble in order to aid expulsion of the drug which:

> ❝ *guaranteed that the patient receives an accurate dosage and that no drug is left in the syringe, making disposal much safer. It also helps prevent leakage from the site.* ❞

It is to be noted that Methotrexate is a cytotoxic drug, hence the need for safe handling. Consider these potentially conflicting issues when discussing the scenario.

As we can see from this example, it is essential that any change in practice is not only considered in an 'evidence-based' way but also that the evidence itself may be contradictory. This is why in later chapters we will be considering what the best evidence is and how you determine this.

Summary

- An awareness of research and the research process is essential to implementing EBP.
- Being able to utilize current and best research evidence is essential to care delivery and development.

- There is a requirement of professional nursing bodies around the world, including the UK's Nursing and Midwifery Council, that in order to be fit for practice that you are able to both interpret and utilize an evidence base to your practice as a registered nurse.

■ Online resource centre

 To learn more about the importance of EBP to the nursing profession and keep up-to-date with new proficiencies for nursing, please now go online to www. oxfordtextbooks.co.uk/orc/holland/ to find more resources.

■ References

Cullum, N. (2002) IMP 2–11 Cullum: *Nurses' Use of Research Information in Clinical Decision-Making: a descriptive and analytical study.* London: DH.

Garbett, R. & McCormack, B. (2002) A concept analysis of practice development. NT Research, 7, 2, 87–100, cited in Gerrish, K. & McMahon, A. (2006) Research and development in nursing: In K. Gerrish & A. Lacey *The Research Process in Nursing* (5th edn). Oxford: Blackwell Publishing, 1–15.

Gerrish, K. & McMahon, A. (2006) Research and Development in Nursing: In K. Gerrish & A. Lacey (eds) *The Research Process in Nursing* (5th edn). Oxford: Blackwell Publishing, 1–15.

Haberman, M. & Uys, I. R. (2005) *The Nursing Process: a global concept.* London: Churchill Livingstone, Elsevier.

Hart, S. (2010) *Nursing: Study and Placement Skills.* Oxford: Oxford University Press.

Hockey, L. (1984) The nature and purpose of research: In Cormack, D.F.S. (Ed) *The Research Process in Nursing* (1st edn). London: Blackwell Science, 1–10.

Lauder, W., Roxburgh, M. Holland, K. Johnson, M. Watson, W. Porter, M. Topping, K. & Behr, A. (2008) *Nursing and Midwifery in Scotland: being fit for practice.* Dundee: University of Dundee.

Macleod Clark, J. M. (2009) *Key note paper: Looking Back, Moving Forward: pursuing the science of nursing interventions.* RCN Annual International Nursing Research Conference: Cardiff.
    (http://www.rcn.org.uk/development/researchanddevelopment/rs/research2009)

National Rheumatoid Arthritis Society (2007) *Why Is There a Bubble in my Metoject Methotrexate Injection?* www.rheumatoid.org.uk

Newell, R. & Burnard, P. (2006) *Research for Evidence-based Practice.* Oxford: Blackwell Publishing.

NHS Executive (1996) Promoting Clinical Effectiveness: A Framework for Action in and through the NHS: In NHS Executive (1998) *Achieving Effective practice – a Clinical Effectiveness and Research Information pack for Nurses, Midwives and Health Visitors.* Leeds: NHS (accessed on DH website).

Nursing & Midwifery Council (2004) *Standards of Proficiency for Pre-registration Nursing Education*. London: Nursing & Midwifery Council.

Nursing & Midwifery Council (2008) *A Review of Pre-registration Nursing Education*: report of consultation findings. London: Nursing & Midwifery Council Parahoo, K. (1997) *Nursing Research*: principles processes and issues (*1st edn*). Basingstoke: Palgrave.

Parahoo K. (2006) *Nursing Research: principles, processes and issues* (*2nd edn*). Basingstoke: Palgrave Macmillan.

Roger, M. A. & King, L. (2002) Drawing up and administering intramuscular injections: a review of the literature. *Journal of Advanced Nursing* 31 (3) 574–582.

Royal College of Nursing (1996) *Clinical Effectiveness: a Royal College of Nursing guide*. London: Royal College of Nursing.

Sackett, D. L., Strauss, S. E., Richardson, W. S., Rosenberg, W. & Haynes, R. B. (1997) *Evidence-based Medicine: how to practice and teach EBM*. Edinburgh: Churchill Livingstone.

Thompson, D., Daly, J., Elliott, D. & Chang, E. (2002) Research in Nursing: concepts and processes. In: Daly, J., Speedy, S., Jackson, D. & P. Darbyshire, *Contexts of Nursing – an introduction*. Oxford: Blackwell Publishing (Chapter 8, 84–100).

■ Further reading

Key influential papers in nursing care

To celebrate the 50th anniversary of the RCN Research Society 12 reports from the 'study of nursing care project' 1970–1975 have been published (all are accessible as the full report in pdf). These reports are classic studies of their time and remain influential pieces of work, most of which have never been replicated. Please see the list below and choose any that you think sounds interesting.

All of these papers can be accessed online by visiting the RCN website and visiting the 'Development' and 'Research and Development section' – see this url *accessed June 2009*.

> http://www.rcn.org.uk/development/researchanddevelopment/rs/publications_and_position_
> statements/rcn_study_in_nursing_care_project

Anderson, E.R. (1973) *The role of the nurse: views of the patient, nurse and doctor in some general hospitals in England.* London: Royal College of Nursing. (The study of nursing care project reports, series 2 no. 1.)

Franklin, B. L. (1974) *Patient anxiety on admission to hospital,* London: Royal College of Nursing. (The study of nursing care project reports, series 1 no. 5.)

Hawthorn, P. J. (1974) *Nurse – I want my mummy!* London: Royal College of Nursing. (The study of nursing care project reports, series 1 no. 3.)

Hayward, J. (1975) *Information –* a prescription against pain. London: Royal College of Nursing. (The study of nursing care project reports, series 2, no. 5.)

Hunt, J. M. (1974) *The teaching and practice of surgical dressings in three hospitals.* London: Royal College of Nursing. (The study of nursing care project reports, series 1 no.6.)

Inman, U. (1975) *Towards a theory of nursing care: an account of the RCN/DHSS research project 'The study of nursing care'.* London: Royal College of Nursing. (The study of nursing care project reports: concluding monograph.)

Jones, D. C. (1975) *Food for thought: a descriptive study of the nutritional nursing care of unconscious patients in general hospitals.* London: Royal College of Nursing. (The study of nursing care project reports, series 2 no. 4.)

Lelean, S. R. (1973) *Ready for report nurse? a study of nursing communication in hospital wards.* London: Royal College of Nursing. (The study of nursing care project reports, series 2 no. 2.)

McFarlane, J. K. (1970) *The proper study of the nurse: an account of the first two years of a research project "The study of nursing care", including a study of the relevant background literature.* London: Royal College of Nursing. (The study of nursing care project reports, series 1 Introduction.)

Munday, A. (1973) *Physiological measures of anxiety in hospital patients,* London: Royal College of Nursing. (The study of nursing care project reports, series 2 No. 3.)

Roberts, I. (1975) Discharged from hospital. London: Royal College of Nursing. (The study of nursing care project reports, series 2 no. 1.)

Smith, S. H. (1972) *Nil by mouth?: a descriptive study of nursing care in relation to pre-operative fasting.* London: Royal College of Nursing. (The study of nursing care project reports, series 1 no. 1.)

Stockwell, F. (1972) *The unpopular patient.* London: Royal College of Nursing. (The study of nursing care project reports, series 1 no. 2.)

Wright, L. (1974) *Bowel function in hospital patients.* London: Royal College of Nursing. (The study of nursing care project reports, series 1 no. 4.)

Useful websites

The Royal College of Nursing UK Development Practice area

http://www.rcn.org.uk/development/practice/

This site has online resources which you will find of value in relation to current evidence in practice. The subjects covered include:

- Clinical guidelines
- NICE consultation gateway
- Clinical governance
- Perioperative fasting
- RCN clinical leadership programme
- Essence of care
- Diabetes
- Social inclusion
- eHealth
- Patient safety

The Joanna Briggs Institute of Evidence-based practice

A leading international institute, the Joanna Briggs institute website is well worth a visit and bookmarking for essay research.

www.joannabriggs.edu.au/about/eb_nursing.php/

2

Understanding evidence and its utilization in nursing practice

Colin Rees

The aims of the chapter are:

➤ To outline the development of evidence-based practice.

➤ To consider the nature of evidence.

➤ To outline the different levels of evidence.

➤ To explore the sources of evidence including non-research-based evidence.

➤ To examine evidence-based guidelines and their use.

➤ To consider examples of evidence-based collaboration centres.

Introduction

Chapter 1 has introduced you to a number of key ideas in nursing that will be examined throughout this book. In particular, it has emphasized that the skills needed to be a nurse are not simply clinical, but also relate to the justification of those skills, and the decision-making process involved in providing care. The global health care system is now influenced by the ideals of evidence-based practice (EBP). As Craig & Smyth (2007) explain, the approach of EBP aims to deliver appropriate care in an effective manner to individual patients. It is not something outside nursing, or an 'add-on' to nursing, but is part of the responsibility of the nurse to ensure that best care is provided to each and every patient. Achieving this, however, requires a certain understanding of what **evidence** is and the various types of evidence that can be used to underpin this care, combined with the knowledge and skills of the nurse as a practitioner. As a student nurse you will need to learn about these in order to become a qualified nurse.

This chapter will focus on the basic principles of EBP and what it has replaced. It will also focus on the hierarchy of evidence because it is important for the student nurse to appreciate different kinds of evidence and gain an understanding of how this is evident in the literature. Evidence obtained from the internet and whether this is a reliable form of evidence will also be considered. Many students now use this resource for assignments but it is important, as you will see in Chapter 9, that the evidence used is not only reliable but also valid in the context of ensuring safe evidence-based nursing practice.

So far we have connected the two concepts of research and EBP together. This is because within the current culture of health services such as the NHS there is a professional obligation to base clinical decision-making on the best evidence available. Although this may come in many forms, as we shall see later on in this chapter, in most cases we are talking about 'research evidence'. The whole topic of EBP is discussed within a clinical practice context as opposed to a completely abstract or theoretical context. In other words, EBP is to do with everyday nursing and what you will be expected to do and participate in as both a nursing student and qualified nurse.

EBP is to do with the standard of care provided by individual practitioners, including nurses, and the knowledge or 'evidence' used to help make clinical decisions.

To gain a better understanding of evidence, we need to be clear on the different types of evidence and identify how we can arrive at decisions that will ensure best practice for your patients. Many writers have acknowledged that in the practice situation the nurse takes information from several different sources. EBP also suggests that support for decisions may come from published research, locally generated data such as nursing or clinical audits, professional clinical experience, as well as the patient's point of view (Dartnell *et al.* 2008).

EBP in action

What are the criteria that should inform a nurse's clinical decision-making with regards to patient care? Imagine you are in a clinical placement and have been caring for a patient with an indwelling catheter who seems to be suffering from depression? What would be on your list of the criteria you would look for in the information to aid your decision-making with regards this patient?

An example of this could be that you think you should know what other practitioners would do in this situation or what information is available to you in the clinical placement itself. Consider this question again when you have read this chapter and determine if there is a difference with your original list.

Given the importance of EBP then, how did it become an essential part of health care in the UK and other countries?

Historical developments of evidence-based practice

Firstly, we must recognize that EBP developed from evidence-based medicine. This developed in both the UK and USA and one man is credited with the inspiration for what can be called the 'movement' or 'philosophy' of an evidence-based approach to clinical decision-making. That man was Archie Cochrane who was an epidemiologist in the UK and who gave his name to the Cochrane Collaboration, the organization responsible for systematic reviews of the literature. Fineout-Overholt *et al.* (2005) pinpoint the event that started the movement as being Cochrane's public criticism in 1972 of the medical profession's failure to act on evidence from a large number of clinical trials on administering corticosteroids to high-risk women in preterm labour. Cochrane believed that if the evidence had been produced in the form of a systematic review (that is a summation and critique of all available evidence) it would have convinced obstetricians to act on it and so save the lives of thousands of low birth weight premature babies.

Cullum *et al.* (2008) identified the first person to use the term 'evidence-based medicine' as Gordon Guyatt and the Evidence Based Medicine Working Group in 1992. This gives the system quite a recent history in comparison to other systems within health care.

One of the frequently mentioned people who has helped to develop the more recently popularity of the concept is David Sackett (a medical doctor) whose definitions are frequently quoted. For example his definition of EBP as '*The conscientious, explicit and judicious use of current best evidence about the care of individual patients*' (Sackett et al. 1997: 2) has already been introduced in Chapter 1.

Sackett makes the point that medicine had gone from a position where there was little evidence for many of the clinical procedures undertaken to (as a result of the explosion of randomized control trials (RCTs) available) a lack of the application of this knowledge. Sackett felt that the main priority was to have quick access to information that needed to be implemented into practice.

As a movement, evidence-based medicine is often traced back to McMaster University in Ontario, Canada, where a group of researchers were trying to overcome the problem of clinical decision-making being based on clinical experience rather than clear evidence (Hamer & Collinson 2005) and they set about changing that view to one which accepted that the only way to make good decisions was to combine evidence with patient preferences and the professional's experience (see http://hsl.mcmaster.ca/resources/ebpractice.htm, which offers access to major resources related to EBP worldwide).

Much of the continued support for EBP in the UK has come from the Cochrane Centre set up in 1992 by the National Health Service Research Programme (see http://cochrane. co.uk/en/about.html/). There are now 12 of these centres worldwide that support the Cochrane Collaboration. You will find a wealth of information on all the websites associated with this development.

The change from evidence-based 'medicine' to evidence-based 'practice' was a natural development, as it was realized that this system was not only relevant to medicine but to all health professional groups. EBP has therefore become a multi-professional issue and, considering the importance of an integrated approach to care of patients, this can only be to the benefit of ensuring best practice is delivered to those who need care.

Evidence-based practice

What is EBP? Is it a system, a movement, a way of thinking, a philosophy, a paradigm or a set of principles? You will already have seen a brief explanation in Chapter 1 and now this section will look at some of the ways writers have examined and promoted EBP.

It is clear from the literature and other sources such as the World Wide Web that it has become a 'movement', in that it is supported worldwide by many different health groups, including doctors, physiotherapists, occupational therapists, as well as all branches of nursing (Craig & Smyth 2007; Pearson *et al.* 2007).

However, it is true to say that EBP was not an automatic success as it also had, and still maintains, its critics who argue that it requires the practitioner to abandon professional knowledge bases and surrender to whatever research evidence suggests as best practice. However, that was never the intention. This is clear from writers such as Fineout-Overholt *et al.* (2005: 335), who define EBP as:

> 66 *A problem-solving approach to clinical practice that integrates a systematic search for, and critical appraisal of, the most relevant evidence to answer a burning clinical question, one's own clinical expertise, patient preferences and values.* 99

This provides us with a system that is a combination of the three factors simplified in Fig. 2.1. This clearly demonstrates that true EBP is the result of an integration of these three elements where published research is firstly carefully evaluated and then taken into account with the practitioner's experience and the patient's voice.

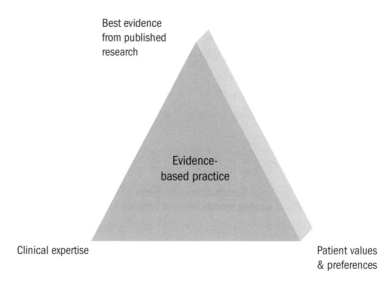

Best evidence
from published
research

Evidence-
based practice

Clinical expertise

Patient values
& preferences

Figure 2.1 The elements of evidence-based practice

It is important to emphasize that the evidence used is collected in a systematic way and it more than just a single study that is used to make clinical decisions. As will be seen in Chapter 6, evidence must be drawn from a careful search of the literature and an evaluation of that literature to form some conclusions as to what is best practice. The reason for such a stringent process is clear from this comment from Brown (2009: 16), who points out that:

> 66 *Findings from many soundly conducted studies are necessary to build a reliable base of clinical knowledge regarding an issue. Insistence on confirmation of a finding from more than one study ensures that a knowledge claim is not just a fluke resulting from the particular patients setting or research methods of that one study.* 99

As with research, there is a process that clinicians should follow in supporting the idea of EBP. The total process can be seen as a series of stages outlined in Fig. 2.2. You will recognize this as the problem-solving process which begins with the statement of a clear question that needs to be answered. In EBP this takes the form of the PICO statement, which we will cover in more detail in Chapter 6 on reviewing the literature. For now you need to know that PICO is an acronym and stands for:

Population—those (patients/clients) who form the focus of the review.

Intervention—that is, the treatment.

Comparison—with an alternative treatment or no treatment.

Outcome—the measurable way that success is measured.

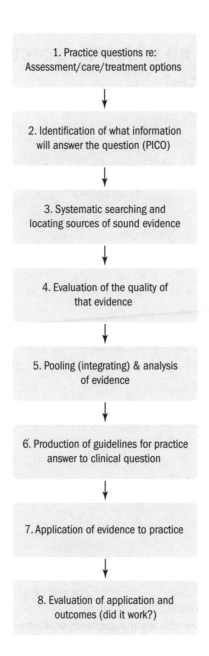

Figure 2.2 The evidence-based practice process

Such a structure helps to consider nursing practice and the question of evidence regarding 'what' will be required to answer a clinical question. The key to this approach is the need to consider how we can demonstrate the outcome of care that is required in a measureable way. This book will follow the major elements in the evidence-based process, as was outlined at the end of Chapter 1. For now, it is clear that the system needs to be supported by principles that will ensure that the outcome is meaningful to patient care.

The principles on which evidence-based practice is based

One of the major principles on which EBP is based is the need for efficiency in the use of health care resources, where the choice of intervention will lead to the best use of resources and the maximum health outcome for the individual. This means clinicians concentrating on those practices that are shown to be successful and abandoning those interventions that have been shown not to work or are less successful for the resources required.

Hamer & Collinson (2005: 9) suggest that 'evidence-based practice is based on the principle of rational decision-making'. That is, that we 'work things out' by looking at possible options, consider the strength of evidence supporting options, and choose the one with the most likelihood to produce the best clinical outcomes.

The medical origins of EBP have left their mark on some of the principles regarding sources of evidence. Unfortunately, this has led some people to believe that some sources of evidence such as randomized controlled trials are the only forms of evidence, instead of realizing that the form of the evidence depends on the question it is trying to answer.

In medicine one frequently wants to answer the question what is the best drug or medical intervention required for this condition, and so the best source of information will be clinical trials that have put the drug to the test against other forms of intervention. This will form the gold standard for medical questions but may not always suit the questions asked within nursing.

✛ ···

EBP in action

You may have been in a clinical placement, in a hospital, or in a health care setting where some patients had agreed to be involved in a drug trial. Considering the various fields of practice (branches) in nursing, what do you think would be challenges for engaging patients in these trials?

If you are an adult or mental health nursing student, you may have been caring for older people with dementia, where new medication may help them to recover some degree of memory but they were unable to consent to see if the drug may have made an improvement. Similarly if you have nursed in a mental health setting with people with severe depression there is no guarantee that if they were entered for a drug trial that they would receive an active treatment or a placebo.

Such issues are difficult to resolve, but the RCN (UK) has some excellent guidelines which may help you to answer the question posed (http://www.rcn.org.uk/development/researchanddevelopment/rs/publications_and_position_statements/informed_consent/).

···

Evidence-based medicine was seen as essential to the principle of high standards of care through a move away from the intuitive and subjective approach of clinicians to a more objective and 'scientific' method of choosing clinical interventions, that is, to apply interventions that are seen to work (Dale 2006). There is also a desire through EBP to reduce wide variations in practice through agreeing to use effective interventions, and to apply consistent practice guidelines (Cohen & Hersh 2004).

The Darzi Report *High Quality Care for All* (DH 2008) has continued the emphasis on setting high standards in health care delivery. This review of the NHS identified a number of principles that were seen as fundamental to continuing positive changes and developments in care. This included the ability of staff to base care on high quality clinical information in order to choose the best of health care options and apply consistent standards throughout the country. It was this report that led to the setting up of the 'NHS Evidence' search engine to provide a quick and easy access point for clinicians to good quality information (http://www.nice.org.uk/nhsevidence/).

When setting it up, the NHS claimed this new access point to health information was to be as easy and simple to use as 'Google' and run by the National Institute for Health and Clinical Excellence (NIHCE). The report also made the following promise:

> 66 *Easy access for NHS staff to information about high quality care: All NHS staff will have access to a new 'NHS Evidence' service where they will be able to get, through a single web-based portal, authoritative clinical and non-clinical evidence and best practice.* 99

> (DH 2008: 12)

+ ....

EBP in action

If you are not a regular user of the NHS Evidence health search engine, take a clinical topic of interest and / or relevance to your field of practice (branch) and visit the website at http://www.nice.org.uk/nhsevidence/ to explore the information available on your topic. In particular, take note of the options on the left of the screen when it provides results for your search, and the way in which you can narrow down the results.

....

What kind of evidence?

It is easy to take concepts like 'evidence' for granted, but in this section we want to consider what is meant by this term within the context of EBP. Within medicine the need for evidence was in relation to the best forms of treatment and medical intervention, often in the form of drugs given to patients. The question frequently asked was: is drug 'A' better than drug 'B'? The evidence most appropriate to answer this is the RCT (see Chapter 5). Although nursing is increasingly involved in prescribing, many other nursing questions requiring evidence are not always of this type however, so RCT research evidence is not always the most appropriate for nursing practice. For questions related to nursing care, and patient experience, it may be surveys or qualitative methods (i.e. those which describe or interpret the quality of something such as an experience—see Chapter 4) that may be most useful in answering such questions. The important issue is to use the best and most appropriate approach to answer what needs to be known.

It is clear, however, that the strength of opinion and indeed practice in relation to EBP is to rely more heavily on quantitative methods (i.e. those concerned with the measurement and analysis of something—see Chapter 5) and in particular the findings of a RCT.

EBP may seem to you to be all about research but this is not quite the case, although there are reasons why research figures so often in relation to this, and this will be clear from later discussions.

✚..

EBP in action

Given that you may have limited knowledge of EBP at this stage in your nursing career, what criteria might you look for in sound evidence? What aspects would you expect to find if the information was going to be accepted as relevant to your hunt for' sound information?

....

Evidence is usually taken to mean information that provides a confirmation of support for something. It has a legal context in that in relation to crime for example, there is duty to collect evidence that will demonstrate whether someone may be guilty or innocent of a crime. As with EBP, in a legal setting, not just any evidence will do, we have to be certain of its reliability and it must be 'fit for purpose'. Drake *et al.* (2001: 179) believe that there must be a connection between research and EBP in the context of patient care:

> ❝ Evidence-based practices are interventions for which there is scientific evidence consistently showing that they improve client outcomes. ❞

The advantage of research as a basis for evidence is that it is usually presented in a way in which the processes that have produced the findings are transparent; we can see and therefore assess the likely strength or accuracy of the evidence. This is usually evident in the methods section, for example in the choice of method used to collect the information or that of processing or analysing the results, we can assess if sufficient control over accuracy have been taken. (This will be considered in the methodology chapters.)

EBP therefore grew out of evidence-based medicine, as it was realized that improvements across health care could not happen if it was left to doctors alone. All of the major health professions had to sign up to this common philosophy of basing care on justifiable evidence. The meaning of evidence, following on from this is high quality research evidence, and this is combined, as we saw in Fig. 2.1, with clinical expertise and patient values and preferences.

What has evidence-based practice replaced?

Cullum *et al*. (2008: 2) provide a definition for evidence-based nursing by stating that it is 'the application of valid, relevant, research-based information in nurse decision-making'. They see it as related to research as the source of the evidence that facilitates decisions. They also say that this information is not used alone but in conjunction with other sources of information such as knowledge of the patient, the context in which the decision is taking place, and professional expertise and judgement.

It is not that EBP is replacing non-evidence-based practice, it is simply that the nature of evidence had been redefined and the process of using evidence on a more consistent and logical basis has been accepted as an essential part of care giving. This is to move closer to a system of more consistent approaches to care based on what has been demonstrated to work, and dropping those things that have been shown to be ineffective or in some cases, unsafe.

One of the problems that led to the implementation of EBP was an over-reliance on the quality of professional judgement and 'experience'. You may still hear some of your tutors or mentors referring back to their early careers as nurses in clinical practice, with comments such as 'well, I just knew that was the best ointment to put on the skin' or 'on our ward we agreed that despite any evidence to tell us otherwise, we would continue to use spirit massaged into patient's heels, followed by powder to help prevent soreness and rubbing of the sheets, when they were on bed rest'.

The problem here was that judgements varied considerably, as did experience, this led to many different 'solutions' and beliefs held about what was 'best practice'. Many of these practices and beliefs were quite clearly either not effective, or could be harmful. A more objective and consistent system was needed rather than an over-reliance on ritual and routine (Walsh & Ford 1989). EBP then can be seen as the opposite of traditional approaches to care. For example, Theroux (2006: 245) states that:

> 66 *EBP de-emphasizes ritual; ungrounded opinion and tradition as a basis for nursing practice and emphasizes the use of research findings.* 99

This allows nursing to play its part in the multidisciplinary team and share the same philosophy and principles when it comes to decision-making.

+..

EBP in action

Some nursing decisions are still influenced by:

    a. tradition and ritual

    b. what you are taught

    c. role models

    d. trial and error

    e. research

Take each of these alternatives a) to e) in turn and list what you consider may be the 'advantages' and 'disadvantages' of each one. Use your own experiences, both personally and as a student nurse, to guide you, as well as other sources.

When you have completed this exercise, either on your own or with colleagues, consider what conclusions you have arrived at and how you can use this to set learning goals for yourself in clinical practice.

You may wish to use the information provided in Chapters 6 and 7 to help you to achieve this, as well as talking to your mentors and tutors about their experiences.

....

Hierarchy of evidence

There has been a huge increase in the number of research studies undertaken in both medicine and nursing. This makes the search for evidence a daunting task where many studies have been completed worldwide on the same topic. Each study will have its strengths and limitations. Any clinician would find it almost impossible to track down and make sense of all the publications under one heading. It would be far better to have someone knowledgeable find and compare them all and come up with some kind of conclusion. This is the purpose of a systematic review. We will be looking at aspects of searching for the literature in Chapter 6, and writing reviews in Chapter 9, so in this chapter we will just make the point that systematic reviews of well conducted studies are highly regarded in evidence-based care and so come high up the hierarchy of evidence.

There are many examples in the EBP literature of hierarchies of evidence. These often take the form of a pyramid showing the rank order of sources of evidence indicating which has the greatest and which the least levels of trust in their use for clinical decision-making (see Fig. 2.3). This is based on the principle that different research designs are open to different levels of accuracy and vary in the ability of the researcher to reduce the risk of errors and bias (Evans 2003). Early hierarchies were developed to distinguish the quality of research examining medical interventions and their effect on clinical outcomes. Therefore, it is not surprising to find that RCTs are the most favoured source of evidence in EBP because of the way they attempt to reduce levels of error and offer alternative explanations for the results. We shall discuss more about this method of research in Chapter 5. At the very top of such hierarchies is the systematic review based on a collection of RCTs such as those produced by the Cochrane Collaboration mentioned earlier in this chapter.

The hierarchy in Fig. 2.3 shows that it is not a single study that is used to influence decision-making as there can be so many limitations to a single study. At the top of the ranking is a review of literature that has been carried out to very high standards in the form of a systematic review undertaken by groups of experts, such as those produced by the Cochrane Collaboration, or the Joanna Briggs Institute (JBI) in Australia. This helps to identify if there is a consensus in the evidence that clinical outcomes have been produced by specific interventions. Lower down this example of a hierarchy are qualitative studies and then expert opinion.

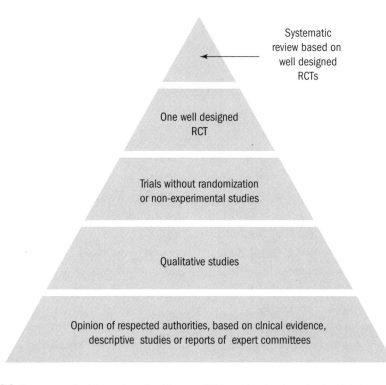

Figure 2.3 Example of a hierarchy of evidence. RCT, randomized controlled trial

This kind of rank ordering of sources is appropriate in deciding which interventions to use, but there is a great deal of debate about the usefulness of such hierarchies for other forms of decision-making. So Dale (2005: 51) warns:

> ❝ The research-based evidence of nursing is complex and therefore a hierarchy of evidence with a gold standard is inappropriate. All research methods have their place and the research question should determine the design and method used to ensure research is relevant to nursing practice. ❞

The existence of such hierarchies has long put nursing research at a disadvantage as it does not try to answer the outcome of drug interventions but more nursing interventions where the input is not as easily defined and controlled as drugs. However, as we saw in Chapter 1, Professor Dame Jill Macleod Clark challenges nurses to undertake research that does measure the direct impact of nursing care. In her review of nursing research at the RCN Research Conference 2009 she urged nurses to develop collaborative programmes of research across the world to begin to develop this critical need for evidence-based *nursing* interventions which would clearly show the benefit they have on patients (You can watch this presentation via the RCN webcast which is available on our online resource centre). This is a challenge for nurses who are not, on the whole, comfortable with approaching nursing in relation to its underlying science base.

Challenges to achieving evidence-based practice

The initial response to EBP was not all positive. Even in the early days of evidence-based medicine, doctors were very suspicious of the principle, even though it had been championed by people such as Archie Cochrane for many years. There was a fear that it would lead to a restriction in choice of treatments, loss of effective traditional approaches to care, and loss of individual preferences (Eisenburg 2002). More recently, even in nursing, there was the feeling that in many situations 'lip service' was paid to the concept of EBP and claims that it was being followed did not stand up to close scrutiny (Leufer & Cleary-Holdforth 2009). The implication of this, they point out, is that the quality of care received by patients is reduced as a result.

There are, however, difficulties to achieving a high level of EBP, not least of which is a lack of available nursing research, particularly in some clinical areas such as dermatology, and also a lack of good quality research. Craig & Smyth (2007: 10) agree that:

> 66 *there are yawning gaps in the robust evidence for much of what nurses do in the course of their daily work.* 99

This has led to the careful vetting of information used in clinical practice as there is no point in ensuring that decisions are based on evidence if that evidence is poor or unreliable.

However, Craig & Smyth (2007: 8) warn that if evidence is not readily available we should not panic or become 'frozen and disempowered by the lack of robust evidence for much of what we do'. A wide variety of sources of evidence may be available when research evidence is not available, but an attempt has to be made to assess which sources and forms of evidence are 'better' or more reliable to use than others. We also need some guidelines as to what we should be looking for in good evidence so that we know it when we see it.

The challenge, therefore, is to integrate the evidence with clinical practice and to change poor practices that might be ingrained in care delivery. This has been high-lighted by Thompson *et al.* (2005: 433), who warn that despite the emphasis on evidence-based health care *'the extent to which research knowledge is transferred to clinical practice in nursing remains unclear'*. This is an important study to consider here, as their aim was to examine the perceived barriers and obstacles to accessing and using research-based information. As part of the data gathering for the study, community nurses were observed and 82 interviews with community nurses working in three different clinical areas were carried out.

The results of the study showed that problems included a perceived lack of time to gather information needed in decision-making. Nurses also felt they lacked com-puter skills to access databases and locate relevant information. Once information was found, one of the big challenges nurses had was in interpreting research findings, particularly when they were in the form of RCTs. There was a feeling that they lacked cri-tiquing skills that would help them assess the quality of the research (see Chapter 7). They also felt that they did not have sufficient knowledge of statistics to understand many of the results in studies (see Chapter 5). On the whole, nurses wanted informa-tion from research written and presented in a plain language and a straightforward way that gave clear directions for practice. Many nurses felt that there was no protected time in working hours to search for information and so could not make use of it, as it was difficult to access out of work time. Information needs were often satisfied by draw-ing on past experiences when decisions had to be made.

It should be stressed that this study was done some years ago, so the situation may have changed, with more nurses qualifying with more advanced computer skills and critiquing skills. However, it is worth taking into account the results of such studies, as you will meet people with a variety of computer and information skills during your clinical experiences and when qualified. The conclusion of the study was that it is important to look at the context in which information behaviour takes place, and that nurses will vary in their ability to access, evaluate and integrate available information into clinical practice.

+ ···

EBP in action

Thinking of your last clinical placement, were you aware of the extent that those around you were accessing information in its different forms as part of nursing practice? Were there ways in your placements where you did make use of information sources, or were there opportunities for you to have made a greater use of information than you did?

You may have found that practitioners did not choose to access evidence-based information during their working hours, due in part to lack of time or accessibility of computer-based resources. There may, however, have been many information packages available to student nurses as part of ensuring the NMC requirements of a good learning environment. It is part of a practitioner's role to ensure that the learning environment provides students with learning resources as well as good supervision, and mentors are expected to assess students' knowledge and use of evidence in their caring for patients and meeting the NMC standards of proficiency (see Chapter 1).

···

Sources of evidence including non-research-based evidence

It is clear from much of the literature that when writers talk about evidence they are referring specifically to research evidence, and in particular quantitative research evidence. For example Swage (2004: 93) states that

> ❝ the evidence for the effectiveness of interventions can be found in research papers. ❞

The source of this information can be from information centres such as the Cochrane Collaboration Centre or the York University Centre for Reviews and Dissemination.

Some nursing writers have argued strongly for a wider definition of evidence within nursing. Dale (2005: 50), for example, is very clear that the nature of nursing and the questions related to clinical practice it needs to answer do not always lend themselves to the quantitative approach. She says that:

> ❝ ...qualitative research is as necessary as quantitative in the generation of research based nursing knowledge and therefore evidence to inform nursing practice. ❞

It is important to recognize that there is controversy in relation to the nature of evidence and some of this is related to the historical background of the topic and its roots within medicine.

The need to embrace evidence in its broadest sense has been acknowledged by NHS Quality Improvement Scotland (2005: iii) in the development of best practice statements. In producing guidance for a whole range of conditions they state that these

> 66 *best practice statements represent a unique synthesis of research evidence, evidence complemented by audit, patient surveys and inputs derived from expert opinion, professional consensus and patient/public experience.* 99

Examples of their guide on the prevention and management of pressure ulcers (NHS Quality Improvement Scotland 2009) can be seen in Table 2.1, which demonstrates how evidence is used to ensure best practice is clear to those involved.

Statement	Reasons for statement	How to demonstrate statement is being achieved
As part of the holistic assessment, all patients/clients have their skin examined regularly, with special attention being paid to bony prominences. In children and neonates, particular attention is paid to the occiput, ears and areas under equipment and devices, eg nasogastric tubes, splints and casts, that may be pressing or rubbing on the skin.	Early identification of skin changes and intervention can prevent skin deterioration. The majority of pressure ulcers are located on the sacrum and heels. In children and neonates, the occiput and ears are the most common site of damage as well as the sacrum and heels. Ulceration is also common secondary to perinenal dermatitis or 'nappy rash'.	Each skin examination is documented in the individual's health record. Findings from skin inspection which indicate that further action is required, along with the subsequent action taken, are documented in the health record.
Regular skin examination takes place at opportune times, for example during assistance with personal hygiene.	Early identification of skin changes and intervention can prevent skin deterioration.	Identification of any skin changes and associated treatments are documented in the health record.
Where an area of redness (erythema) or discolouration is noted, further examination is carried out.	Further examination may help in the identification of the early stages of pressure ulcer development.	Erythema/discolouration and subsequent examination is documented.

Taken from: NHS Quality Improvement Scotland (2009) *Best Practice Statement March 2009*: prevention and management of pressure ulcers

Section 1: Skin examination, assessment and care

Key points:

1 All individuals should have their skin assessed. If changes are observed, preventative strategies should be initiated.

2 Darkly pigmented skin requires particular vigilance. Discolouration of the skin, warmth, oedema, induration or hardness may also be used as indicators.

Table 2.1 Prevention and management of pressure ulcers

However, in the practice area there are likely to be other sources of evidence that you can call on; these include:

- Local clinical guidelines
- National guidelines
- Government White Papers
- National Service Frameworks
- Local and national audits on specific service issues

Clinical practice guidelines

In reading about EBP, it is easy to believe that each nurse must develop their own clinical practice by finding and evaluating all the evidence for all the nursing interventions they carry out. This is clearly impossible and simply just not feasible. As Dartnell *et al.* (2008) observe, the alternative to trying to do everything yourself is to use clinical guidelines for specific procedures or patients, where all evidence has not only been sifted but has been turned into action points for clinical practice.

Guidelines were seen as one of the early goals of EBP and at the turn of the 1990s a lot of activity was centred on developing the principles and skills of writing guidelines. So, one of the early definitions of clinical guidelines was that they were

> 66 systematically developed statements to assist practitioner decisions about appropriate healthcare for specific clinical circumstances. 99

> *(Field & Lohr 1990:38)*

The source of evidence for guidelines for clinical interventions is usually RCTs. This is because of the level of control over accuracy of the results. If guidelines are to be sound, they should be based on the form of research that is strongest in relation to being able to make predictions on their results. RCTs, then, form the best available evidence to support this kind of activity (Evans 2003).

According to Timmermans & Mauck (2005):

> 66 non-adherence to practice guidelines remains the major barrier to the successful practice of evidence-based medicine. 99

This has been seen as a general problem wherever EBP exists. For example Grol & Buchan (2006: 301) suggest that one problem is that EBP:

66 *assumes that professionals are rational decision makers who will act on convincing information about the pros and cons of specific routines.* 99

and this may not be the case. There may be a multitude of reasons why practitioners decide not to follow best practice, or are blocked from doing so because of conditions in the clinical area.

Challenges with clinical guidelines

There are a number of issues relating to guidelines that have to be faced, including the lack of evidence or good quality research on which to base guidelines.

Grol & Buchan (2006: 301) also draw attention to the way in which guidelines do not take into account the challenges that the uses of guidelines might have in being translated into practice. They state that:

66 *Many current programs for guideline development seem to be 'science-driven', rather than scientifically based but 'customer-driven'. Guideline developers would do a far better job if they focused on the needs of the end user and provided clear statements, decision aids, patient education materials and practical tools to manage difficult problems in practice.* 99

This is an important aspect that requires thought. It is the health professional who needs to use the guidelines: that requires help to put them in the context of current practice. Once qualified as a nurse, this will be you! Therefore, learning about clinical guidelines and their application in a clinical situation would be a very valuable skill for you to gain.

+ ....

EBP in action

Find one clinical guideline that is relevant to your field of practice using the websites that are included at the end of this chapter. Consider the evidence base for it and how you can use this to inform your learning outcomes regarding use of evidence underpinning care. It may also be an excellent reference source for an assignment you may have which asks you to consider the use of evidence in the care of a patient you have met in practice.

....

Summary

- EBP is a philosophy and movement designed to improve nursing practice and the quality of care received by patients. It has a clear structure and purpose.
- The role of evidence is to reduce bias and inaccuracies in the source of knowledge we use for decision-making.
- Nursing has traditionally used knowledge from a wide range of sources and valued the personal sources of knowledge such as professional experience.
- Learning about the different kinds of evidence and EBP is an inherent part of learning to be a registered nurse.
- Nursing needs to increase the research evidence available with regards to impact and outcomes of nursing interventions.

You may find it interesting to revisit the first 'EBP in action' box in this chapter and reconsider your answer.

■ Online resource centre

 You can watch the webcast of Jill Macleod Clark's keynote speech on nursing research from the RCN Research Conference 2009 on our online resource centre. You can also access several key websites which will help you to explore the utilization of evidence in nursing practice and find excellent sources of evidence quickly. Please now go online to **www.oxfordtextbooks.co.uk/orc/holland/**

■ References

Albanese, M. & Norcini, J. (2002) Systematic reviews: What they are and why should we care. *Advances in Health Sciences Education* 7 (2) 147–151.

Brown, S. (2009) *Evidence-Based Nursing: the research-practice connection*. Sudbury: Jones and Bartlett.

Cohen, A. & Hersh, W. (2004) Guest Editorial: Criticisms of evidenced-based medicine. *Evidence-based Cardiovascular Medicine* 8 (3) 197–198.

Craig, J. & Smyth, R. L. (2007) *The Evidence-Based Practice Manual for Nurses (2nd edn)*. Edinburgh: Churchill Livingstone.

Cullum, N., Ciliska, D., Haynes, R. & Marks, S. (2008) *Evidence-Based Nursing: an introduction*. Oxford: Blackwell.

Dale, A. (2005) Evidence-based practice: compatibility with nursing. *Nursing Standard*. 19 (40) 48–53.

Dale, A. (2006) Determining guiding principles for evidence-based practice. *Nursing Standard* 20 (25) 41–46.

Dartnell, J., Hemming, M., Collier, J. & Ollenschlaeger, G. (2008) EBN notebook: Putting evidence into context: some advice for guideline writers. *Evidence-Based Nursing* 11 (1) 6–8.

Department of Health (2008) *High Quality Care for All: NHS next step review final report (Chair of the Review Lord Dazi)*. London: DH.

Drake, R., Goldman, H., Leff, H., Lehman, A., Dixon, L., Mueser, K. & Torrey, W., (2001) Implementing evidence-based practices in routine mental health service settings. *Psychiatric Services* 52 (2) 179–182.

Eisenburg, J. (2002) Globalize the evidence, localize the decision: evidence-based medicine and international diversity. *Health Affairs* 21 (3) 166–68.

Evans, D. (2003) Hierarchy of evidence: a framework for ranking evidence evaluating healthcare interventions. *Journal of Clinical Nursing* 12 (1) 77–84.

Field, M. & Lohr, K. (1990) *Clinical Practice Guidelines: directions for a new program*. Washington: National Academy Press.

Fineout-Overholt, E., Melnyk, B. & Schultz, A. (2005) Transforming health care from the inside out: advancing evidence-based practice in the 21st Century. *Journal of Professional Nursing* 21 (6) 335–344.

Grol, R. & Buchan, H. (2006) Editorials: Clinical guidelines: what can we do to increase their use? *Medical Journal of Australia*185 (6) 301–302.

Hamer, S. & Collinson, G. (eds.) (2005) *Achieving Evidence-Based Practice: a handbook for practitioners (2nd edn)*. Edinburgh: Bailliere Tindall.

Leufer, T. & Cleary-Holdforth J. (2009) Evidence-based practice: improving patient outcomes. *Nursing Standard* 23 (32) 35–39.

Machin, D., Day, S. & Green, S. (eds.) (2006) *Textbook of Clinical Trials (2nd edn)* Chichester: John Wiley.

NHS Quality Improvement Scotland (QIS) (2004) *Best Practice Statement: working with dependent older people to achieve good oral health*. Edinburgh: NHS QIS.

NHS Quality Improvement Scotland (2009) *Best Practice Statement March 2009: prevention and management of pressure ulcers*. Edinburgh: NHS Quality Improvement Scotland.

Pearson, A., Field, J. & Jordan, Z. (2007) *Evidence-Based Clinical Practice in Nursing and Health Care: assimilating research, experience and expertise*. Oxford: Blackwell.

Sackett, D. & Rosenberg, W. (1995) On the need for evidence-based medicine. *Journal of Public Health Medicine* 17 (5) 330–34.

Sackett, D., Strauss, S., Richardson, W., Rosenberg, W. & Haynes, R. (1997) *Evidence-Based Medicine: how to practice and teach EBM*. Edinburgh: Churchill Livingstone.

Swage, T. (2004) *Clinical Governance in Health Care Practice (2nd edn)*. Edinburgh: Butterworth Heinemann.

Theroux, R. (2006) How to bring evidence into your practice. Association of Women's Health, *Obstetric and Neonatal Nurses* 10 (3) 244–249.

Thompson, C., MCCaughan, D., Cullum, N., Sheldon, T. & Raynor, P. (2005) Barriers to evidence-based practice in primary care nursing – why viewing decision-making as context is helpful. *Journal of Advanced Nursing* 52 (4) 432–444.

Timmermans, S. & Mauck, A. (2005) The promises and pitfalls of evidence-based medicine. *Health Affairs* 24 (1) 18–28.

Walsh, M. & Ford, P. (1989) *Nursing Rituals, Research and Rational Action*. Oxford: Butterworth Heinemann.

■ Further reading

Logan-Sinclair, P. and Coomb, K. (2006)Science in Nursing or nursing science? a preliminary report, https://www.aare.edu.au/06pap/log06165.pdf/

Endacott, R., Jevon, P. and Cooper, S. (2009) Clinical Nursing Skills - Core and Advanced. Oxford University Press: Oxford (This book has evidence underpinning the clinical skills).

■ Useful websites

Cochrane Collaboration

> http://cochrane.co.uk/en/about.html/

McMaster's University

> http://hsl.mcmaster.ca/resources/ebpractice.htm/

NHS Evidence:

> http://www.nice.org.uk/nhsevidence/

NHS Scotland - Health on the web:

> http://www.show.scot.nhs.uk/

NHS Quality Improvement Scotland:

> http://www.nhsqis.org.uk/

WHO Health Evidence Network:

> http://www.euro.who.int/hen/

NHS Education Scotland: NHS Flying Start

> http://www.flyingstart.scot.nhs.uk/Waysofovercomingbarrierstoimplementingevidence.htm/

Understanding the research process for evidence-based nursing practice

Colin Rees

The aims of this chapter are:

➤ To outline the research process.

➤ To provide an overview of each step within the research process.

➤ To examine some of the ethical issues involved in research studies.

➤ To identify some of the main issues faced by the researcher when designing research studies in relation to outline the concepts of reliability, validity, bias, and rigour.

➤ To identify why student nurses need to understand the research process.

Introduction

Understanding how and why research is carried out is essential to your understanding of evidence-based practice because in order to be able to read a research paper or report on new evidence that might lead to a change in nursing practice, you need to understand what it is saying, and most importantly, whether the research follows a rigorous and ethical process.

This chapter covers one of the most important structures in research: that of the research process. This can be defined as the stages or steps the researcher follows in carrying out a research project and is sometimes referred to as the research design. The research process is the backbone of a study, as it supports and gives purpose to many of the activities carried out by the researcher. Before starting a study, the researcher outlines the way it will be structured in the form of a research proposal. This is the written plan of action for the study and is used to apply for ethical approval and to gain permission to gain access to any participants or data. This proposal includes the justification for carrying out the study, as well as providing a clear plan of the research process the researcher will follow.

Knowledge of the stages in the research process is beneficial to you in two ways:

- It provides you with a guide to evaluate (critique) how well a researcher has structured their study, which in turn will influence the quality of the outcome of the study.

- It will allow you to construct your own outline of a study (research proposal), either as part of an assignment or as an activity in the clinical setting.

If we start by looking at research as an activity, one of the distinctive characteristics of research is the careful and systematic way it is carried out. Just as an architect must draw up and follow accurate plans concerning all the elements that go to make up a house, office block, or other building, so the researcher must plan in detail exactly how a study will unfold.

This is to ensure that the study runs smoothly and reaches its objectives. It has to be fit for purpose, so the fine points involved in research cannot be left to chance or decisions made on an ad hoc basis. Clearly, one of the most important criteria of successful research is that it should be accurate and meet its objectives. However, as research is a complex activity, the researcher needs to anticipate some of the influences that can affect the accuracy of the outcome. An essential part of developing your understanding of research then, is to have a clear understanding of how a researcher designs and follows the research process to produce sound information that can be used in deciding on best practice.

EBP in action

Although we have not yet explained the steps of the research process, it will be useful if you can follow these in an article of your choice. Use a research article from your area of practice (perhaps you have to read one for an assignment or placement anyway?), or find one of the examples used in Chapters 4 and 5. Make a note of all the headings within the article, and as you progress through this chapter make a note of any additional stages in the research process that may have left out (you can highlight sections or write on a printed copy of the article or jot them down from your electronic copy). This will also help you with the exercises in Chapter 7.

The research process

Research studies come in several different types. The way each of these is structured will be influenced by a number of choices and decisions made by the researcher, for example the research approach that will be used. Writers such as Bryman (2008: 22) use the term research strategy to refer to the same element. He defines this as 'a general orientation to the conduct of social research'. In general, the research approach can take two forms, either a quantitative research approach, where the main emphasis is on measurement and the search for relationships between variables, or a qualitative approach, where the main emphasis is on description through words or narratives and the interpretation of personal experiences either of individuals or groups or possibly even documents. Each approach has variations in the main features of the research process that will affect how it looks, and the research principles it follows. More detail on some of the distinctions between these two approaches will be given later in this chapter, and there will be more in-depth information in Chapter 4, which looks at qualitative approaches and Chapter 5, which looks at quantitative approaches.

As you become familiar with different examples of research, you will notice a basic order and structure of elements used in the description of all research. This is the research process that forms the subject of this chapter, and which is made up of a number of steps or stages. It is helpful to see these stages diagrammatically before we go on and consider each stage in detail. As can be seen from Fig. 3.1, the process can be compared to the spine of a skeleton where everything is connected to this central structure running through the body that is the research study. You will also see that certain decisions made early on have important implications for the choices that are made later in the process.

✚ ....

EBP in action

Reflect on how closely the stages in the research process can be compared to those in the nursing process, i.e. assessing, planning, implementing, and evaluating. One other stage often used after assessment is that of the nursing diagnosis.

....

Using the stages in the nursing process, you can see that:

Assessment can be compared to selecting a problem area or assessing an area that can be researched. Reviewing the literature is another part of assessment.

Diagnosis of a patient or nursing need can equate to the development of a research question or aim, where once these have been set a method of answering these has to be developed.

Planning can be compared to choosing how to do this, through a plan of care, or, in the case of research, through choosing the right approach and methods, the sample size, and so on.

Implementing a nursing intervention is similar to carrying out the research itself and involves the researcher gathering information and data.

Evaluating the care or effectiveness of the nursing interventions is similar to the analysis of the data obtained and developing some conclusions about the findings of the research and the implications they have for patient outcomes or practice.

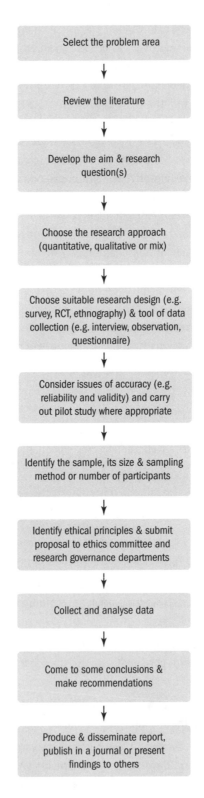

Figure 3.1 The research process. RCT, randomized controlled trial

Although the steps are presented in Fig. 3.1 in a vertical progression, when the researcher plans the study, and indeed carries it out, there will be a blurring and overlapping between some of the stages. Some of you, prior to starting your course, may have already undertaken some research or have been involved in gathering data and will be familiar with this overlapping. If you are undertaking a post-graduate pre-registration programme, you may have to undertake a small research study as part of the course, or as in some undergraduate programmes, you may have had to write a research proposal. Understanding that research is not a linear process is important also when you come to critiquing a research paper in Chapter 7. The steps can now be outlined in more detail.

Step 1: Selecting the problem area

The first stage of research is to identify the area that needs to be researched. In nursing, this is usually a situation seen as 'problematic' or an area where clear information is lacking. Burns & Grove (2009: 68) define a research problem like this:

> 66 *A research problem is an area of concern where there is a gap in the knowledge base needed for nursing practice.* 99

It is worth pointing out that this definition brings together two important aspects: firstly, the problem area identified by the researcher, and secondly, the practice of nursing. This highlights that research is a way of producing evidence to improve nursing practice or other areas such as nurse education. From your clinical experiences and your theory sessions, you will have already discovered that there are so many issues within nursing that need solutions or evidence to support nursing interventions, so clearly there is a need for nurses to be involved in clinical research. The introduction of Clinical Academic Careers for nurses, midwives, and allied health professions, which focuses on research, is testament to the importance of being placed on this by the Department of Health (see **http://www.nccrcd.nhs.uk/nursesmidwivesandahp/** for further details).

EBP in action

There are so many topics that could be researched in nursing, so what is it that makes some topics more suitable for research than others? List what you consider might influence whether a topic is more or less likely to be chosen to be researched. Consider the patient care experiences you have had in clinical placements in deciding these, and also what you know from reading about health priorities such as the impact of smoking in causing health problems.

Firstly, we should be clear that not all topics or problems are researchable. Some problems can only be answered through debate or discussion; research may not tell us what the best course of action is in all situations. For example, should nurses use secondhand cars to travel to their workplace? Such topics cannot be 'answered' by research, it is more a case of developing an argument for why there might be any disadvantages to this and convincing others with evidence to support the argument. This type of question does not fit the definition of research—that of increasing our understanding of a particular phenomenon.

To help us work out what is researchable, consider how Wood & Ross-Kerr (2006: 5) talk about the nature of the research question:

> 66 *Research deals with facts—that is, with observable phenomena in the real world. A question that will provide answers that explain, describe, identify, substantiate, predict or qualify is a researchable question.* 99

This not only helps us see what we should expect from research findings, but also helps to distinguish research from **audit**. This is a process for collecting information to assess current performance in a local area to gain feedback on the output or performance of that area. This information can then be compared to an organizational or clinical target or standard, or to a previous audit result from the same area to monitor improvements over time. It is not used as a way of obtaining generalizable knowledge that will explain or allow us to predict relationships between aspects of care or nurse education. Although EBP requires audit to provide evidence and data on performance, it is different from research. It does not increase our understanding of the topic itself, or allow us to transfer the results to other situations in the same way that we look for in research findings.

So we might undertake an audit of how many patients in a clinical setting are self-medicating prior to discharge from hospital, so that it can be compared with a target of at least 80% self-medicating before going home. This will not provide us with evidence on the extent to which self-medication leads to greater levels of drug adherence or concordance, or if some patients are better candidates for self-medication. That would require a research study. As a student nurse you may have seen examples of a nursing audit or decided to learn more about it during your clinical placement. You can see a student example at **www.nottingham.ac.uk/nursing/students/prereg-docs/portfolio/annotated-bib.doc/**. This student conducted an audit of nursing documentation under the supervision of the nursing team and linked it to the NMC Standards of Proficiency.

Once a researcher has a researchable question, there are a number of factors that will influence which topics are suitable for research. On a practical level, there is the cost of resources needed to answer a question, such as research staff, paper resources, travelling, and computer hardware and software, and the time required to complete it. There may also be ethical issues raised concerning the appropriateness of the research and its possible negative impact, both physical and emotional, on those taking part.

A further consideration in selecting researchable projects is the extent to which change may be possible once we have the answers. If we found that taller women found it easier to swallow tablets compared to those not as tall, there is little we could do to increase the height of this latter group. The conclusion is that perhaps we need to consider the priority of the topics that are researched and ensure that studies that can contribute the greatest knowledge or usefulness, and require the least resources, may be placed higher than those with a lower utility. However, that again is a matter for debate.

> ## ! Key points
>
> If you are asked to construct a research proposal of your choice, for example for an assignment or group project, remember, not everything is 'researchable'. Ask yourself 'would knowing the answer to this question increase our general understanding of the topic?' If it will only answer a limited question or it can only be answered by debate and discussion, it may not be a topic suitable for research.

One of the first things the researcher must do in designing a research proposal is to be clear on the rationale for the choice of topic selected. Just because it is something a researcher is interested in, does not make it a worthy topic for research. The researcher must have good reasons for pursuing a particular topic and should ensure that the answer to the research question does not already exist. One of the ways in which the researcher can develop a rationale is by examining the available research literature on the topic.

Step 2: Review of the literature

Each research study has the potential to increase our knowledge and understanding of a nursing issue or problem. It is clear that this new knowledge should not simply be a repeat of sound knowledge we have already gained, so one way of avoiding this is to examine the literature on the topic. Polit & Beck (2008: 106) make the point that a researcher carries out a review of the literature in order to provide a foundation and context for their own study. In particular, they say, the researcher should critically examine the existing body of knowledge looking for gaps that their research might fill.

More detail on the methods used to search for and locate the literature will be found in Chapter 6, and the methods of critically examining, or critiquing, the literature will be covered in Chapter 7. Here, it is important to state that the researcher, particularly in the case of quantitative research carries out a thorough and complete review of the research literature in order to establish the current level of knowledge on their topic. The review will also reveal valuable information on how the topic has been researched by others.

This will help in determining the research design that will be most valuable to follow, and those aspects that should be avoided.

> **! Key points**
>
> Any research study does not stand in isolation from the body of knowledge already existing on that topic; it must be placed within the context of current knowledge. This is the function of the review of the literature. Often the researcher will use this to point to a gap in the literature or evidence available that the study will help to close.

The review of literature may also help the researcher to develop a clearer wording of their research question, or help to develop the content of the tool for data collection, for example the kind of questions to include in a questionnaire. However, such an in-depth review of the literature is not always conducted at the start of a study. As we will see later in regard to qualitative research, sometimes the qualitative researcher may avoid a comprehensive review of the literature. This is to ensure that their thoughts and interpretations of the data are not influenced or biased by the ideas that already exist, as this may prevent new insights from emerging from their findings.

+ EBP in action

If you have chosen a research article to use throughout this chapter, now would be a good time to consider the content of the early stages of the research process. What you should find is that the title gives some clue as to the topic and that the introduction sets the scene for 'the research problem' and the nature of the problem. You should find that this supports the choice of topic as a research study. You may find there is a specific subheading 'review of the literature' or 'literature review' where previous studies of the topic are examined. Other articles may incorporate the literature as part of the introduction to the study. At the end of these sections you should be clear as to why the topic has been chosen and whether the researcher has justified their choice. Check your article now and notice how the study has been justified.

All you are doing at this stage is reading the article, developing the skill of critiquing or evaluating an article will be covered in Chapter 7. It is important for students to learn to read articles, not just to see what they are saying but also to learn how to paraphrase their content. This is an important skill which we will discuss in Chapter 9.

Step 3: Developing the research aim and questions

Perhaps the most important part of the research process is writing the research aim. This is because it identifies the variable, or variables, that will form the focus of the study

(Burns & Grove 2009). The aim will also identify what the researcher wants to find out about the variable, and this will influence and provide direction for the whole study. So, for instance in Table 3.1, which contains a number of research aims, the first aim by Robson *et al.* (2009) looks at the rate of wound healing (variable) and questions if the choice of treatment (variable) between honey and conventional treatment has a direct effect on the rate of wound healing. This type of question is usually answered by a randomized control trial (RCT) where one form of treatment is tested against another in terms of the effect they have on a particular clinical outcome. Here the outcome, which is called the dependent variable, is rate of wound healing. The intervention introduced or controlled by the researcher (here the difference between honey and conventional treatment) is called the **independent variable**. More information will be given on RCTs in Chapter 5.

The second aim in Table 3.1 by Banbury *et al.* (2008) looks at the variable 'attitudes and experiences of analgesic use' in a particular patient group. As the wording of the aim starts with 'to explore' this is an indicator that rather than precise measurements, this study will be a qualitative study as this type of study is undertaken where little is known about the topic and the data will be broader than the more narrow numeric or quantitative study. Here patients were asked about their experiences of taking analgesics for back pain in an interview setting where their responses were taped and later analysed looking for common themes.

The statement of the aim in quantitative research will lead to measurable aspects of the variable or variables that form the focus of the study. The more precise the researcher makes the wording of the aim, the easier it will be to design a suitable approach to measuring it. So, it is difficult to have an aim such as 'to examine does sunshine affect mood'. It is better to have an aim such as 'to establish if the number of hours exposed to direct sunlight produces a reduction in the depression scores of community patients suffering from clinical depression'. When you look at an aim it should conjure up a picture of how it would be possible to answer that aim.

Aim	Source
To compare a medical grade honey with conventional treatments on the healing rates of wounds healing by secondary intention.	Robson, Dodd & Thomas (2009)
To explore the attitudes and experiences of analgesic use of patients who are experiencing low back pain and who have been referred to a back pain programme.	Banbury, Feenan & Allcock (2008)
To determine if the provision of computer-aided scoring could increase the accuracy and efficiency of early warning score calculations, when compared with the traditional pen-and paper method.	Mohammed, Hayton, Clements, Smith & Prytherch (2009)
To compare patient and staff perceptions of phase III cardiac rehabilitation delivered in a hospital versus community setting.	Blake, Tsakirides & Ingle (2009)

Table 3.1 Example of research aims

+···

EBP in action

Consider the list of aims in Table 3.1 and determine what the possible objectives to meet that aim could be. Use the following examples to help you.

Research question: What are midwives' attitudes towards fathers being present at the birth of their child?

Research aim: To determine the attitudes of midwives working in a community hospital towards fathers being present at the birth of a child.

Research objectives:

1. To ask student midwives about their attitudes towards fathers being present at the birth.

2. To ask qualified midwives about their attitudes towards fathers being present at the birth.

···

! Key points

The research aim is the pivot around which everything else rotates. The researcher must be very clear about the aim of the research and ensure that all the other aspects of the design of the study will answer this aim in the most efficient way. When you read an aim you should be able to anticipate the way in which the researcher will set about answering it.

Related to the aim of a study is the question that was in the researcher's mind when they developed their ideas about the study. In the example of the fictitious depression and sunlight study suggested above, we can see that the question may have been 'does the amount of sunlight improve a patient's level of depression?' Here the key variable is level of depression, which is an outcome measure and so forms the dependent variable, and the variable that may be associated with that is the amount of sunlight; this is the variable that the researcher may control access to, so forms the independent variable. Some studies will state both the aim and the research question as in the example of the midwives attitudes, but they may be so closely linked that only the aim is shown.

In some studies, particularly RCTs, there may also be a hypothesis. This is a statement that the researcher wants to test through the study. So in the study above a hypothesis may be:

> " Those patients exposed to at least 3 hours of sunlight a day for one week will have a lower depression score than those who have been exposed to sunlight for less than 3 hours a day for one week. "

Here, we can see a hypothesis is a statement, not a question. It does allow us to think of how the study may be answered by taking one group exposed to this amount of sunlight in comparison to a group not exposed to that level of sunlight, and using a depression scale to see if the difference is evident, usually using statistical tests to rule out the possibility that any differences are due simply to chance.

A hypothesis statement regarding midwives attitudes could be:

> 66 *Midwives do not have a positive attitude to fathers being present at birth in any circumstance.* 99

✛ EBP in action

Return to your research article and see if you can identify the aim of the study. This may well be headed 'Aim' in the abstract, and also be written either at the end of the literature review, at the beginning of the methods section, or in the introduction. Does the aim allow you to 'see' what the researcher would have to do to answer that aim?

Step 4: Choosing a suitable research approach

There are two main research approaches used in nursing research, both of which have already been mentioned; these are the **qualitative approach**, which examines from a broad point of view people's experiences or interpretations of a situation, and the **quantitative approach**, which concentrates on the measurement of variables and the possible relationship between different variables. These approaches are sometimes referred to as a 'paradigm' or world view, as they are based on the researcher's beliefs about the purpose of research and the nature of variables.

The research question will give clues as to the research approach used by the researcher. Anything that suggests measurements or quantification of variables using some kind of measuring tool, or quantifying how much or how many of something there is, will indicate a quantitative approach. Anything that would require talking to someone in depth and recording verbatim answers, or observing a situation and broadly describing what was said or done, rather than counting it, would suggest a qualitative approach.

One easy way to tell if a study is qualitative or quantitative is to look at how the results are presented. If there are a number of tables with numbers, percentages, or graph and bar charts it is a quantitative study. If there are no tables, or only one showing the characteristics of the sample and a number of quotes from individuals linked to key themes from the data then it is likely to be a qualitative study.

You will discover more about these approaches in detail in the next two chapters. For now, the main point is that, depending on the approach, there will be some quite noticeable differences in the way the study is designed and the way it looks when presented as a research report.

+ ··

EBP in action

You may like to return to Table 3.1 and look at the examples there and see if you can categorize each study as either qualitative or quantitative. Then check your research article to see if it takes a qualitative or quantitative approach in its design.

Once you have identified the design in your article, consider whether you feel that was an appropriate choice given the aim of the study.

··

Can a study be both qualitative and quantitative?

The answer is that it can use a mixed method approach to answer a research question or study aim, as in a case study. You may also see the word triangulation also used in such studies, where evidence is considered from a range of sources to come to a conclusion. It could also be a quantitative study, such as a survey, that also includes some open questions from a questionnaire. This stays in the quantitative paradigm where the main aim is to numerically present most of the results. The qualitative data included are likely to add depth to the main quantitative results. In some studies however even the qualitative data can be represented as numerical data, for example by counting the number of times an issue or statement is made by the participants.

Step 5: Choosing a suitable research design and tool of data collection

Once the broad methodological approach has been chosen (qualitative or quantitative) the researcher must then decide on an appropriate design of the research within that approach. The research design can be compared to the situation in architecture where the design plan will follow a different format depending on whether the aim is to produce a house, a bungalow, or factory. Each category differs from the other, and follows certain recognizable 'type' characteristics that help to identify it as belonging to one category rather than another.

For qualitative approaches there are a number of designs or strategies, the most frequently used ones include:

- Phenomenology
- Ethnography
- **Grounded theory**
- A more general qualitative design that is less restrictive than the above options

Each of these options is structured in certain ways that will be outlined in Chapter 4. For quantitative designs the options include:

- Surveys (these may be descriptive or correlation designs)
- RCTs
- Non-randomized trials such as quasi-experimental designs

The choice of design will lead the researcher to choose the research method or data collecting tool. You will recognize many of these as they are familiar ways of collecting research data:

- Questionnaires
- Interviews (focus groups or individual interviews)
- Observation
- Documentary methods
- Assessment scales or physiological measurements

Some of these can vary in structure depending on whether the methodological approach is qualitative or quantitative. So, for instance, interviews may feature in quantitative research, but will be very structured by offering a number of choices in the answers that can be selected. In qualitative research interviews will tend to be more open and unstructured. This will have implications for the method of analysis. For example, the answers selected in interviews in the quantitative study will be turned into a number or numeric value (for example a 'yes' answer will equal '1' and a 'no' answer equal '2'. The number of ones and twos will then be counted to give a score), in qualitative interviews they will be analysed in terms of the themes emerging from the interview.

As you will see in Chapter 4 on qualitative data gathering, questionnaires are not a common feature of qualitative research, as it is difficult to conform to one of the principles of qualitative research, which is that the method should be flexible and start from the perspective of the respondent. Questionnaires are designed from the perspective of the researcher and so are likely to reflect their preconceptions about the important issues in the situation. This means that questionnaires frequently leave the respondent to choose something that fits in with the researcher's ideas on a topic rather than the respondent's own ideas or experiences.

This is an example of some of the methodological issues faced by the researcher at every step of the way in the research process. For each of the methods there will be advantages to their use, and also limitations. When you are reading someone's study or designing one yourself, it is important to consider both these strengths and limitations in making assessments about the quality of a study.

Step 6: Issues of reliability and validity

While we are considering the tools of data collection, it is worth introducing two closely related concepts that are fundamental to talking about research. These are the concepts of reliability and validity. As they often appear together, it can be difficult to be clear on the difference between them, or even be sure if a difference exists. However, they are fundamentally different, so it is worth clarifying their meaning and use here.

Reliability

Reliability is used when talking about the tool of data collection in a quantitative study. It relates to the accuracy and consistency of the measuring tool, such as a depression scale, or type of thermometer, anything that is used to produce a number to be used as a measurement of a variable. Polit & Beck (2008) refer to the extent to which a measuring tool in research is consistent in the way in which it measures a particular variable. In the case of an attitude scale, or pain scale, would it give the same measurement when used by one person and then re-applied either by the same person, or a different person? Reliability, then, can be defined as the extent to which the tool of data collection measures accurately and consistently the variable under consideration.

A researcher will often demonstrate reliability of the tool of data collection by either using a method that has been used in a previous study, or at least piloting the tool to ensure that it measures in a consistent way. A pilot study is a small scale version of the larger study that is used to test the tool of data collection and to ensure that any practical problems that may be encountered in a study are discovered and reduced before the main study commences.

Validity

Validity is a different concept from reliability as it is related to the nature of the result and not the measuring ability of the tool of data collection. The idea of validity is to check the extent to which the researcher can demonstrate they have measured what

> **! Key points**
>
> The terms **reliability** and **validity** are part of the language of research. Although they cover somewhat different aspects they are often used together and the similarity in the way they are written can lead to confusion. Illustrating you can show the difference between these two concepts will demonstrate your understanding of research and its language.

they think they have measured. Bryman (2008) elaborates on this by suggesting that it relates to the extent to which the result of measuring a variable truly reflects that concept or variable. So for instance, with a pain scale, is it pain that has been measured, or is it anxiety? It is more difficult for the researcher to convince us of the validity of the results and often will draw on the similarities of their results to other studies to argue that the same concept has been measured.

In quantitative research, a tool of data collection should be both reliable, that is measuring consistently, and also a true measure of the variable being considered. It is possible to have a measuring tool that is consistent, for example a tape measure could produce exactly the same measurement independent of who was using it, but it may not be a true measure of say the degree of pain in a patient's foot if the circumference of the foot is measured with that tape. So a tool can be reliable but not valid.

The challenge for the researcher then is to select a tool that both measures consistently, accurately and can be relied on to measure what the researcher intends it to measure, and not some other variable.

In qualitative research it is still important to consider rigour of the research, and words often associated with this are credibility and trustworthiness. Ensuring that any research evidence is trustworthy is as important as reliability and validity in quantitative research, especially when considering changing nursing interventions or practice as a result of the research.

+..

EBP in action

If you return to your research article, what tool of data collection is used in the study? Do you consider it was a good choice in relation to the aim of the study? If it is a quantitative study, are issues of reliability or validity talked about, or is anything done to give you some reassurances about these two concepts? If it is a qualitative study how does the researcher explain the trustworthiness of the research?

....

There are a number of principles related to the tool of data collection, and a particular problem shared by questionnaires and interviews is the issue of self-report. This concerns the assumption we make when we gather information through these two methods about the accuracy or truthfulness of the answer. In other words, just because people say they drink a particular number of units of alcohol per week does not mean it is true or accurate. This is a self-report figure and it may differ if a more objective method was found to measure it.

Related to this last issue, we must also consider that when we ask people questions about their behaviour or their beliefs, there may be good reasons why they may not give an accurate answer.

Firstly, this may be to do with the nature of the activity, such as excessive smoking or drinking and the level of disapproval that an individual may feel they would receive if they told the truth. Here, people may give an inaccurate answer to ensure they are seen in a positive light by others, even themselves. Secondly, people may be asked to provide information on the frequency of something where it is difficult to give a completely accurate answer.

An example would be to ask on 'average how many times a day do you yawn?' Or 'how many times a day do you feel hungry?' In these examples, the activity is not usually carefully monitored or recorded, so at best any answer is likely to be an estimate and may be an over or under estimation of the real number of occasions something happens. Yet in all these examples, many people will hear or read the results of surveys collecting this type of very inaccurate data and regard it as 'fact'. We need to be aware that the accuracy of research findings can vary from study to study, and we need to consider the possible inaccuracy of some kinds of data collected in studies.

Step 7: Identify the sample and the sampling method

We now turn to the people (or things and events) in a study from whom information is collected. Here we need to consider the two concepts of the study population and sample. The study population is the people, things or events the researcher wants to say something about. This could be the elderly who suffer a fall in hospital, types of compression bandages, or the number of lecturers assigned to nursing students in a semester. It is unusual in one single research study to include the entire study population, the researcher will usually take a proportion of these to include in the study. That proportion will form the study sample. The goal of most researchers, particularly in quantitative research, is to select a study sample that will represent the study population as closely as possible, to ensure that generalizations can be made. In other words, the researcher will want to be confident that they can assume that what was found in the sample will be found in the study population as a whole.

In a qualitative research study, however, the researcher is not attempting to make generalizations about what they discover, but may nevertheless ensure that participants are representative or have knowledge of the topic being researched (see Chapter 4 for further details).

In order to get as close a fit as possible between sample and population, there are a number of aspects of sampling we need to consider. These include:

- Sample size
- Sample inclusion and exclusion criteria
- Sampling selection method (sampling strategy)

Sample size

Most research texts agree that in quantitative research, the larger the sample size the closer the results will fit the study population (e.g. Wood & Ross-Kerr 2006: 161/2). Where the researcher wants to plan the size of an experimental and control group for a RCT, there are statistical formulas called 'power statistics' that will give some guide to the sample size needed. Burns & Grove (2009) feel that nursing research pays too little attention to the calculation of the sample size required to show clear differences between groups in correlation and experimental studies, and they suggest that the accuracy of experimental nursing studies suffer as a consequence.

   On the whole, however, and particularly in the case of surveys, most researchers follow Polit & Beck's (2008: 348) advice that '*you should use the largest sample possible*'. However, this principle is not true of qualitative studies, where the sample size should be sufficient to capture the depth of the topic. There are also other considerations that affect sample size, such as the variability of the factor being studied: the wider the variability, the larger the size of the sample needed to capture that variability (Parahoo 2006: 277). Sample size, then is not a straightforward part of planning a study. This is another case where the researcher will turn to the experiences of other researchers found in the review of the literature on the topic.

Sample inclusion and exclusion criteria

If the sample is to be representative, then the researcher will need to consider who should be included in the sample, and who may need to be excluded. A sample should reflect the major characteristics that are typical within the large study population, factors such as the spread of ages, gender, type or severity of illness, previous treatments, and so on. These would form the *sample inclusion criteria*. The *sample exclusion criteria* would be anything that would make the individual, item, or even event untypical or unsafe to include. Examples of this might include those with serious illnesses, untypical experiences, or characteristics that might put individuals at risk within the study, such as those with cardiac conditions or on certain kinds of drugs. There can also be practical criteria leading to exclusions such as those with communication difficulties or unable to speak the same language as the researcher.

Methods of selecting the sample (sampling strategy)

This is the technical side of sampling where a number of options exist for the way the sample is selected for the study. The more accurate the results of the study have to be, the more stringent the method of selecting the sample in order for them to stand a reasonable chance of being typical and representative.

There are two broad categories of sampling strategy:

i) Probability methods: these are used where the sample must represent the total population as closely as possible. A probability sample has a high likelihood of matching the results that might have existed in the total sample.

ii) Non-probability methods: where the intention is to explore a topic and it is not clear who might be 'typical' or the intention is to get a rough idea that still may be reasonable enough to be useful. However, there is no way of estimating how probable the results may match those in the total population.

Table 3.2 shows some of the sampling strategies and a description of how they are carried out. These are shown for both probability sampling methods where there is likely to be a close fit between the results for the sample and the population as a whole, and strategies for non-probability sampling methods, where it is more difficult to say how close the results in the sample will fit the larger population.

+···

EBP in action

Look at your research article where the sample is discussed and the beginning of the results or findings. What details are given of:

i) Number of people/things/events making up the sample on whom the results/ findings are based.

ii) Is there a clear statement of inclusion and exclusion criteria?

iii) Is there a statement and description of the sampling strategy?

In this exercise you are reading the paper and not critiquing or evaluating whether these were the best criteria or approaches to take.

···

The quality of a studies results or findings will be influenced by those included in the sample. Usually, the more representative the members of a sample, the more accurate the results will be. The more unrepresentative those included, the more likely the study is to be flawed by bias, where the results will be unrepresentative as those included are not typical of those in whom the researcher is interested. Although we are using the term bias here in relation to the sample, such a distortion can occur at many stages of the research process. For this reason it is worth remembering the definition of bias given by Burns & Grove (2009: 689):

❝ *Any influence or action in a study that distorts the findings or slants them away from the true or expected.* ❞

Probability methods	Description
Simple random sample	Each person/item/event must have an equal chance of selection. This requires each person to be numbered in a sampling frame or list of those from the study population, a proportion of the total number of individuals is then selected using a table of random numbers or computer generated numbers.
Stratified random sample	Instead of one sampling frame there may be several dividing the study population into criteria, such as gender or nursing grade, clinical area, that might influence the outcome of the research.
Proportionate random sample	This is similar to a stratified sample except instead of there being an equal number drawn from each strata, they are selected to represent the ratio that exists in the larger population, e.g. if females outnumbered men in the sample by 4 to 1 then the sample would draw four from the female group for every one male.
Cluster (or multi-stage) sample	This is where there is a large number or large geographical spread of the study population. Instead of individuals being numbered, units in which they 'cluster' such as hospitals, or first sampled, then perhaps wards/clinical areas, then every person within that selected unit is inclusion.
Cohort	All of those falling into a specified group or time period are taken as the sample, e.g. all those discharged from a clinical area in the month of November.
Non-probability methods	
Convenience/opportunity/ accidental/	All these terms describe the situation where the researcher uses those people, things, or events that are easily accessible and relate to the inclusion and exclusion criteria. There is no guarantee they are typical but they will provide quick access to information. People waiting in an outpatient clinical would be an example of this sampling strategy as they are easy and convenient to include.
Quota sample	This is an attempt to make the previous example more typical by looking for representatives from various groups who need to be included in such a sample. For instance different genders or age groups may be seen as influencing the results, so a 'quota' or amount from each of these groups is included.
Snowball/chain/nominated sample	This method is often used in qualitative research where it is difficult to find members of a group as they may not be that visible, or part of a record system. It consists of locating a small number of representatives and asking them to name or nominate others like themselves who might be willing to take part.

Table 3.2 Common sampling strategies

All the elements in this section will allow you to consider the way in which the researcher has planned the sample for their study, and the way that this has influenced your confidence in the study results. In EBP, a great deal of importance is placed on the extent to which the findings of a study are likely to be representative of similar situations. For this reason, studies that use probability sampling methods are favoured as they are more likely to be sound and capable of being applied elsewhere, in comparison to studies that have used non-probability sampling methods. However, we have to acknowledge that in some situations it is not possible to use such intricate sampling methods and other, simpler, methods will need to be used.

Step 8: Ethical considerations

The principle of EBP has committed health professionals, including nurses, to using research as a major source of information. However, should this information be collected regardless of cost, and the affect it may have on those providing the information? Will the end result of 'good evidence' always justify the way that evidence is collected. The answer is clearly 'no'. Data gathering is not a right of the researcher but an activity that first of all needs permission and careful scrutiny to ensure that the activity of data gathering is justified, and, secondly, carried out in an acceptable manner to all those concerned. These judgements come under the heading of 'ethical considerations'.

+···

EBP in action

Imagine you are receiving treatment for a chronic health problem at your local hospital on an outpatient basis every 6 months or so. At one visit you are informed that there is a treatment trial about to start and you are asked if you would like to take part. List some of the questions that you might like answered before you make a decision on whether to take part or not.

···

Just as the activity of nurses is carefully scrutinized and follows a number of ethical principles outlined in *The Code: standards of conduct, performance and ethics for nurses and midwives* (NMC 2008), so researchers follow a code of practice (see for instance RCN 2007). Nurse researchers have an obligation to ensure that their research is 'safe, robust and ethical' (RCN 2007). Research ethics cover similar aspects to professional ethics in that the nursing code ensures that those in a nursing capacity are appropriately trained and accept responsibility for their actions. Researchers must also contribute to an individual's positive health, and avoid causing them harm, so research ethics follow similar principles. They are there to protect those who take part in research, including nursing staff, from harm, and ensure that those carrying out the research are appropriately qualified to undertake the work.

Ethical principles have been built up over time and are written guidelines that are updated from time to time and are based on a number of important agreements such as the Helsinki Declaration of 1964 developed by the World Medical Organisation and have been influential in providing the basis for subsequent guidelines (see web links at the end of this chapter).

The management of research activity is guided at a national level by the National Research Ethics Service (NRES), which is part of the National Patient Safety Agency (NPSA), both of which are part of the Department of Health (DH). If a researcher plans to collect information from patients, service users, carers, or care professionals, or carry out research using human tissue, or on health care premises, then they must apply to a local research ethics committee (LREC) for ethical permission. A summary of their intended research along with their tool of data collection, patient information sheet where relevant, and consent form is sent to the LREC. This is an ethics committee, comprising health professionals and members of the lay public, whose role is to consider the ethical issues raised by the study and the precautions researchers intend taking to protect those involved. This includes not only the safety of the individual but also the security of any data collected, particularly where this may be stored electronically. Such security arrangements will come under the 1998 Data Protection Act. In addition to this committee each NHS Trust in the UK will also have a Research and Governance Committee of its own that offers an additional layer of protection to research participants (see www.dh.gov.uk for further information).

Table 3.3 illustrates some of the key ethical principles that all researchers must follow when undertaking research.

+···

EBP in action

Which aspects identified in Table 3.3 can you see addressed in your research article? Are there any other issues from reading the paper that have not been identified by the researcher that you feel could also be an ethical issue? Where such issues are identified consider why the researcher has not included them in the article. You may be reading this article as part of a critique assignment, discuss with your tutor why the researcher may not have considered this aspect.

···

Research is not simply a matter of technique in collecting information; it also has implications for the way in which the researcher carries out the research. This relates to two important time periods, firstly getting people to take part in a study or 'recruiting' them into the research, and secondly, to the relationship with those taking part while the study is being carried out. So, at the beginning of the study the individual must feel that they have been in a position that recognizes their right to decide for themselves whether to take part in a study without being manipulated or forced into agreeing to take part. In this they should feel that the researcher has been honest with them and described exactly what will happen as part of the research (Polit & Beck 2008). Throughout the study, those involved should continue to feel that their human rights are being respected and the researcher is protecting them from any hazards that arise as a result of participation.

> **❗ Key points**
>
> The ethical aspects of a study are some of the most important considerations in designing a study. Unless the researcher has thought carefully how the principles of ethics may affect their study and built in safe guards and ways of demonstrating they have followed ethical principles, they will not get permission to carry out the study. Avoiding getting ethical permission may result in journals refusing to accept the study for publication. For all these reasons, it is important that you spend some time on this topic.

Although this section has drawn on the process in the UK, similar principles are followed elsewhere. In the USA instead of LREC, the corresponding body is an Institutional Review Board (IRB) which will review the ethical aspects of a study.

Priniciple	Description
The dignity, rights, safety, and well-being of those taking part must be protected	Individuals should not be forced or coerced to take part in the study. They should only take part of their own free will and can decline to take part, or cease to take part at any time without any consequences for their treatment, care or, in the case of students, their education. As part of this, individuals will be given time to think about participation and not have to make a quick decision. They will also be able to ask any questions about the study in addition to having full written information on the study.
Do good (beneficence) and avoid harm (non-maleficence)	The researcher must protect anyone involved in research from all forms of physical, psychological, social, or financial harm. Taking part in a study should have the potential to benefit the individual directly or society generally, and not expose them to unacceptable risks or harm.
Informed consent	Those taking part in research should be given an explanation in plain English (preferably written) that explains important details about the study. Special protection should be given to vulnerable groups such as the young and those who lack mental capacity. Where appropriate consent can be given by those with legal responsibility for such individuals.
Anonymity and confidentiality	Individuals should not be identified, or be identifiable, in the results of the study. This will also extend to locations that might identify individuals. The identifying information gathered in the study will not be shared with other people and will be kept securely. It will be destroyed after a suitable time period.
Justice	All those taking part in the study will be treated in with the same respect and will not be disadvantaged on any grounds.
Conform to the principles of research governance	The principles laid down in the principles of Research Governance Framework (DH 2005) should be followed particularly in respect to the involvement of an ethics committee (LREC) who will judge the ethical suitability of the study.

Table 3.3 Main Ethical Principles Involved in Research

Step 9: Collect and analyse data

Once a study has been given ethical approval, the researcher is ready to start data collection. The first stage may be a *pilot study*, referred to above in the section on issues of reliability and validity. This is where the researcher will test the tool of data collection to ensure the method does work accurately with this particular sample. In qualitative research you may note that the researcher has undertaken a pilot interview; this is not the same as a pilot study but is where the researcher may be new to undertaking an interview and wanted to gain experience of the process itself rather.

The data collection part of the main study is exciting for the researcher as this will provide the basis for the findings of the research. It is also, as Serrant-Green (2008: 4) observes, *'one of the most important phases in completing any research'*. This is because it provides an 'answer' to the research question and so the success or failure of the whole study will depend on how well it is managed. Everything depends on the accuracy of the data collected and the researcher's interpretation of it. In the case of qualitative research, data collection and analysis may take place in parallel, whereas in quantitative research the data analysis does not usually start until data collection is complete.

Data analysis, according to Burns & Grove (2009: 44) is the process used by the researcher to reduce, organize, and give meaning to the data collected. This makes the results or findings easier for the reader to grasp, and also provides a way of enabling the research question to be answered in the light of the study findings.

The method of analysis is different for the two research approaches, as Chapters 4 and 5 illustrate. In qualitative research, the researcher looks for ways of coding or grouping the themes or categories emerging from the descriptions or interview data collected. Computer programs can be used to make this activity easier. The researcher will search the findings for suitable examples that might be used to illustrate the categories and themes identified. The concern of analysis here is to suggest the broad pattern that the topic examined appears to fall into when the study findings are carefully considered. So, for example, in the qualitative study by Banbury (2008) identified in Table 3.1, the data analysis resulted in five main headings that the interview comments could be grouped under. These were:

1. Knowledge and understanding of analgesia
2. Benefits of analgesia
3. Patterns of analgesic use
4. Side-effects
5. Analgesics that do not treat the pain

Depending on the focus of the article you have chosen to use in reading this chapter you will be able to determine similar headings.

In quantitative research, the researcher will analyse the numeric results of the study. These may be processed with the help of a computer onto which data such as questionnaire responses or experimental data sheets are be entered. These will be subjected to statistical analysis. This can take two forms, using either descriptive statistics or inferential statistics.

i) Descriptive statistics

The aim here is to describe the pattern of the results in terms of frequency of the numbers (how many people said 'yes' and how many people said 'no' to a particular question. Percentages may be used to indicate the proportion of people saying yes or no to allow comparisons to be made with groups of different sizes. Measures such as averages can be used in the form of the mean, or median, which are different ways of calculating the average, and the standard deviation, which is how closely or widely spread are the results from the mean of a particular question.

ii) Inferential statistics

These process the numeric results in a study and look for relationships between the results. These can be 'correlation' where there is a pattern or association between variables such as the amount of exercise taken and social class. They can also be in the form of a 'cause and effect' relationship, where one variable always has a direct effect on another, such as the level of a certain drug on the amount of stress hormones in the blood.

> **! Key points**
>
> The planned method of analysing the data produced by the tool of data collection is frequently examined very carefully by those judging whether to grant the researcher permission to carry out the study. This is because it will indicate the researcher's knowledge and expertise in the technical aspects of research. The time and effort of those who have provided data will only have been worthwhile if the researcher can get the best from the data through the correct method of analysis.

In qualitative research, you will note that in the section called findings that the data analysis has discovered major themes and these are often illustrated by actual quotes from the research participants to support an explanation of what they mean. Examples of these can be found in Chapter 4.

Whatever the type of analysis, perhaps the most important aspect is the researcher's interpretation of the results. Here the researcher has to be confident that their interpretation is supported by the results or findings of the study, and that, as far as possible, they have ruled out other interpretations. It is always difficult to be absolutely certain that the right interpretation has been reached, so the researcher is always hesitant to say this is 'the answer' to the question, or they have 'proved' something. They will usually say the results 'supports the view that' something is the case.

Step 10: Conclusions and recommendations

The final stages of the research process will include a conclusion that provides an answer to the aim of the study. This should return to the wording of the aim and so be written using many of the same words that have been used to state the aim. If it is an experimental study or perhaps a correlation study that started with a stated hypothesis, the conclusion should also say whether the hypothesis has been accepted or rejected on the bases of the results. It is usually only quantitative research that includes a hypothesis.

Following the conclusion the researcher will consider the possible recommendations for practice that would follow from the results. This should indicate who should do what now on the basis of the study.

These last two sections form the resolution to the study and will form a loop back to the beginning in the way in which they offer a possible solution to the 'problem' or issue giving rise to the research, and answer the aim of the study.

The skill used by a researcher to design and carry out a study to the highest standard is referred to as *rigour*. A clear definition of this is provided by Burns & Grove (2009: 720), who state that it describes a:

> 66 Striving for excellence in research through the use of discipline, scrupulous adherence to detail, and strict accuracy. 99

A small point worth noting is that the UK spelling of rigour is used in this book, which differs from the American spelling, which is 'rigor'.

! Key points

The concept of 'rigour', along with the earlier concepts of 'bias' and 'reliability' and 'validity' adds to your research 'fluency', that is the way you talk professionally and accurately about the important aspects of any research study. These four concepts are foremost in the researcher's mind at the design stage, and are frequently used by those who evaluate research studies. They are important words, then, for you to use when talking and writing about research.

Step 11: Produce a report and disseminate findings

Once a study has been completed, the researcher has an obligation to communicate and disseminate the findings and so make a contribution to our knowledge on the topic. This can take the form of a report, article, poster presentation (see Chapter 10), or conference paper. The format is very similar in that it covers:

- What was the problem?
- What does the literature say?
- What is the aim?
- How was it done?
- What was found?
- What does it mean?
- What can we say now?
- Who should do what now?

This is the logical and straightforward structure that reports follow. Some of the key features of such reports should be accuracy throughout, followed by transparency of the processes that have been used and truthfulness in the way all the details have been presented. Research should be clearly structured and the stages of the research process are frequently used as the basis for headings throughout a research report.

As research does take many forms you will find some variations to the way research is conducted, but the more contact you have with research articles, the more familiar you will become with the underlying structure of the research process.

+ EBP in action

Finally, returning to your article, check if you can identify the stages of the research process in the article. Note any differences or deviations and see if you can think why there may be variations from the structure given in this chapter.

As part of the analysis and presentation of any report, the researcher should consider possible limitations to the study and draw the reader's attention to these. A statement of limitations should be seen as a strength of the researcher in demonstrating rigour in the way in which they have objectively assessed the quality of their own work, and should not be seen as a weakness.

Dissemination, as you will see in Chapter 10, is not just about writing a research report. One of the most frequent forms of dissemination is the publication of a research article, as this makes the results available to others in the nursing or healthcare professions to enable them to gain new knowledge and most importantly decide whether the findings could be used to underpin or change their practice.

So, we have now come to the end of this chapter and a very broad description of the research process the researcher follows in planning and conducting a research study. This chapter has contained many of the major building blocks not only in constructing research, but also in critically evaluating research. The following chapters will now elaborate further on some of the details covered in this chapter, in particular the differences between qualitative and quantitative research in the stages of the research process. Learning about these will help inform the use of various types of evidence that are used to underpin the practice of nursing and nursing interventions.

Summary

- Good research is a carefully planned and executed activity.

- Although each study will have variations, there is a broad process of research followed by all researchers. This is the research process.

- The research process allows the researcher to think through each stage of the study that will need to be completed to a high standard.

- At each stage in the process, there will be a number of options open to the researcher and decisions that have to be made.

- The research process varies somewhat depending on whether the research is quantitative or qualitative in its approach.

- The process is not just about technique but also about how those from whom data are collected are treated by the researcher. This is covered by the ethical issues in research; the key principle is that the researcher should do no harm.

- Knowing the research process will help you in understanding the structure of research studies and the skills displayed by researchers in designing and completing their studies. It will also help your research design and critique skills.

■ Online resource centre

 To help your understanding of the research process, please go online to
www.oxfordtextbooks.co.uk/orc/holland/

■ References

Banbury, P., Feenan, K. & Allcock, N. (2008) Experiences of analgesic use in patients with low back pain. *British Journal of Nursing* 17 (19) 1215–1218.

Blake, E., Tsakirides, C. & Ingle, L. (2009) Hospital versus community-based phase III cardiac rehabilitation. *British Journal of Nursing* 18 (2) 116–122.

Bryman, A. (2008) *Social Research Methods (3rd edn)*. Oxford: Oxford University Press.

Burns, N. & Grove, S. (2009) *The Practice of Nursing Research: Appraisal, Synthesis, and Generation of Evidence (6th edn)* St Louis: Saunders.

DH (2005) *Research Governance Framework for Health and Social Care (2nd edn)*. London: DH.

Mohammed, M., Hayton, R., Clements, G., Smith, G. & Prytherch, D. (2009) Improving accuracy and efficiency of early warning scores in acute care. *British Journal of Nursing* 18 (1) 18–24.

NMC (2008) *The Code: standards of conduct, performance and ethics for nurses and midwives*. London: NMC

RCN (2007) *Research Ethics: RCN guidance for nurses*. London: Royal College of Nursing.

Robson, V., Dodd, S. & Thomas, S. (2009) Standardized antibacterial honey (Medihoney™) with standard therapy in wound care: randomized clinical trial. *Journal of Advanced Nursing* 65 (3) 565–575.

Parahoo, K. (2006) *Nursing Research: principles, process and issues (2nd edn)*. Houndmills: Palgrave Macmillan.

Polit, D. & Beck, C. (2008) *Nursing Research: generating and assessing evidence for nursing practice (8th edn)*. Philadelphia: Lippincott Williams and Wilkins.

Serrant-Green, L. (2008) Commentary: Data gathering. *Nurse Researcher* 15 (4) 4–6.

Wood, M. & Ross-Kerr, J. (2006) *Basic Steps in Planning Nursing Research: from question to proposal (6th edn)*. Boston: Jones and Bartlett.

■ Further reading

Gerrish, K. & Lacey, A. (2006) *The Research Process in Nursing*. Oxford: Blackwell Publishing Ltd. Brown, R. B. & Saunders, M. (2008) *Dealing with Statistics—what you need to know*. Maidenhead: Open University Press.

■ Useful websites

Declaration of Helsinki

http://www.wma.net/e/policy/b3.htm/

National Research Ethics Service (NRES)

http://www.nres.npsa.nhs.uk/

Royal College of Nursing Research ethics

http://www.rcn.org.uk/_data/assets/pdf_file/0004/56695/researchethicsmay07.pdf/

National Institute for Health Research

http://www.rddirect.org.uk/

4

Research evidence
Qualitative methodologies and methods

Karen Holland

The aims of this chapter are:

➤ To explain what a qualitative approach within research is.

➤ To explore how a qualitative approach (methodology) can be used to answer questions relating to nursing and health care practice.

➤ To discuss various research methods (tools) which can be used to answer questions relating to nursing and health care practice.

➤ To discuss how data obtained from using the methods can then be analysed to be meaningful.

➤ To discuss ethical issues related to using a qualitative approach in nursing research.

➤ To explain the nature of qualitative evidence and how it can be used to underpin nursing practice.

Introduction

The rationale for including this chapter in a book on evidence-based practice (EBP) is to help you as a student to understand how the evidence gained from qualitative research can be used to underpin nursing practice, as well as helping you to understand in more detail the stages of the qualitative research process when critiquing an article or evaluating the relevance of the actual research for your practice.

It is important to stress at the outset that this chapter does not offer detailed explanations of various research approaches which other books will cover, instead it offers you a broad introduction to the key aspects of qualitative research. We will recommend additional reading at the end of the chapter to direct those of you who wish to learn more or have to examine in depth one methodology for an assignment or student seminar.

You will have seen in Chapter 2 that qualitative research has not always had the same 'status' in health care research as that of quantitative. However, that has significantly changed in the past 10 years in nursing and in other fields of health care research, to the point where it could be argued that nurse researchers are no longer confident in undertaking what Macleod Clark (2009) calls the research which measures the effectiveness of nursing interventions, through conducting for example randomized controlled trials. The importance of qualitative research is also being recognized as important to the body of evidence on specific topics, with researchers now undertaking systematic reviews of qualitative research using appropriate frameworks for doing so. An example being McDermott *et al,* (2004) review on the experiences of being a teenage mother in the UK.

Whatever the debate it remains important for you understand the differences between qualitative and quantitative research and how their findings can both combine to offer the best possible evidence on which to base our practice as nurses and also combine with other health care research findings to establish an integrated collaborative approach to ensuring the best possible outcomes for patients.

Qualitative research in nursing knowledge

The main purpose of nursing research can be said to increase knowledge in relation to what nurses do in the context of their work, whether it is in education, management, or practice. The knowledge that we shall be talking about in this chapter is that gained by undertaking qualitative research. It is important to remember however that knowledge gained through undertaking research is not the only kind of knowledge that nurses can gain, and the framework identified by Carper (1978) illustrates this. She noted that there were four patterns of knowing which nurses may use in their practice:

- Knowledge associated with 'empirics' or 'empirical' knowledge, which is gained through observation or testing out theories in a systematic way. This is the type of knowledge associated with a certain kind of research.

- Knowledge that is associated with moral decision-making and ethics, that is with how nurses make judgements about what is right or wrong. Ethics and ethical issues are also important when conducting research.

- Knowledge that is related to the art of nursing, called 'aesthetics', and includes what Benner (1984) calls the intuitive knowledge of the expert nurse, as well as empathy and compassion.

- Knowledge that is related to the personal self, which is unique to you as an individual. It is knowledge that includes self-awareness and how you relate to others.

+··

EBP in action

Consider these types of knowledge or 'patterns of knowing 'and your experience in a practice placement. Did you use these yourself in any situation? If yes, how did you experience the first type of knowledge, i.e. that associated with a research base?

The use of research-based knowledge in practice is probably not as easy to see as the other types of knowledge, but is nevertheless an important part of nursing practice. Consider, for example, if you were caring for someone with a mental illness what you would need to know in order to help that service user understand how a new treatment might work and the possible impact on their life.

'Empirical' knowledge would be gained from the information about the particular drug or treatment, and linked to what has been 'scientifically' tested. However, there is another essential aspect to the care of this client/patient with a mental illness and that is the experience of that individual themselves and how they live. It is in relation to this that we can see the difference between what is qualitative or interpretive research and that of quantitative or positivistic research (discussed in Chapter 5). The latter is very much linked to the testing of a theory about something (hypothesis), in other words the drug given to the patient may well have been tested and outcomes measured, using a hypothesis such as: if we give the drug to people in a certain age group they will experience fewer side-effects than if given in another age group. If this turns out to be right, it can be generalized (generalizablity) to the wider public, then the doctor can then prescribe it for your client who is in the right age group, and he is less likely to be affected.

In the former example it could be a theory which developed from the client/patient point of view (inductive), i.e. from their insider perspective (emic) and not the researcher's outsider perspective (etic).

Your client may experience certain life situations that impact on him taking that prescribed medication and you need to be able to understand these in order to ensure that he takes the medication which is helpful to his condition. There may be (research-based) evidence from others who have experienced similar life situations which can help you with your own client/patient, and although their experiences will be individual, the collective similarities have enabled a common understanding to emerge which can then be applied to your client and help you to manage his care. This can be considered as **typical (typicality)** for the kind of experience your client is going through.

+··

EBP in action

Find two different research papers where you can see these words:

> **qualitative, inductive,** and **emic** and

> **quantitative, hypothesis,** and **generalizablity.**

What was the focus to the research? Make a note of other words found in the different papers and find out their meaning. A selection of words can be found in the Glossary of terms and in the Further reading list. We will be returning to some of these terms related to qualitative research later in the chapter and those related to quantitative research can be found in Chapter 5.

What is qualitative research?

As you will already have seen in the above example, qualitative research can be related to an individual's experience. Parahoo (2006: 63) offers this very comprehensive explanation:

> 66 *It is an umbrella term for a number of diverse approaches which seek to understand, by means of exploration, human experience, perceptions, motivations, intentions and behaviour. They are based on the belief that interpretation is central to the exploration and understanding of social phenomena. They use interactive, inductive, flexible and reflexive methods of data collection and analysis in order to do so. Their findings are presented in a variety of formats including descriptions, themes, conceptual models or theories.* 99

A word very often used in relation to qualitative research is '**explore**', much in the same way as an **explorer in a strange land or in uncharted territory** (Parahoo 2006: 63). Qualitative research is often used as a methodology to answer research questions when there is very little known about the subject (phenomenon).

EBP in action

Consider the following article titles which are focused on the student nurse and mentor and determine which one is the qualitative study (the answer is at the end of the chapter).

Pearcey, P. & Draper, P. (2008) Exploring clinical nursing experiences: Listening to student nurses, *Nurse Education Today,* 28, 595–601

Pulsford, D., Bolt, K. & Owen, S. (2002) Are mentors ready to make a difference? A survey of mentors' attitudes towards nurse education, *Nurse Education Today*, 22, 439–446.

To take your learning one step further you could obtain a copy of both papers and consider them in relation to the stages of the research process outlined in Chapter 3.

Qualitative research is often used when there is little known about the area or phenomenon being studied. Another word associated with research of any kind is a paradigm, which is a set of basic beliefs about the world, what constitutes reality in that world, and what counts as knowledge (Kuhn 1970). Qualitative researchers aim to try and understand the social world from the viewpoint of those who live in it, or from observing them in that world. There are however many different ways of doing this, through the use of research methodologies, which are also based on the researchers' *'assumptions that they hold about the nature of the research they carry out'* (Holloway 1997).

Different methodologies in qualitative research

The main approaches or methodologies in qualitative research are:

1. Ethnography
2. Phenomenology
3. Grounded theory

Other methodologies which can be also be considered as related to qualitative research are:

4. Action research
5. Historical research

Each of these will be considered in turn, and how they can be used to understand nursing practice and nurses will be explored. There are however other research methodologies such as case study research and feminist research which incorporate elements of the 'world view' associated with qualitative research and further reading will be provided with respect to these.

Ethnography

Ethnography is according to Roper & Shapira (2000) *'a research process of learning about people by learning from them'*. Van Maanen (1988), an eminent American ethnographer, also tells us that an ethnography is a written representation of a culture (or selected aspects of a culture). Ethnography then is both a methodology for research, i.e. the process but also the written story of the research. The main methods of collecting data in ethnographic research are: participant and non-participant observation, semi-structured and unstructured interviews together with informal interviewing, depending on the cultural group or aspect of the culture being studied. Ethnographers may also review documents related to the group and historical accounts of the culture. This approach has its foundation in the discipline of social anthropology when anthropologists such as Bronislaw Malinowski and Margret Mead studied the lives and patterns of behaviour in different tribal groups in non-western culture. However, many of these early cultures began to either disappear or change and anthropologists started to research their own cultures. Being an ethnographer in true anthropological tradition however does mean having to consider yourself a 'stranger' to the culture being studied, and a modern version of the kind of experience was that of Nigel Barley (1990), an anthropologist and ethnographer, who studied various aspects of English life, such as the ritual, tradition, and ceremony that exists in everyday life. One example was the village wedding, where he looked at the giving of wedding gifts, going on a honeymoon, and who was invited and why. Many of his other books offer a very humorous view of what it is like to undertake research in different cultures (see further reading list).

Holloway (1997: 61) explains however that there are what she calls two types of ethnography: descriptive and critical. The first one which is more akin to the traditional approach of studying cultures:

> 66 *focuses on the description of cultures or groups through analysis, uncovers patterns, typologies and categories.* 99

The second one

> 66 *involves the study of macro-social factors such as power, and examines common-sense assumptions and hidden agendas. It is meant to generate change in the setting it investigates or in the researcher who studies it.* 99

An example of this approach can be seen in a study by Manias & Street (2001: 442), who studied 'nurse–doctor interactions during critical care ward rounds'. They found that

> 66 *... by challenging the different points of view that doctors and nurses might hold about the ward round process, the opportunity exists for enhanced participation by nurses.* 99

Ethnographic research and nursing practice

So how can ethnographic research help us change nursing practice or understand what happens in day to day nursing activities? From a personal viewpoint I had always been interested in learning about different cultures and also what happened on a hospital ward, especially why we did things in certain ways and why some of the practices we undertook seemed to have always been done without any change. I decided to combine these interests and I undertook an ethnographic study of nursing culture to explore whether there was a system of ritual in place (Holland 1993). Ritual was a term often ascribed to some of these common practices. It was a different topic to study at that time as there were not many nurse researchers studying the culture of nursing nor indeed using ethnography. Two of these were Madeline Leininger, an American nurse anthropologist, who developed **Transcultural Nursing** and Zane Robinson Wolfe (1988), who explored nursing rituals in a hospital. One nursing practice that both she and I found evidence to suggest that it was a ritual in an anthropological sense was the nursing handover or as she called it 'the change of shift report'.

Over the past 20 years ethnography has developed as a research methodology and there are many nurse researchers now using it to look at different aspects of nursing. Savage (1995) is one such example with her study on relationships between nurses and patients on hospital wards.

Nurse ethnographers therefore have a 'world view' which considers nursing and nursing practice in terms of a culture, with aspects of it relating to the way in which we live and work and how things around us contribute to making it different wherever we work. An example of that would be how nursing on an adult intensive care unit is very different from that on a unit caring for older people with dementia.

EBP in action

The following are some examples of ethnographic studies. Consider the nature of the culture that has been explored. What were the research questions that initiated the studies? What did the researchers want to find out? And did they succeed? You may wish to discuss one of the papers with your mentor or personal tutor, as part of your achieving one of your goals to either critique a paper related to EBP or as part of a module assessment looking at care of a patient in one specific placement.

> Cole, E. & Crichton, N. (2006) The culture of a trauma team in relation to human factors. *Journal of Clinical Nursing*, 15, 1257–1266.
>
> Hopkins, C. (2002) But what about the really ill, poorly people ? (An ethnographic study into what it means to nurses on medical admissions units to have people who have harmed themselves as patients.) *Journal of Psychiatric and Mental Health Nursing*, 9, 147–154.
>
> Hunter, C. L., Spence, K., Mckenna, K. & Ledema, R. (2008) Learning how to learn: an ethnographic study in a neonatal intensive care unit. *Journal of Advanced Nursing*, 62 (6) 657–664.

Obtain copies of these papers and consider their findings in relation to the focus of the study being undertaken. This will help you to understand the way in which different kinds of ethnographies are undertaken and will also help you to begin to read research papers which you can use as critique papers in Chapter 7. We will return to some of these later when discussing data collection methods.

Phenomenology

Phenomenology, when used as a research approach, focuses on the lived experience of an individual and how that individual expresses it. It has its origin in the philosophical movement. There are different approaches that can be taken, dependent on which philosophical view you take (further reading on this will be identified for you). Newell & Burnard (2006: 90) explain that:

> 66 *Phenomenological research is concerned with how an individual views the world and how she or he lives his life from **inside**. While many approaches to research look for commonalities of human experience..... phenomenological research considers what it may be like to **this** person, living **this** life at **this** time.* 99

Phenomenological research and nursing practice

We can see from this why phenomenology has possibly become more popular in nursing research, because it focuses on the individual experience and this is in keeping with the major change towards asking the client or patient what their needs are and what they think of services and care. It also links very much to nurses' holistic view regarding patient care. The focus in health care generally has moved from a practitioner-centred perspective to that of the patient's. Phenomenology as a research methodology will enable us for example to see what having cancer means to the patient and their family, what is it like for an individual to have to live with a long term mental illness or how chronic pain affects a person's life.

Some studies that have used or been influenced by this approach are: Ramsamy (2001) in his work called **Caring for Madness—the role of personal experience in the training of mental health nurses;** Taylor (1994) in her work **Being Human—the ordinariness in nursing**. A collection of research studies can be found in Madjar and Walton's (1999) book on nursing and the experience of illness, where examples such as living with chronic leg ulcers, living with schizophrenia, and nurses' 'experience' of inflicting and relieving pain can be found.

These and other research studies can be of immense value when both caring for people and also enabling you find evidence that can support your practice. Understanding the patient's perspective through research will enable you to translate that into your learning to be a nurse.

+..

EBP in action

The following articles are examples of phenomenology as a research approach. Obtain a copy of one of these articles according to your branch or programme of study and area of interest, read it and consider what the researcher has learnt about the people whotook part in the study (participants). The articles can also be used to critique the whole research study undertaken (often **used in student assignments**) and also help you to understand the different aspects of the research process described in Chapter 3.

Cashin, G. H., Small, S. P. & Solberg, S. M. (2008) The lived experience of fathers who have children with asthma: a phenomenological study. *Journal of Paediatric Nursing*, 23 (5) 372–85.

Coombs, L. & Wratten, A. (2007) The lived experience of community mental health nurses working with people with a dual diagnosis: a phenomenological study. *Journal of Psychiatric and Mental Health Nursing*, 14, 382–392.

Donovan, J. (2002) Learning Disability nurses' experiences of being with clients who may be in pain. *Journal of Advanced Nursing*, 38 (5) 458–466.

Santy, J. & Mackintosh, C. (2001) A phenomenological study of pain following fractured neck of femur. *Journal of Clinical Nursing*, 10, 521–527.

....

Grounded theory

Grounded theory has according to Holloway & Todres (2006) many similarities to other qualitative approaches. Its main aim however is the generation of theory from the data collected and analysed. It has its origins in the discipline of sociology and in particular the field of symbolic interactionism (Holloway 1997). This way of looking at the world considers that how people interact may involve using symbols in order to communicate with one another and also that these then have an effect on behaviour when they socially interact with each other. Researchers using grounded theory are then specifically interested in investigating these 'interactions, behaviours and experiences as well as individuals' perceptions and thoughts about them' (Holloway 1997). Examples of the use of grounded theory to inform their research include Pam Smith's (1992) study on the emotional labour of nursing and Jocelyn Lawler's (1991) study on how the body is managed and viewed by nurses in their work. Both of these studies have been influential in developing our nursing knowledge, and although some of you will be considering that these are very dated pieces of research, that does not mean that they are not relevant to the evidence base of nursing (see Chapter 9).

Although it can be considered an overarching methodology it is often used just as an approach to collecting data and its analysis. An example of this is in a study by Fallon (2003: 395), who used phenomenology as the main research approach to exploring 'the lived experience of people with borderline personality disorder in contact with psychiatric services' but then used a grounded theory approach to data collection and analysis. He chose this because it combined 'qualitative discovery and the generation of theories about the subject under investigation'. The key category of 'travelling through the system' as a journey was determined as a way of explaining the participants' experience.

+ ··

EBP in action

The following are examples of studies where grounded theory has been used either as a methodology or a data collection and analysis method.

Pick one paper and consider how you could use the findings in practice.

> Edwards, B. & Sines, D. (2007) Passing the audition – the appraisal of client credibility and assessment by nurses at triage *Journal of Clinical Nursing* (doi:10.1111/ j.1365–2702.2007.01970.x)

> Granskar, M., Edberg, A. K. & Fridlund, B. (2001) Nursing students' experience of their first professional encounter with people having mental disorders, *Journal of Psychiatric and Mental Health Nursing* 8 249–256.

> Higgins, A., Barker, P. & Begley, C. M. (2008) 'Veiling sexualities': a grounded theory of mental health nurse response to issues of sexuality, *Journal of Advanced Nursing,* 62 (3) 307–317.

> Woodgate, R. & Krisjanson, L. J. (1996) 'Getting better from my hurts': towards a model of the young child's pain experience, *Journal of Paediatric Nursing,* 114 (233–242). (although it is 12 years since the study undertaken it is used here to illustrate the methodology only).

··

Action research

Action research is a research methodology which usually involves collaboration between researchers and practitioners. It is used to create change in the area being investigated and is usually the result of initially identifying a problem situation. One of the first people to use this was a social psychologist named Kurt Lewin. Speziale & Carpenter (2007: 331) said that:

> ❝ ... for a change to occur individuals would need to unfreeze—give up their ideas about something or give up the dominant structure. They would then need to change. The change would require the acceptance of new ideas or a new structure. Finally once the new ideas were formally in place, the individuals involved in the change would refreeze, or hold the new ideas or structure as permanent. ❞

A key component of action research is evaluation of any change implementation as a result of research findings, and this then can initiate a further cycle of actions. Parahoo (2006: 201) believes that

> ❝ ... action research has the advantage that researcher and practitioner can enter into a dialogue, discuss their different interpretations and produce more valid findings by drawing from each other's special knowledge and experience. ❞

He continues by stating that because of this immediate decision and interaction that findings can be acted upon immediately rather than waiting as in 'conventional research 'for anything' up to two years before any findings are published (Parahoo 2006: 201). Although much of action research has a qualitative element, there can be quantitative data collection activity depending on the questions to be answered and the best possible way for data to be collected to answer them. The benefits of action research, other than immediate implementation of ongoing findings, is the potential for enhancing collaboration in research, often between those working in universities and those from practice. Action research is also considered to be empowering and emancipatory, because there is this collaborative approach to resolving a problem (Meyer 2006). For example, a study by Jones *et al.* (2008) looking at how service users could be engaged in developing stroke services resulted in informing 'the work of four collaborative workgroups to lead developments in the stroke pathway'.

+ ....

EBP in action

Here are some articles which report action research studies. Consider from the titles who was involved in these studies and what change took place as a result of the research. You may wish to use one of these papers to critique or use as evidence in an assignment. You could also share this with your mentors in practice as part of your learning outcomes.

Bellman, L., Bywood, C. & Dale, S. (2003) Advancing working and learning through critical action research: creativity and constraints. *Nurse Education in Practice* 3 186–194.

Dickinson, A., Welch, C. & Ager, L. (2007) No longer hungry in hospital: improving the hospital mealtime experience for older people through action research. *Journal of Clinical Nursing* 17 1492–1502.

Payne, J. (2002) An action research project in a night shelter for rough sleepers. *Journal of Psychiatric and Mental Health Nursing* 9 95–101.

Price, J. (2003) A parent in the classroom-a valuable way of fostering deep learning for the children's nursing student. *Nurse Education in Practice* 4 5–11.

....

Historical research

Although not an extensively used qualitative research methodology, historical research is nevertheless important to our understanding of nursing as a profession and nursing and health care practice. To be able to understand the present it is often necessary to be able to understand the past, and it is to this past that historical researchers turn to in their task of representing historical events and experiences in a valid and accurate way as possible.

One such history was undertaken by Peter & Mary Birchenall (2001) in their research of nursing in Guernsey during its occupation by Germany during the Second World War. They used the narratives of ten people, nine women and one man, through which to understand what nursing was like during this period of time. This historical research used 'living people' rather than documents to illustrate living history. This is one kind of primary source of evidence and is biographical in that it is their story of an experience. Others may be actual letters or a diary written by a person (Speziale & Carpenter 2007). Other historical researchers may use analysis of documents which were written by others but are interpretation of events rather than directly experienced. These are known as secondary sources of evidence and examples include newspaper accounts. You will come across these words in Chapters 6 and 9, when discussing the different types of reference sources. The most important aspect for the historical researcher is to confirm the genuineness and authenticity of the primary source if it is a document, in other words that the document is not forged and that 'it provides the truthful reporting of a subject' (Barzun & Graff 1985 cited by Speziale & Carpenter 2007).

EBP in action

Using the content of Chapter 6 as a guide, search and retrieve other papers explaining these methodologies described. Consider how you could discuss these papers within what is called a 'journal club', where a group of you could come together, choose a paper for discussion beforehand, and then meet to discuss different aspects of the paper and its value for practice. You may find a journal club already set up in your main placement locality. Find out if there is and see if you can join in. If not, consider talking to your tutors in the university about setting one up in the clinical environment. Your link teacher may be able to help there as well.

Data collection methods associated with qualitative research

As with any research methodology chosen to answer research questions, you will have already seen in Chapter 3 on the research process that all research involves collecting data and then analysing it. Choosing data collection methods will depend on what question you are attempting to answer. For example:

The aim of a possible study could be:

To explore decision-making between doctors and nurses in an intensive care unit.

The main research questions may be:

How are decisions made between doctors and nurses in an intensive care unit?

What do doctors and nurses believe their role is in decision-making in an intensive care unit?

+

EBP in action

How would you find out the answer to these questions? What would you need to do?
You may have considered that in order to determine the answer to how they made decisions that you could observe them in the intensive care unit. To find out what they believed their role was in making decisions you may have thought to ask them directly. Both these types of collecting data are to be found in qualitative research. To enable you to decide however on the most appropriate method of finding out the information required a number of these will now be considered in more detail.

We will consider the main methods used to collect data:

- Interviews
- Observation
- Documentary sources
- Vignettes

Interviews

Interviews can be used in both qualitative and quantitative research. In the latter however these are usually very structured. A very popular example of this kind of interview is when you are stopped in the middle of a visit to town and asked for 5 minutes of your time in answering some very quick questions. The 'interviewer' then asks you a number of set questions to which she/he may just tick a choice of responses, such as:

Which of the following cars are you familiar with: Ford, Vauxhall, Renault, Audi, Jaguar, Peugeot.

Which of these do you own? (a tick would be made against one or none)

If none of these what is the make of your car?

Through asking such questions to large numbers of people in different towns and cities, a picture would be built up of the numbers of people who know a specific make of car from a selection but most importantly the numbers who drive them. Other questions would also be asked on different aspects of the topic. From the responses a complete set of numerical data can then be obtained on usage, popularity, male or female drivers, colour, etc enabling some statistical findings to be produced.

In qualitative research however interviews are undertaken for different reasons and information. Consider again the question: 'What do doctors and nurses believe their role is in decision-making in an intensive care unit?'

To understand this fully we need to have a method that would give us more than just a simple response, and ensure also that we give those that are asked an opportunity to tell us in detail what they believe in. We need more 'depth' in particular if there is not much known about the topic being researched. It is important if our practice is to change as a result that in the above question we explore as much as possible what the doctors and nurses in intensive care units believe their role to be in decision-making.

So what kind of interviews are there to answer such questions and what skills are needed to undertake them? The main types of interview found in qualitative research are: face to face interview with one person (unstructured or semi-structured), a face to face interview with more than one person (focus group), and a telephone interview.

Unstructured or semi-structured interview

In an unstructured interview the researcher will have a focus but will not have specific areas to explore with the interviewee. For example if we use the research question: 'What are service user experiences of mental health services?' The focus is on the experience of mental health services. In an unstructured interview the researcher would simply ask that as a question: 'Tell me about your experiences of mental health services' or 'What is your experience of mental health services?' and the general organization and any further questions would then depend entirely on the interviewee's or **participant's** point of view and perspective (Tod 2006).

These kinds of interviews are often difficult to manage and very often even in these kinds of interviews the researcher has a 'mental guide' of what he/she wants to know. The interviewer in this kind of interview has less control over the format of it but is often rewarded with very rich data. It is a very useful method if there is little known about a topic or if someone wishes to ask someone to relate their life history. Holloway (1997) however explains that in this type of interview you are more inclined to get material that is of no use to the research whatsoever (this is called **dross**).

In a semi-structured interview there is much more focus but as in the unstructured the participants answer the questions from their point of view. The researcher however will have a number of questions around which others may arise, but the important issue here is that all participants will be asked those same set of questions. For example if you were trying to determine a service user perspective of mental health services you may ask these questions (these are only for illustrating possibilities):

1. How did you come to use mental health services for the first time?
2. What and how many members of the mental health team have you met?
3. How did the mental health team members help you?

4. What are your views on how the mental health team members work together in your care?

5. What would you consider are the most important factors in ensuring that you receive the care you need?

As you can see these questions are linked to the same issue set out in the unstructured interview, but it is clear that the researcher is focusing the main questions here on the mental health team members themselves.

+···

EBP in action

To explore the use of both kinds of interviews discussed above, plan an interview schedule for yourself using one of the following topics below. This would include at least five key questions for a semi-structured interview. Remember when doing this to consider what information you want to elicit from the interviewee with regards to the overarching aim of your study area. Ask a colleague if they would agree to be asked the questions. Consider how you would also record their responses and also what the ethical issues of asking the questions and conducting the interview are. All the topics are related to the student experience (see later section Ethical Issues in Qualitative Research).

Topic 1: Research aim: To explore the student learning experience in practice

Topic 2: Research aim: To explore the experience of being a student nurse in a problem-based learning group

Topic 3: Research aim: To explore the student experience of multidisciplinary working in practice

···

Focus group interviews

A focus group interview involves one or more researchers and a small number of participants, usually no more than 12 (Goodman & Evans 2006: 357). They state that 'the group must be large enough to ensure diversity of perspectives and be small enough to ensure everybody has a chance to participate'. In a focus group not only is there an interaction between the researcher and participants but also between participants. It is because of this that a focus group needs careful management. It is important that everyone has the opportunity to contribute and also, for the purpose of ensuring that any recording of the interview can be understood, that only one participant speaks at any one time. A focus group usually lasts for about 1 hour and it is essential that there is some structure to the questions, either two or three broad discussion areas or a semi-structured format (Goodman & Evans 2006). An example of the use of a focus group can be seen in Box 4.1.

Box 4.1 Focus groups

Interviews in focus groups (Kreuger & Casey 2000) were used as a means of studying DNs'[District Nurses'] experiences, perceptions, attitudes and values. Focus groups were selected because group interaction was supposed to provide authentic accounts of actual care situations. The study concentrated on daily care of chronic pain sufferers-regardless of underlying causes and diagnoses. An interview guide with open questions was used to focus on key topics of interest. For example District Nurses were asked to explain how they perceived the encounter with patients with chronic pain conditions in everyday practice. The key questions were subsequently moderated according to the information gained in the focus groups. For example, they were asked to give examples of when the pain care worked well and when it did not. The first author moderated the focus groups and an observer took field notes during the interviews which were then summarised to the group at the end of each interview. The interviews were audio taped and transcribed verbatim.

From: Blomberg, A.M., Hylander, I. & Tornkvist, L. (2008) District nurses' involvement in pain care: a theoretical model., *Journal of Clinical Nursing*, 17, 15, 2032–2041.

You will have noted from the earlier exercise of interviewing a colleague that you need a certain set of skills to establish an effective interaction that enables you to gain the information you require as well as develop a positive relationship between you and your colleague. Tod (2006: 338) notes that although nurses have very good skills with regards to interviewing patients 'to obtain information' to do so in a research capacity requires a different set of skills. Let us consider these differences in the EBP in action box.

+···

EBP in action

During your clinical placement you will have an opportunity to interview a patient/client, either as part of their admission to hospital or as an ongoing evaluation of their needs and care in a variety of health care settings.

Consider one of these experiences and answer the following questions:

a. What kind of information were you obtaining?

b. What was the purpose of finding this out?

c. What kind of questions did you ask?

d. How did you know what questions to ask?

e. How much talking did you do and how much did the patient/client?

f.   What did you record during this interview and where did you record it?

g. What issues were considered when you recorded the information obtained, for example with whom did you share it?

h. Could you have obtained the information in another way?

i. How long did the interview last?

Now consider the differences with interviewing your colleague.

j. What kind of information were you obtaining?

k. What was the purpose of finding this out?

l. What kind of questions did you ask?

m. How did you know what questions to ask?

n. How much talking did you do and how much did your colleague?

o. What did you record during this interview and where did you record it?

p. What issues were considered when you recorded the information obtained, for example with whom did you share it?

q. Could you have obtained the information in another way?

r. How long did the interview last?

In considering both these different kinds of interviews, reflect on what the importance differences were and what have you learnt from the exercise. For instance, you may have noted that the main difference is the purpose of the asking questions, although both are interviews and are assessing experiences and gathering information on which to make decisions. Recording of responses would also be very different, as would where they would be recorded and who would share in this knowledge.

Both sets of data (another word for the evidence collected) would require the issues of data protection and confidentiality to be considered. Discuss some of these issues and others with your colleagues or with your tutors. You could agree to consider this exercise as a goal in achieving a better understanding of gathering information as well as a communication skill.

Recording interview data

Three ways of recording data at interview are:

• tape or digital recording

• note taking during the interview

• note taking after the interview.

It is important to record as accurately as possible what is being said by those being interviewed. They are not always reliable however as a colleague and I found out to our cost on a recent study when we thought we had enough tape for the interview but because of the excellent and detailed responses we were getting from the participants we suddenly ran out of tape! As we were both present at the focus group interview I took responsibility to write down as fast as I could what the responses were in more detail than I would normally, as it was important to have their exact words so meaning was not lost. We eventually developed a system whereby we used one tape recorder and one digital in order to ensure that the responses were captured. This not only allayed our fear of losing valuable data on a major national study but also meant that we could both listen to and review the data at the same time for different reasons.

> **! Key points**
>
> Before undertaking an interview you need to prepare, prepare, and prepare again! You should have a thoroughly prepared set of questions, with enough copies for everyone involved. The participants need to be invited with plenty of advance notice and always bring an extra set of batteries for your digital recorder or tapes for a tape recorder!

EBP in action

In order to be able to understand some of the issues just discussed, and in turn appreciate the researcher experience when reading a research-based article, consider undertaking a very simple exercise in interviewing someone. For example, a member of your family or a colleague could be asked the following questions related to viewing television:

1. What kind of programmes do you watch on the television?
2. Why do you like watching these? (a possible next question may arise from this one)
3. Having explained what kind of programmes you like to watch, do you watch films on the television?
4. If yes what kind of films and tell me about one of the recent films watched and what it was about?
5. Why did you decide to watch this film in particular?
6. If no please tell me do you watch films anywhere else?

As you can see there are many possible avenues to explore in asking questions and I am sure you can think of many others. However for the purpose of this exercise you just need to focus on these and write down their answers in as much detail as you can. If you have a tape recorder to hand try asking the questions and recording them and then write out their answers through listening to the tape (transcribing). Following this you can then consider the answers and can begin to see that if you had more of the same how you can begin to build up a picture of what the data are telling you about what people watch on the television and why. We can consider more of this in the section on data analysis.

You can also begin to appreciate what the researchers in any study you are reading about have experienced in their data collection.

Telephone interviews

One other form of interviewing that is becoming increasingly used is that of the telephone interview for both structured and semi-structured interviews (Tod 2006: 342). This can be recorded through a simple connection between the telephone and tape recorder. It does have advantages such as less cost and less travel for the researcher but also disadvantages in relation to not being able to pick up possible cues by the interviewee which would lead to other questions or the interviewee themselves might not find that an easy way to respond to questions. If a sensitive subject was going to be discussed however an interview by telephone might be a preferred option, as in the study on the experiences of sexuality for individuals living with multiple sclerosis (Gagliardi 2003), although it was not stated as such in the article because of this reason. An interview of NHS managers (Williamson & Webb 2001:) on the subject of supporting students in practice was however undertaken via telephone for practical reasons, including the managers workload and also 'the difficulty of assembling groups together to hold a focus group'. It is also evident that telephone interviews tend to be shorter in length than a face to face interview, with between 20 and 30 minutes being an average (Persenius *et al.* 2008; Gagliardi 2003). This could affect the depth of the data obtained.

+..

EBP in action

A study is being carried out to understand the needs of an elderly person using a health centre. During your community placement an elderly person you are caring for as part of your caseload asks you should they take part. They have been sent a letter explaining the study, a form to sign, send back with a request for their telephone number, and a request for best time to call. What would be the main issues to consider in your response?

....

A study undertaken by Worth & Tierney (1993) on conducting research with elderly people by telephone following their discharge home from hospital may give you some ideas. As well as reporting some of the difficulties they had such as hearing impairment which caused both interviewee and researcher some stress, there were also issues around memory recall, the researcher being asked questions unconnected with the study, and 'occasionally telephone calls revealed patients to be in real physical or emotional distress', which resulted in the researchers feeling obliged 'to contact carers or health or social work professionals directly to express concerns about the patient's well-being'(Worth & Tierney 1993: 1082).

Your answer may have considered some of these issues but also others such as whether the patient had been given information about the study, could they actually read it and understand it. It may also be a question of whether or not they had a telephone that they felt able to use. This would also be the case if they had been sent a questionnaire through the post. As a student nurse you may not actually have to undertake research but here we have an excellent example of why it is important to understand the principles of different kinds of research activity and applying them in a practice context.

Observation

Observation is the other main method of gathering data in qualitative research. As with interviewing it is also a skill that student nurses have to develop as part of their learning to be a nurse, for example observing patients in various ways such as taking patient's blood pressure, temperature, and respirations following surgery or observing their speech if they have experienced a stroke. Observation in research is usually associated with the sense of sight but the other senses of hearing, touch, smell, and taste can also be involved (Parahoo 2006: 347), especially when the observer actually participates in the 'cultural scene' being observed (**participant observer**). Speziale & Carpenter (2007: 42) point out that there are four types of observation:

- the complete participant
- the participant as observer
- the observer as participant
- the complete observer

These are a very useful way of considering the role of observation in research, but the main description in many research papers are of participant or non-participant observation.

+···

EBP in action

Find two papers which describe these two kinds of observations and determine the issues that arose, if any, from undertaking the observer role.

···

You may have found papers which talked about telling people they were being observed and gaining their consent, gaining permission to undertake observations from what are known as 'gatekeepers' to the area where the observation was to take place or having to decide whether a complete observer role could be achieved. This latter observer role is where the observer cannot be seen by those being observed, much as the children were in the BBC series Child of our Time, where Professor Lord Robert Winston observes the different behaviour of children completing different challenges in a studio setting and then the audience itself becomes the observer when the children are filmed in their normal environments. In all cases permission must be obtained for this to happen, in this situation not from the child but from the parent. Although in some situations this may also involve permission from the child (see **section on ethical issues later in this chapter**).

So what happens in participant and non-participant observation? Complete participant observation is when the observer conceals what they are doing from the people they are researching. They become a member of the group (Speziale & Carpenter 2007). This also has serious ethical implications and is called undertaking 'covert' research.

Real experiences of observation in nursing research

I undertook a participant observer role in my first ethnographic research study (Holland 1993) and adopted an active participant role in ward activities but ensured I acted within my professional code as a nurse. Everyone also knew I was undertaking research, including any patient I came into contact with, but the focus was talking to the students and qualified nurses as they went about their daily activities. I also undertook a non-participant observer role where I observed from the nurses' 'station' in the middle of the ward who came into the ward and what they were apparently doing. I had to treat what I was seeing as if I did not know what I was looking at. This is called adopting a 'stranger' approach within the area under study. This non-participant 'stranger' role in observing was not an easy one, as I was often interrupted to ask my professional opinion on either equipment use or by the students who knew me in my teacher role and needed help with answers to questions concerning aspects of patient care.

I had a similar experience when undertaking an ethnography of the student nurse in transition to becoming a qualified nurse (Holland 1999). The type of observation here was also participant but it also enabled me to ask the students questions immediately after I observed them doing something.

One such event that comes to mind was when following the morning **handover**, a mentor had decided the student was to look after Mr EJ and asked the student to read his care plan and then plan his care for the day. She began to write out a care plan for the patient and once completed I then asked her how she knew what to write. She said that she knew from the care plan and the previous nurse's report about the patient. Included in this was her decision to give the patient a bowl and to assist him with a wash. Her mentor, when she returned to check on this however, thought that a bed bath might be better for him given what he had experienced and that he was still in a great deal of pain. She had of course visited with the patient and observed this, whilst the student nurse had only read the care plan and had not anticipated that other issues may be having an impact on his needs. She had in fact not undertaken her own 'observation' of the patient in order to gather her data in order to write an up-to-date care plan.

This was an important learning experience for the student. For myself as a researcher it gave me a valuable insight into the way the mentor helped the student learn and what a good role model she was for the student through her patient-focused care.

The unpopular patient by Felicity Stockwell

A study which utilized non-participant observation and which still has relevance today is that of the Unpopular Patient undertaken by Felicity Stockwell (1972: 33) (see Chapter 1 for access to this report on the RCN website). She undertook 'observations of incidents, conversations and comments relevant to the aims of the study' and had told the staff only 'that the researcher was studying interpersonal relationships on the ward'. Her observations were selective as well, as she had a different focus to her observations during her observation periods. If possible obtain a copy of her study and decide whether her findings are still valid from your experience in clinical practice. In other words is the evidence that she talks about still valid in relation to patients you have come into contact with. Some studies such as this undertaken over 35 years ago may still be valid today but have never been replicated to determine for definite. You may also wish to critique her study as part of an assignment (see Chapter 9).

EBP in action

How many of you have played the 'let's consider what people do for a living' type of game when sitting in a pub? In fact there was a television programme based on this kind of activity in the 1980s called Watching. What kind of observation is this? Is it covert or non-covert? If you were asked to watch a film and then write a review of the film, what kind of observation would this be and could either of these activities be called research?

There will be various answers to these questions and they are used to illustrate that not every activity can be called research, although both have aims and objectives and will contribute in various ways to our understanding of observation and the skills required to undertake it and with film watching, how what we observe is then written down. Do we write down everything we observe in the film as it happens or do we summarize our observations and write down what we think the film is about? In research observation we cannot rely on this kind of summary, as it may not accurately reflect what we observe. Observation notes in research have to be written down as it happens or as they are seen, and is particularly important when a nurse is observing something that is familiar. An example of observation notes in a study on how both nurses and adolescents use the ward space on a purpose built ward (Hutton 2007) can be seen in Box 4.2.

> **Box 4.2** Observation notes (ward layout)
>
> Each bed space equals a patient area; these areas hold a bed, locker, wardrobe and a chair (sometimes two) and a soft felt board in navy-blue at the head of the bed. Additionally, the bed area is demarcated by curtains, which are suspended by curtain rails from the ceiling (Observation 35, Paragraph 2–155)
>
> From: Hutton, A. (2007) An adolescent ward: 'in name only'? *Journal of Clinical Nursing* 17 3142–3149.

Documentary sources

Although documentary methods are not used as extensively as interviews and observation there is a place in nursing research for using documents as data rather than the person. Appleton & Cowley (1997) for example used *'official guidelines to assist health visitors in identifying and prioritising vulnerable families requiring increased health visitor support'* and analysed them using various criteria. This kind of evidence was categorized as secondary source data and also a document and not a record, which was defined using a cited reference by Guba & Lincoln (1981: 1010) as:

> 66 *any written statement prepared by an individual or an agency for the purpose of attesting to an event or providing an accounting.* 99

It is clear however that there are varied interpretations of what constitutes documents in documentary research. Some researchers such as Mason (1999), who investigated how nursing care plans were being used, ask research participants to keep diaries in which they record various activities depending on the focus of the research. Others such as Heartfield (1996) analysed patient case notes in order to understand aspects of nursing practice, and Scholes *et al.* (2000) analysed a large number of nursing curricula focusing on critical care.

+ ··

EBP in action

Consider the various documents or records that you use in nursing practice or are given to you as part of your programme of study. Think of two examples and consider what the documents could tell you if you were to look at them as a source of research evidence.

··

You may have considered your student portfolios where you are required to keep reflective diaries, records, and analysis of significant events, or records of clinical skills undertaken. If this was considered in the context of wishing to understand the student experience of learning to be a nurse in clinical practice then all these records could be viewed as giving an insight into this. If you were to then gather together the same from other students, then these could all be analysed (using agreed criteria) to give not just an insight into your experience but that of a group of students undergoing the same programme. There would be no need in this kind of research to actually undertake any data collection activities involving people.

Vignettes

Vignettes are often used in research where there is a need to explore people's beliefs beyond that raised in a question. Holloway (1997: 163) notes that:

> ❝ *A vignette is an illustration or simulation of a typical event or phenomenon in the researcher's area of study It is a brief description or an outline which demonstrates what is happening, and it is presented in a story form.* ❞

For example, if you were a mental health student and wanted to understand how your adult nursing colleagues viewed mental illness you could write some short vignettes from your experience and ask them questions about the scenario. An example of a vignette in this instance would be:

+··

Case study Vignette: Mr J

Mr J, a 45 year old man has recently started to experience some chest pain which has resulted in his attending the accident and emergency department. He arrives in the department clearly agitated, he is not making himself clear when being asked questions and he keeps telling the nurses that he is being followed. When told that there is no one there he starts shouting and telling the nurses and the doctor who has been called to see him that they are also involved in spying on him and refuses to let them examine him or take observations. Other people in the waiting area are becoming disturbed by his actions. Some tablets fall out onto the floor from his jacket and when the nurse checks what they are for she finds that they are normally given to patients with schizophrenia.
Questions could then include:

1. What do you think is happening in this scenario?
2. How would you manage the situation?
3. What would your priorities be?

··

It is clear from these questions that the researcher (you) needs to find out more about how nurses manage the care of someone who is exhibiting behaviour which may or may not be attributed to mental illness. Using vignettes will already have been decided as one of the ways in which to answer the research question (see Chapter 3). Vignettes can also be photographic material and although used widely in social science research have not been as widely used in nursing research (Hughes & Hugby 2002). As in the scenario above Hughes & Hugby (2002: 385) believe that they can:

> **66** ... *also provide a focused uniform response base that can be used whether or not participants have detailed knowledge of the topics under consideration* **99**

You may also see a similarity to scenarios called 'triggers' used in problem-based learning and again have a similar purpose which is to generate discussion. Vignettes have both advantages and disadvantages but a full discussion of these are beyond the scope of this chapter (see Further reading for additional sources).

Sampling in qualitative research

A sample in research is normally the number of people who can represent or have knowledge of the topic being researched (see Chapter 3). In qualitative research the participants in the sample are those who have knowledge and/or experience of the research topic. They are usually purposely sought out and this sampling is called purposive (Holloway & Todres 2006). In ethnography for example, participants in the sample 'are usually called informants because they inform the researcher about issues in their world' (Holloway & Todres 2006: 214).

Some studies such as Holland (1993) have key informants who have 'special knowledge about the history and culture of a group, about interaction processes in it and cultural rules, rituals and language' (Holloway 1997). The sample size is relatively small in qualitative research and as a result research findings cannot be generalized (Generalizability). This is often a criticism of qualitative research. The key outcome in qualitative research is to have depth and richness to the data rather than large numbers of responses. Another word associated with sampling in qualitative research is convenience, where participants are selected because they are easily accessible. For example if I was undertaking research exploring the student nurse experience in clinical practice I would more than likely choose to invite students from my own university. However not everyone agrees with this, although Roberts (2007) makes a good argument for doing so.

✚ ....

EBP in action

Using the skills gained in Chapter 6 find three papers which illustrate both purposive and convenience sampling as well as the key informants of ethnographic research. Some of the papers already offered as examples in the methodology section may help here.

....

Data analysis methods associated with qualitative research

Certain methods of analysing data are very much linked to the specific approach taken and the data collection tool used. In qualitative research it means 'breaking down' the data (i.e. the information that the researcher collects and in which the findings originate) and searching for codes and categories which are then reassembled to form themes (Holloway 1997: 43). In general terms the basic steps in data analysis follow some or all the elements and these can be seen in Box 4.3.

Each of the qualitative methodologies previously discussed will have variations in relation to those steps in Box 4.3. In grounded theory, for example, 'researchers collect, code and analyse data from the beginning of the study' (Speziale & Carpenter 2007) and there are three levels of coding, followed by concept development, which is a stage that begins to refine the theory that is beginning to emerge and followed by determining the core category which eventually leads to the theory which is grounded

---

Box 4.3 Steps in the process of data analysis in qualitative research

1. Ordering and organizing the collected material
2. Re-reading the data
3. Breaking the material into manageable sections
4. Identifying and highlighting meaningful phrases
5. Building, comparing, and contrasting categories
6. Looking for consistent patterns of meanings
7. Searching for relationships and grouping categories together
8. Recognizing and describing patterns, themes, and typologies
9. Interpreting and searching for meaning

From: Holloway, I. (1997) Basic Concepts for Quantitative Research Oxford: Blackwell Science, 44.

in all the data. Fallon (2003) in his study concerning the lived experience of people with personality disorder used grounded theory as his method of data analysis.

The data obtained from some interviews may well be considered as narratives and Holloway (1997: 106) tells us that:

> 66 ... the researcher lets the participants develop their tales and gives them long continuing stretches of time. The interviewer asks very few questions and encourages the participants to tell their own story, reconstruct it and relive their experiences. 99

The interviewer may ask only a few questions, or possibly only one main question is asked such as: 'Tell me about your experiences of caring for patients who are dying'. Narratives are often found in phenomenological research and the method and stages of analysis will vary depending on the actual philosophical approach taken to the research.

Management of data analysis can also be undertaken through the use of computer software packages such as QSR NUD-IST, NVivo, and Ethnograph. They facilitate the management and analysis of the text arising out of the data collection. They will have a way of coding the data and help you to organize it into different themes and groupings. However, it is considered that the researcher should be 'perceptive and experienced in the analysis of qualitative data' (Parahoo 2007: 397) if choosing this approach. Webb (1999: 323) in her paper exploring qualitative data analysis also highlighted an important issue when it came to data analysis and one which is often a criticism in the use of computer packages for all aspects of data analysis and that is:

> 66 ... that the intellectual work of actually conceptualising can only be done by the brain of the researcher. The computer may be able to assist, but there is a risk of becoming so concerned with the technical aspects that this interferes with the 'artistic' aspects. 99

(Webb 1999: 329)

You may have your own views about this and if you have an opportunity it would help you to understand some of the debate if you were to access one of these packages as an exercise and insert the data sets about John and Peter given below. Undertake the same exercise but using the software. Compare both experiences and discuss with your tutor. For some of you undertaking programmes of study at Master's level this may well be part of your programme.

EBP in action

In order to appreciate the researcher's experience of analysing data please consider the following data set and using the basic principles of data analysis seen in Box 4.3 make an attempt to analyse the data. The data are based on actual student experiences in practice and were developed initially to explore practice issues with student nurses. It has been revised for the purpose of this exercise. What does it tell us about the students and their experiences? Can you relate to this experience? Note that there is no indication of what 'branch' of nursing the student is studying.

Data Set 1: John

John was a 43 year old gentleman whose only close living relative is his elderly mother. John was also a self confessed alcoholic. He had felt unable to refrain from drinking for personal reasons and was aware of the severe impact that his continuous heavy drinking had had on his health. John had been admitted to the ward several days before and had had many previous admissions, all related to his condition. John's medical diagnosis was chronic renal failure and he was in the later stages.

John's condition had deteriorated throughout the afternoon, he had become agitated and at times disorientated. His blood pressure was elevated and he appeared quite distressed. I reported John's condition to the staff nurse in charge, who instructed me to monitor his blood pressure and pulse at regular intervals. This I did informing her each time. I also voiced my concerns regarding his anxiety emphasizing that he did not appear to be coping very well. I suggested that it may be helpful for John if he was not already prescribed any hypertensive medication to either be prescribed some or at least a mild sedative to help him cope a little better by reducing his anxiety and the symptoms related to this. Throughout the following hour I continued to monitor John's condition, charting his vital signs and reporting them to the staff nurse. I requested that the consultant who was treating John be informed of the changes in his condition.

Once again I reported John's condition, stressing that John was distressed and that John had in fact appeared to me at this moment very anxious and frightened. I was instructed to go and sit with John whilst she contacted the doctor and informed him of John's deterioration. On returning to John I tried to reassure him and make him as comfortable as possible. After sitting with John for a short while I noticed a marked change in his colour and breathing. I suspected that he was dying and immediately pressed the nurse call bell. The staff nurse arrived and whilst she was checking his pulse John died.

+ ···

Data Set 2: Peter

I met Peter with my assessor on a clinical placement with a team of community psychiatric nurses. He is a 45 year old man living with his partner in a council house near to the centre of town. Peter has a long history of contact with both inpatient and community psychiatric services of over 20 years and has received visits from my assessor, an experienced CPN for over 5 years. Peter had a diagnosis of severe anxiety/depression with a history of self-harm, by cutting himself and taking overdoses of medication, and a number of suicide attempts; he is also dependent upon and abuses benzodiazepines.

The aims of the nursing interventions and the significant event were to reduce Peter's level of anxiety and to educate him to the dangers of abuse of benzodiazepines. These interventions were agreed with Peter for his care plan review for the Care Programme Approach. My involvement with Peter was as part of the learning outcomes I had to achieve as a student nurse, that is to demonstrate the ability to assess, plan, implement, and evaluate a patient's care under minimal supervision. With Peter's and my assessor's agreement an anxiety management package was commenced. The aims of this were to enable Peter to be better able to recognize his stressors and to provide coping strategies such as relaxation and breathing technique so he could better access the available community resources such as day centres, college, and possibly in the future a return to some employment.

···

Validity and trustworthiness in qualitative research

These are very important aspects of any qualitative research study (see Chapter 3). According to Holloway (1997: 159):

> ❝ validity is the scientific concept of the everyday notion of truth' and that 'in qualitative research it is the extent to which the findings of the study are true and accurate. ❞

Trustworthiness is a term often used instead of validity, and Koch (1994) in an excellent paper exploring the establishment of rigour in qualitative research cites Guba & Lincoln's (1989) view that to establish it one needs to consider how credible it is. She notes that they claim:

> ❝ that a study is credible when it presents faithful descriptions and when co-researchers or readers confronted with the experience can recognize it ❞

(Koch 1994: 976)

Despite the fact that these references are 15–20 years old, the points made by the authors are still valid in the context of today's research.

Another way that researchers establish the trustworthiness and therefore the credibility of the research is to return their analysis of the data back to the participants and they recognize the findings as their own experiences. These issues are often the subject of debate (Rolfe 2006) and you will see when you read research papers that not every researcher acknowledges this in the same way.

Ethical issues and management of data in qualitative research

The ethical codes which now guide research are a direct result of abuse of human rights such as those that occurred in the Nazi biomedical experiments in Germany at the time of Adolph Hitler. This resulted in the Nuremberg Code (1949), which is concerned

> 66 *with the adequate protection of human subjects, the rights of participants to withdraw from a research study and the importance of conducting research only by qualified individuals* 99
>
> *(Speziale & Carpenter 2007: 61)*

All researchers therefore who involve human beings in their research must consider the ethical aspects of their study. Individuals have the right to determine whether or not to be involved in research and this is why it is essential that they have the right information about the research study and their potential involvement to enable them to do so.

You will see when reading and critiquing research papers (see Chapter 7) key words that relate to ethical aspects of any study:

- informed consent
- confidentiality
- anonymity
- Ethics committees
- Research governance

These will be found in both qualitative and quantitative research studies and elements of them all should be reported in any published study. They assure us that all participants had been protected from harm by the researcher or the research being undertaken. Some papers will also report on the need to ensure safety for the researcher when conducting research, especially if they are placing themselves at risk, such as visiting someone they do not know in their own home to conduct an interview. In those kinds of situations it is essential that the researcher makes it known where and when they are going and to leave contact details with someone. This is part of managing risk associated with any research study.

A brief overview will be given of the key issues that follow, as they relate particularly to qualitative research studies. It is not the purpose of this book to give full details but enough to enable you to understand the key issues when reading or critiquing research in order to be able to determine its value for EBP.

Informed consent

This is quite simply consent that is given following the giving of information and often explanation by the researcher of what the study is about and why they would wish for the individual to be involved. This is sometimes difficult to be precise in qualitative research as sometimes because of data collection and analysis the researcher may wish to explore different issues not initially considered. However, that can be managed by returning for further permission from the participants. So when undertaking research it is important that any information gives as full an explanation as possible, and also that it is easy to read and understand. Of course when the participants are unable to read the language it is then that translation is required; it is also important not to assume that the participant can read in any language. Polit & Beck (2004: 151) cited in Speziale & Carpenter (2007: 63) have an excellent definition which explains clearly what informed consent is:

> 66 Informed consent means that participants have adequate information regarding the research; are capable of comprehending the information; and have the power of free choice, enabling them to consent voluntarily to participate in the research or decline participation. 99
>
> *(Polit & Beck 2004: 151)*

Consent to be involved in research must be informed and in writing. Two issues to be considered alongside consent which will need to be guaranteed to a participant are anonymity and confidentiality. Anonymity means that the participant should not be identifiable at any time by anyone reading the publication of the research. The same applies to organizations where the research took place, unless with written agreement by that organization. In qualitative research this is not always easy to achieve, especially with small clearly defined groups or situations. Giving people pseudonyms (made up names) is usual practice, as is giving people a specific number or letter such as Student23AB— (which relates to a student, number 23, in the adult branch) when reporting research.

Confidentiality is essential in order to protect people, especially if they are disclosing sensitive information as part of the research. Again this is important when needing to use quoted material, and consent should be given in relation to using the research in a publication. Security of gathered data is essential as is the safe disposal of data once used (Johnson & Long 2006).

✛ EBP in action

Consider situations or groups of people in society who may need additional consider-ations with regards to informed consent. Access the National Research Ethics Service (NRES) site for further information on informed consent and other ethics-related issues. (http://www.nres.npsa.nhs.uk/).

You may have considered people who are not capable of giving consent and the Men-tal Capacity Act 2005 regulates research on adults where this is concerned. Children of 16 and below are deemed not to be competent to consent to be involved in re-search, although there are circumstances when they can. A very useful presentation on the issues of children's involvement in research can be found at **www.liv.ac.uk/law/cscfl/docs/2Christina_Lyon.ppt/**.

Others who you may have considered are older people, people with mental illness, and people with learning difficulties. However, all adults are assumed to be competent to give consent unless there are clear reasons otherwise. This may be related to the complexity or nature of what they are being asked to participate in. Anyone who had originally consented has the right to withdraw from the study. This level of information is not always present in a published research paper but will have been considered through a Research Ethics Committee of either the University (in the case of research where students are involved or that staff undertake) or the Health or Social Care Service if undertaken with either patients and staff in those organizations. Sometimes research-ers undertake research where there is no committee to protect the interest of the par-ticipant, for example research involving volunteers from the community at large. It is expected however that the researcher adheres to an ethical code of practice.

Ethics committee

An ethics committee is made up of 'a group of professionals and lay people who scru-tinize any research projects that involves patients or clients or their relatives' (Hollo-way 1997: 59). Researchers are required to complete documentation relating to their proposed research, including in the case of NRES applications examples of participant information documents and informed consent forms. Researchers are often required to attend the meeting at which their research application is being considered. Most countries will have ethics committees, e.g. New Zealand **http://www.ethicscommittees.health.govt.nz/**.

+ ···

EBP in action

For further information on the work of Ethics Committees related to nursing and health care in your country undertake a search on the internet. Read the documents and compare them to those in a different country. What are the similarities and what are the differences?

···

Research governance committee

In order to ensure that research undertaken in the National Health Service in the United Kingdom, the government in 2001 set up the Research Governance Framework for Health and Social Care (DH 2001; revised 2005 in England). It means that in addition to approval from the Ethics Committee described above, that if the research is taking place in the NHS then research governance approval is also required to ensure good quality research. Further information can be seen in the document above at www.doh.gov.uk/.

+ ···

EBP in action

See an example of an abstract from a qualitative study below. Can you identify what the study was about; why it was undertaken; what the methodology was; how were the data collected and what did the findings demonstrate? To be able to understand the conclusion and the title you may need to identify the meaning of hegemony (basically it means predominance of power of one group over another). The structure of the abstract does make it easier for you to identify each of these. Having read this chapter what does the abstract **not tell you** about the conduct of the research?

···

Abstract of a qualitative study

Background. Health care policy in the United Kingdom identifies the need for health professsionals to find new ways of working to deliver patient-focused and economic care. Much debate has followed on the nature of working relationships within the health care team.

Aim. This paper reports on an ethnographic study that examined the nursing role in clinical decision-making in intensive care units. This was chosen as a case for analysis due to the close doctor–nurse relationships that are essential in this acute and complex care setting.

»

Methods. Data were collected during two stages of fieldwork using participant observation, in-depth ethnographic interviews and documentation across three clinical sites.

Findings. The findings revealed the different types of knowledge used for, divergence of roles involved in and degree of authority in clinical decision-making. Furthermore, conflict arose between doctors and nurses due to these differences and in particular because medicine dominated the decision-making process.

Conclusions. The nursing role, whilst pivotal to implementing clinical decisions, remained unacknowledged and devalued. Medical hegemony continues to render nurses unable to influence substantially the decision-making process. This has fundamental ramifications for the quality of team decision-making and the effectiveness of new ways of inter-professional working in intensive care

(Coombs, M. & Ersser, J. 2004 Medical hegemony in decision-making – a barrier to interdisciplinary working in care? *Journal of Advanced Nursing*, 46 3 (245–252)

Summary

- Qualitative research encompasses different ways of looking at the world and this is seen in the various approaches taken by researchers in order to answer specific research questions.

- Central to most qualitative research is the involvement of people, which brings with it a number of research management issues to consider, such as how many participants to include and ensuring that they understand what their involvement will entail and that they give their consent after being fully informed.

- Qualitative research findings enable us to understand how people live, what their experiences of life in various situations is like as well as offering us a valuable insight into how they view nursing care and our practices as nurses. This being essential if we are to ensure that this is of the best quality and standard.

- This chapter should give you a broad understanding of qualitative research in order to be able to understand other chapters which will refer to it and its value to support EBP.

Answer to 'EBP in action' box on page 71. Which is the qualitative study?

Pearcey, P. & Draper, P. (2008) Exploring clinical nursing experiences: listening to student nurses, *Nurse Education Today* 28 595–601.

■ Online resource centre

 To help your understanding of the qualitative research, please now go online to www.oxfordtextbooks.co.uk/orc/holland/ where you will find online resources.

■ References

Appleton, J. V. & Cowley S. (1997) Analysing clinical practice guidelines. A method of documentary analysis. *Journal of Advanced Nursing* 25 1008–1017.

Barley, N. (1990) *Native Land.* London: Penguin Books.

Barzun, J. & Graff, H. F. (1985) The modern researcher (*4th Edition*) Harcourt Brace Jovanovitch, San Diego, California: cited in Speziale H. J. S. & Carpenter D. R. (2007) *Qualitative Research in Nursing, Advancing the Humanistic Perspective (4th edn).* Philadephia: Lipincott Williams & Wilkins.

Benner, P. (1984) *From novice to expert: excellence and power in clinical nursing practice.* California: Addison-Wesley Pub. Co.

Birchenall, P. & Birechenall, M. (2001) *Occupation Nurse. Nursing in Guernsey 1940–45,* Bognor Regis: Woodfield Publishing.

Blomberg, A-M., Hylander, I. & Tornkvist, L. 2008 District nurses' involvement in pain care: a theoretical model. *Journal of Clinical Nursing* 17 (15) 2032–2041.

Carper, B. (1978) Fundamental patterns of knowing in nursing. *Advances in Nursing Science* 1 (1) 13–23.

Coombs, M. & Ersser, S. J. (2004) Medical hegemony in decision-making—a barrier to interdisciplinary working in intensive care? *Journal of Advanced Nursing* 46 (3) 245–252.

Department of Health (2001) *Research Governance Framework for Health and Social Care.* London: Department of Health.

Fallon, P. (2003) Travelling through the system: the lived experience of people with borderline personality disorder in contact with psychiatric services. *Journal of Psychiatric and Mental Health Nursing* 10, 393–400.

Gagliardi, B. A. (2003) The experience of sexuality for individuals living with multiple sclerosis. *Journal of Clinical Nursing* 12 571–578.

Goodman, C. & Evans, C. (2006) Focus groups. In: K. Gerrish & A. Lacey (eds) *The Research Process in Nursing,* Oxford: Blackwell Publishing 353–366.

Guba, E. G. & Lincoln, Y. S. (1981) *Effective Evaluation,* Jossey–Bass Publishers, San Francisco cited in Appleton, J. V. & Cowley, S. (1997) Analysing clinical practice guidelines. A method of documentary analysis. *Journal of Advanced Nursing* 25 1008–1017.

Guba, E. G. & Lincoln, Y. S. (1989) *Fourth Generation Evaluation.* Sage Publications, Newbury park, California cited in Koch T. 1994 Establishing rigour in qualitative research: the decision trail. *Journal of Advanced Nursing* 19 (5) 976–986.

Heartfield, M. (1996) Nursing documentation and nursing practice: a discourse analysis. *Journal of Advanced Nursing* 24 (1) 98–103.

Holland, C. K. 1993 An ethnographic study of nursing culture as an exploration for determining the existence of a system of ritual. *Journal of Advanced Nursing* 18 (9) 1461–1470.

Holland, K. (1999) A journey to becoming: the student nurse in transition. *Journal of Advanced Nursing* 29 (1) 229–236.

Holloway, I. (1997) *Basic concepts for qualitative research.* Oxford: Blackwell Science.

Holloway, I. & Todres, L. (2006) Grounded Theory. In: K. Gerrish & A. Lacey (eds) *The Research Process in Nursing.* Oxford: Blackwell Publishing, 192–207.

Hughes, R. & Huby, M. (2002) The application of vignettes in social and nursing research. *Journal of Advanced Nursing* 37 (4) 382–386.

Hutton, A. (2007) An adolescent ward; 'in name only?' *Journal of Clinical Nursing 17* *3142–3149.*

Johnson, M. & Long, T. (2006) Research Ethics. In: K. Gerrish & A. Lacey (eds) *The Research Process in Nursing.* Oxford: Blackwell Publishing, 31–42.

Jones, S. P., Auton, M. F., Burton, C. R. & Watkins, C. L. (2008) Engaging service users in the development of stroke services: an action research study. *Journal of Clinical Nursing* 17 (10) 1270–1279.

Koch, T. (1994) Establishing rigour in qualitative research: the decision trail. *Journal of Advanced Nursing* 19 (5) 976–986.

Kuhn, T. S. (1970) *The structure of Scientific Revolutions, (2nd edn).* Chicago: University of Chicago Press.

Lawler, J. (1991) *Behind the Screens, Nursing, Somology and the Body.* Edinburgh: Churchill Livingstone.

Mac Leod Clark, J. (2009) *Looking Back, Moving Forword: pursuing the science of nursing interventions.* Key Note presentation RCN Nursing Research conference, March 2009, Cardiff. London: RCN.

Madjar, I. & Walton, J. A. (1999) *Nursing and the Experience of Illness.* London: Routledge.

Mason, C. (1999) Guide to practice or 'load of rubbish'? The influence of care plans on nursing practice in five clinical areas in Northern Ireland. *Journal of Advanced Nursing* 29 (2) 380–387.

McDermott, E., Graham, H. & Hamilton, V. (2004) *Experiences of being a teenage mother in the UK: A Report of a Systematic Review of Qualitative Studies. Lancaster University:* Institute for Health Research (http://www.msoc-mrc.gla.ac.uk/Evidence/Research/Review%2010/SR%20 Executive%20Summary.pdf - accessed June 15th 2009).

Meyer, J. (2006) Action Research. In: K. Gerrish & A. Lacey, *The Research Process in Nursing, (5th edn).* Oxford: Blackwell Publishing Ltd, Chapter 18, 274–288.

Parahoo, K. (2006) *Nursing Research, Principles, Processes and Issues (2nd edn).* Basinstoke: Palgrave Macmillan.

Persenius, M. W., Hall-Lord, M. L., Baath C. & Laarson, B. (2008) Assessment and documentation of patients' nutritional status: perceptions of registered nurses and their chief nurses, *Journal of Clinical Nursing* 17 (16) 2125–2136.

Polit, D. F. & Beck, C. T. (2004) *Nursing Research: methods, appraisal and utilization* (7th edn) Lippincott Williams & Wilkins, Philadelphia, cited in Speziale H. J. S. & Carpenter D. R. (2007) *Qualitative Research in Nursing, Advancing the Humanistic Perspective,* (4th edn) Philadephia: Lipincott Williams & Wilkins.

Ramsamy, S. (2001) *Caring for Madness: the role of personal experience in the training of mental health nurses.* London: Whurr Publishers Ltd.

Roberts, D. (2007) Ethnography and staying in your own nest. *Nurse Researcher* 14 (3) 4–6.

Rolfe, G. (2006) Validity, trustworthiness and rigour: quality and the idea of qualitative research. *Journal of Advanced Nursing* 53 (3) 304–310.

Roper, J. M. & Shapira, J. (2000) *Ethnography in Nursing Research.* Thousand Oaks: Sage Publications

Savage, J. (1995) *Nursing Intimacy – an ethnographic approach to nurse-patient interaction.* London: Scutari Press.

Scholes, J., Endacott, R. & Chellel. (2000) A formula for diversity: a review of critical care criteria. *Journal of Clinical Nursing* 9 382–390.

Smith, P. (1992) *The Emotional Labour of Nursing.* Basinstoke: The Macmillan Press Ltd.

Speziale, H. J. S. & Carpenter, D. R. (2007) *Qualitative Research in Nursing, Advancing the Humanistic Perspective (4th edn).* Philadelphia: Lipincott Williams & Wilkins.

Stockwell, F. (1972) *The Unpopular Patient. The Study of Nursing Care, Series 1, Number 1.* London: Royal College of Nursing.

Taylor, B. J. (1994) *Being Human—ordinariness in nursing.* Edinburgh: Churchill Livingstone.

Tod, A. (2006) Interviewing. In: K Gerrish & A Lacey (eds) *The Research Process in Nursing,* Oxford: Blackwell Publishing 337–352.

Van Maanen, J. (1988) *Tales of the Field—on writing ethnography.* Chicago: The University of Chicago Press.

Webb, C. (1999) Analysing qualitative data: computerized and other approaches. *Journal of Advanced Nursing* 29 (2) 323–330.

Williamson, G. & Webb, C. (2001) Supporting students in practice. *Journal of Clinical Nursing* (10) 284–292.

Worth, A. & Tierney, A. J. (1993) Conducting research interviews with elderly people by telephone. *Journal of Advanced Nursing* 18 (17) 1077–1084.

Wolfe, Z. R. (1988) *Nurses' Work, the Sacred and the Profane.* Philadelphia: University of Pennsylvania Press.

■ Further reading

A general excellent resource is the Nurse Researcher series of the RCN as a journal website to look at papers available:

www.nurseresearcher.co.uk

Case Study

Yin, R. K. (2009) *Case study research—Design and methods* (4th edn). Thousand Oaks, CA: Sage Publications.

Ethnography

Barton, T. D. (2008) Understanding practitioner ethnography. *Nurse Researcher* 15 (2) 7–18.

Seymour, J. E. (2001) *Critical Moments—death and dying in intensive care*. Buckingham: Open University Press.

Feminist issues in nursing research

Chesney, M. (1998) Dilemmas of interviewing women who have given birth in Pakistan. *Nurse Researcher* 5 (4) 57–70.

Grounded theory

Series of papers in *Nurse Researcher* - 2003 11 (2) 7–60.

McCann, T. & Clark, E. (2003) Grounded theory in nursing research -Part 1 - methodology, 7–18

McCann, T. & Clark, E. (2003) Grounded theory in nursing research -Part 2 - Critique, 19–28.

McCann, T. & Clark, E. (2003) Grounded theory in nursing research -Part 3- Application, 29–39.

Narrative research

Holloway, I. & Freshwater, D. (2007) *Narrative Research in Nursing. Oxford:* Blackwell Publishing.

Phenomenology

Koch, T. (1999) An interpretive research process: revisiting phenomenological and hermeneutical approaches. *Nurse Researcher* 6 (3) 20–34.

Ramsamy, S. (2001) *Caring for madness: the role of experience in the training of mental health nurses*. Oxford: Wiley Blackwell (Phenomenological approach).

Vignettes:

Richman, J. & Mercer, D. (2002) The vignette revisited: evil and the forensic nurse. *Nurse Researcher* 9 (4) 70–82.

■ Useful websites

http://www.trentu.ca/admin/library/help/subjectguides/nursing/websites.html/
Offers a range of resources including research and evidence-based practice links world wide.

http://www.blackwellpublishing.com/researchproject/weblinks.asp/
A site created by Colin Robson—A Guide to How to do a research project—A guide for undergraduate students—very useful links for key chapters in this book.

Research evidence
Quantitative methodologies and methods

Colin Rees

The aims of this chapter are:

➤ To define key features of a quantitative research design.

➤ To outline a range of a quantitative approaches to research.

➤ To consider the advantages and disadvantages of the main quantitative research methods.

➤ To illustrate how a quantitative approach can be used to answer questions relating to nursing and health care practice.

➤ To outline methods of quantitative data analysis and presentation.

➤ To highlight ethical issues related to using a quantitative approach in nursing research.

➤ To explain the nature of quantitative evidence and how it can be used to underpin nursing practice.

Introduction

The rationale for including this chapter (as with Chapter 4) in a book on **evidence-based practice (EBP)** is to help you as a student understand how the evidence gained from quantitative research can be used to underpin nursing and health care practice, as well as helping you to understand in more detail the stages of the quantitative research process when critiquing an article or evaluating the relevance of the actual research for your practice.

The previous chapter on qualitative research demonstrated the way nursing knowledge can be increased by exploring people's experiences and interpretations of their health care or, in the case of you the student, your student experience. Qualitative research transforms descriptions and ideas into more general statements in what is known as the 'inductive process' of analysis. This is similar to taking pieces of a jigsaw puzzle and putting them together to form ideas on the possible picture on the box lid (in other words if I have these fragments of meaning, what is the picture they may represent?). For example, you may have noticed from personal experience that communicating with patients in pain, together with helping their relatives understand what the reasons are for the pain, seems to help them to manage this. However, what you do not know is how the patient actually feels or experiences this. You have the jigsaw pieces but need to put them together.

The quantitative approach to research uses the reverse of this process. It actually starts with the picture on the box lid of a jigsaw puzzle, and uses this along with the collection of jigsaw pieces in the box itself (along with possibly related jigsaws) to produce or confirm that picture. This is the deductive approach, in other words if I have this overall picture or general idea, will these fragments of meaning confirm/support that picture? Again using an example as above, you know from the literature and other studies that communicating with patients about their needs is important to their progress. This is what is on the jigsaw box lid—you have the picture. However, what you do not know is the extent to which this occurs in a specific group of patients; let us say patients with rheumatoid arthritis or if in fact if it is true in this group of patients. In quantitative research this is what you set out to find out; do all the pieces of the jigsaw actually make up that picture on the box?

This explanation of these two research approaches is important, as it explains why different research studies can look so different. The variation in approach also illustrates the contrasting beliefs about research and the way that researchers can think very differently about the nature of research, and the way it should be undertaken. As we have seen, one approach starts with evidence and moves to the bigger picture that may lie behind it, while the other starts with the bigger picture and demonstrates how it can be confirmed by gathering the pieces of the picture.

The relevance of this explanation is that in gathering research evidence to underpin practice, you can expect to see research articles vary considerably in their appearance and the thinking behind them. Some of the variations in appearance will be very noticeable, for instance the sample size will vary from quite small numbers in qualitative research with perhaps half a dozen individuals, to large samples of hundreds or even thousands in quantitative research. Other visible variations will include the methods of data collection, the way the results are analysed, and the way they are presented, all of these can be very different depending on the research approach.

As with qualitative research, one of the main challenges is learning the language used in these types of research, not unlike most of you having to learn the language used in nursing and health care. Unlike qualitative research however, where you see words, in quantitative research it is mostly about numbers. Both are of equal importance in nursing, however, as you will experience for example in giving out medication to patients, where you have to use words to communicate and reassure them but at the same time know that you are giving them the correct amount of medication.

+ ....

EBP in action

As you work through this chapter it will be useful to follow the main features of quantitative approaches in a research article of your choice. Identify one that you consider is a quantitative study from reading Chapter 3. You may wish to use an article chosen from one of the exercises. Alternatively, there are a number of studies in this chapter that you may wish to consider. The references for these are listed at the end of the chapter. You might like to stop here and collect an article now, so that you can apply the points below to your example.

....

What is quantitative research?

The first step to understanding this research approach is to clarify what is meant by quantitative research? Why do we need it? And what are some of the principles that we should look for in this kind of study?

Quantitative research is a form of study design examine numerically the features or frequency of a variable, for instance the percentage of patients with post-operative 'pain' in a particular setting or group of individuals. In correlation research the researcher examines whether a pattern can be seen between two variables, such as the 'social class' of individuals and the 'likelihood of taking regular exercise' or 'eating a nutritionally balanced diet'. Correlation is the 'link' between one variable that seems to be related to another variable, but does not necessarily happen in all cases. This can be contrasted to a different kind of relationship between variables that of a cause and effect relationship (as demonstrated through a randomized control trial (RCT)), where one variable has a direct effect on another, such as taking analgesia and pain levels, and will happen in almost all cases. We will return to this later in the chapter.

Quantitative research displays results as numbers. This can be in the form of percentages (e.g. 20% of patients were found to be in pain), raw figures (e.g. 17 of the 85 patients were found to be in pain) or in the form of a statistical statement that is the result of a statistical calculations ('lavender oil was found to reduce pain levels in patients $p < 0.05$', the reason for this type of figure will be explained later). In this way it considers variables in the form of quantities or amounts and their statistical relationships to each other.

There are four major types of descriptive research designs (Fig. 5.1). They are presented here as a hierarchy as they usually 'step-up' in terms of the degree of statistical depth and complexity used to analyse and give meaning to the results.

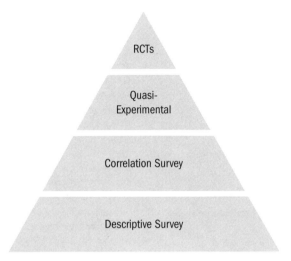

Figure 5.1 Types of descriptive research

Where little knowledge already exists on a variable, a descriptive study, usually in the form of a survey, will be conducted to establish its frequency, type, and amount. More in-depth surveys may try to establish patterns between variables in a situation, such as factors associated with teenagers who contract sexually transmitted infections. This might include variations in age, sexual activity, and gender.

Attempts to increase knowledge in regard to possible treatments or methods of interventions may use a quasi-experimental design where individuals are not randomly allocated to treatment and control groups. Finally, there is the RCT, where individuals are randomly allocated to an experimental group or a control group. The experimental group receive an intervention and the control group allow us to see what would have happened to the experimental group had they not received the intervention. The result is a study that permits us to conclude if an intervention 'works' and does have an effect on important clinical outcomes. A description of each of the four major types of designs is outlined in Table 5.1.

In terms of its place within EBP, quantitative approaches are seen as a major source of reliable evidence and within these categories, RCTs are placed high in the hierarchy of evidence (see Chapter 2).

Quantitative research represents the positivist paradigm of research, that is, one that applies the 'scientific' or systematic and objective approaches of the natural sciences such as physics and chemistry to the study of human behaviour. This approach believes human behaviour follows a set pattern that is predictable, as it follows what in physics or biology would be called 'scientific laws' or principles. That is to say they follow a set pattern because of the relationships that influence the outcome in clearly describable and set ways. Bryman (2008: 13) warns that it is not easy to provide an exact meaning

Purpose of research	Research approach	Description
Describe a situation	Survey	Involvement of a reasonably large group of respondents to create through numbers a picture of a situation. Involvement can be face-to-face or use methods such as postal questionnaires.
Look for patterns in a situation	Survey incorporating correlation analysis	As above, but in the analysis the researcher looks for patterns of relationships between some of the variables collected in the survey. The existence is confirmed statistically through the use of a correlation coefficient.
Look for cause and effect relationships	Experimental study using RCT design	Researcher uses random allocation to divide participants into an experimental and control group. The experimental group receive a different intervention than the control group.
The search for relationships where randomization is not possible or easily achieved	Quasi-experimental study	Very much like the above but differs in that the two groups are not randomly allocated but are likely to be already in two groups. A cause and effect relationship cannot be confirmed, but can indicate a correlation between variables.
The search for possible relationships retrospectively	Ex-post facto study or retrospective study	Similar to a quasi-experimental study but instead of the study being set up prospectively, the researcher examines a situation where the event the researcher is interested in has already happened and is not introduced by the researcher, e.g. development of a condition such as anorexia.

Table 5.1 Quantitative approaches

of positivism but suggests that it centres on a number of beliefs and principles about ways of gathering data through our senses, so that we can objectively test hypotheses rather than rely on our beliefs or assumptions.

Positivism also believes that research involving human behaviour and experiences should aim to establish naturally occurring laws in much the same way as other sciences such as physics and chemistry look for ways of explaining and controlling relationships between phenomena occurring in nature.

Such explanations in the natural sciences are taken to have a 'factual' nature to them and are 'universal', that is, they will be similar wherever they are applied. It is worth remembering that such ideas are constantly disputed by opponents of this view who believe in a more flexible interpretation of the forces that shape human behaviour. However, these principles still influence many of the ideas surrounding EBP. For example, it is recommended that knowledge for practice should be based on sound objective information that has been accurately and objectively gathered, and which can be applied in general to a wide range of situations and is not dependent on the personalities of those carrying out interventions. In other words, EBP values knowledge that holds true in general, and not just in a single setting. This is highlighted in Chapter 1 with regards to nursing interventions (Macleod Clark 2009).

> **! Key points**
>
> For a quick confirmation that a study is quantitative, look at the results section. This should contain tables, or figures such as bar charts and pie charts. It will also give quantities or frequencies of variables in raw figures or percentages. Although qualitative research may have a table, this will usually only relate to characteristics of the sample, and not represent numeric findings

Study designs in quantitative research take a number of forms depending on the purpose of the research question. The major types are shown in Table 5.1.

Why quantitative approaches?

As stated in Chapter 2, a quantitative research design is seen as the major contributor to EBP; indeed Burns and Grove (2009: 33) say that quantitative approaches are essential to develop the body of knowledge needed for EBP. Quantitative research can be used in evidence-based practice to:

i) Identify where, when, and how changes to practice are needed because current forms of intervention are inadequate or where patient needs are not being met. In addition there is a related need to evaluate if any changes that took place were successful and produced a closer fit between care and patient needs.

ii) Identify the most effective form of intervention in care where options exist (this may include the option of no intervention). Quantitative approaches are appropriate as they are based on the production of accurate information using sound methods of collecting data. They also have the ability to test the outcome of alternatives such as interventions in care.

The principles of quantitative research

In order to assess the quality of this type of research, you will need to understand some of the principles on which quantitative methods are based. You will also need to know some of the different forms that quantitative methods can take.

Some of the basic principles of quantitative methods include:

• Clear and unambiguous definitions of concepts being measured.

• Transparency (clear descriptions) of the data collection process.

- Ethical principles applied by the researcher throughout the study.
- Accuracy of the measurements used in data collection assured.
- Ability to generalize from the findings.
- Objective standpoint of the researcher and the process of research.
- Numeric display of results that have been statistically processed.
- Honest and clear representation of findings.
- Interpretations of findings that are clearly based on the data collected and that are unlikely to be explained by chance occurences, or other variables not included in the study.

Although all quantitative research may have these as goals, they will achieve them to different extents, so when you read research articles you will need to consider how well each study has achieved these goals. If you are 'critiquing' research (see Chapter 7), some of the things to look for as indicators that these principles have been followed include:

- A clear and supported definition of key variables on which data are collected (concept definitions).
- Where studies involve data gathering on health premises, patients, staff, that an ethics committee (LREC or IRB if an American study) has been approached to assess the ethical rigour of the study.
- Clear description of what is used to measure the variables (*operational definition*).
- Detailed outline of the method of data collection.
- Detailed description of the sample selection and an indication of the extent to which they may be represent ative.
- Information on the accuracy of the tool of data collection (reliability), its origins if used in previous studies, or the extent to which it has been tested in a pilot study.
- Details of the methods of data analysis with descriptions of statistical processes and tests applied to the data.
- Clear display of key numeric and statistical data with an explanation or highlighting of key points by the researcher to accompany any tables or figures.
- Assessment of the extent to which findings may be due to chance circumstances (probability levels, i.e. 'p values') or suggestions of alternative explanations.
- Description of any limitations that may have affected the results of the study (often in the discussion section).
- Declaration of any interests or relationship in regard to any drug companies or commercial organizations related to the interventions examined in the study.

+ ....

EBP in action

Using your research article, which of the above indicators of good quantitative research does your study illustrate, and from reading the article what would have helped you understand some of the explanations better?

You will find as you continue to read more research articles that you will begin to look for tell-tale signs that the author has produced a sound study. These will often be found in the description of the methodology used to structure the research.

....

Research methods used in quantitative studies

The research methods (or tools) covered in this chapter have a common aim of producing measurements of some kind to answer the research question that forms the focus of the study. The accuracy of the measurement is always a prime methodological issue and the researcher will take steps to convince you through the use of a pilot study or the use of a tool of data collection that has been used in previous studies that the method of collecting the data is accurate.

As we saw in Chapter 3, there are several frequently used methods of collecting data in quantitative research. Each research method (also referred to as the tool of data collection) will have its advantages and disadvantages. The researcher must select an appropriate method for the sample in the study, and the nature of the research question. The method must be one that will produce the most accurate numeric results. A summary of these methods or tools is shown in Table 5.2 along with an indication of some of the advantages and disadvantages that can be associated with them.

It is clear that all methods of data collection will have their advantages and disadvantages. Researchers must ensure that they anticipate possible disadvantages and compensate for them as much as possible. When examining studies it is the kind of issues raised in Table 5.2 that will help you assess the quality of the study.

+ ....

EBP in action

Looking at your research article or another you may be using for a critique assignment, to what extent do you feel the researcher has chosen the tool of data collection wisely? Is there an indication that they have recognized possible disadvantages with this method and have tried to overcome them, at least to some extent?

....

In the following sections we will examine how these methods of data collection are used in the various research approaches starting with descriptive studies.

Research method	Advantages	Disadvantages
Questionnaires	Cheap and rapid method of collecting a lot of numeric data from a widespread sample.	Poor response rates in many studies. Depends on 'self-report', that is what people say they do, or how they rate themselves. This may not always be accurate. Possibility of people misunderstanding questions, or leaving questions blank. Where there is a problem with literacy, language differences, or physical problem relating to eyesight and the ability to write, the range of people participating may not be representative.
Interviews	Better response rate than questionnaires. Interviewer able to clarify questions and their meanings. Answers can also be checked on the spot where accuracy may be a problem.	Still dependent on 'self-report', which may vary from actual situations. Respondents may be influenced by characteristics of interviewers and conform to a 'socially desirable' image and answers.
Observation check lists	Objective method not dependent on 'self-report'. A number of observers can be trained to collect data and 'inter-rater' reliability can be established through training.	Time consuming and can be costly. Can be difficulties of interpretation unless supplemented by other forms of data collection. Suffers from 'observer effect', where behaviour influenced by being observed.
Assessment scales	These can provide numeric values for abstract concepts such as 'pain', 'anxiety', and opinions or attitudes in the form of 'Likert Scales' where you have to rate your views on a scale of some kind.	The validity of some scales can be difficult to demonstrate. Some element of interpretation is implicit in some scales. Individuals can vary in responses depending on a number of variables outside the control of the researcher, e.g. time of day, memory, 'social desirability' factor. Different assessors may produce different 'measurements' (inter-rater reliability problems).
Documentary summary lists	This kind of data taken from e.g. patient records, and similar documents are not subject to social influences especially where collected retrospectively.	Problems with missing, inaccurate, or inconsistently recorded data. May not be recorded in ways which relate to the study. May be difficult to confirm accuracy of information. Can be difficult to source, and time consuming and costly to extract information.

Table 5.2 Frequently used research methods illustrating advantages and disadvantages

Descriptive studies

Burns and Grove (2009: 45) describe the role of descriptive research as 'to explore and describe phenomena in real life situations'. This is different from research that might take place in a laboratory or other protected environment. It can describe a current situation or one from the past, as in the case of a retrospective study, that is where the data lie in the past at the start of data gathering (this will be discussed in more detail later). An example would be looking at patients' past experience of trying to quit smoking using an intervention such as nicotine patches or a quit-smoking group at a local health centre.

Unlike experimental or quasi-experimental designs (described later), descriptive studies do not involve the researcher intervening in the treatment or care received by individuals. This makes such research easier from an ethical point of view, although there are always issues of protecting privacy and the possibility of harm through being confronted with painful or anxiety provoking memories, even through questionnaires. However, it can also be easier to get people to take part in descriptive research compared to experimental studies as they are not physically invasive.

The advantages of this research approach are emphasized by Polit and Beck (2008: 278), who point out that:

> 66 Descriptive studies can be invaluable in documenting the prevalence, nature, and intensity of health-related conditions and behaviours, and are critical in the development of effective interventions. 99

Descriptive research then 'maps out' the nature of a topic or variable of interest. An example of a descriptive study is provided in Example 5.1 below.

! Key points

Throughout this chapter there are some detailed extracts of published research to illustrate the various research approaches. These are designed to focus on the kinds of issues you will find useful to raise in your discussions or critiques of specific research articles. Do take the time to read through these illustrations, reflect on the content, and link them to the information covered in this chapter.

The Australian study in Example 5.1 examines variations in the type of nursing activity carried out by different groups or grades of nurses using observation as a method of data collection. It has been chosen to demonstrate some of the issues that arise in carrying out this kind of study. Its relevance to EBP is that it allows current behaviour to be documented and described so the need for any improvements on what is 'best practice' can be decided. The choice of method, as with all methods, has in-built challenges for both the researcher and the reader of this kind of study, and these have been highlighted in the description below.

EBP in action

Obtain a copy of this paper if possible and consider the issues noted in Box 5.1. Consider what you learnt from reading it. As well as informing practice it is an important exercise for a student to read articles and learn how to identify the key messages from them. You will also find examples of quantitative studies in the further reading section at the end of the chapter.

....

Example 5.1 Example of a descriptive observational study

Title: A comparison of activities undertaken by enrolled and registered nurses on medical wards in Australia: An observational study

Authors: Chaboyer, *et al.* (2008)

Aim: The aim of the study was to describe and compare the activities undertaken by different categories of nursing staff in four medical wards in two acute care public hospitals in Australia.

Method

An observation check list of 25 activities was used to identify the categories of work carried out by three different categories of staff. The observations were carried out by research assistants using a time sampling method. Two-hour time periods were chosen using random sampling methods and activities recorded at intervals of 10 minutes by research assistants in the study. In all 120 hours of observation took place over several weeks in each ward.

Within randomized 2 hour periods, work activities were sampled every 10 minutes. Research assistants were limited to 2 hour periods of observation to ensure that tiredness did not affect accuracy of observation. These 2 hour periods commenced on the hour and the research assistants recorded participants' activities every 10 minutes.

Methodological issues

There are a number of design issues that have to be identified and overcome by researchers when carrying out this kind of study. These include:

i) Sample

Two medical wards in each of two different hospitals volunteered to take part in the study. A total of 114 staff were included giving a reasonable sample size. Details of the age, sex, experience, and hours worked (full time/part time) are provided to indicate the extent to which the sample may be judged as representative or typical.

ii) Observation time periods

The sampled 2 hour periods were drawn randomly from a list of hours between 7.00 am to 7.00 pm Monday to Friday to ensure busy periods of activity were included in the sample and there was no researcher bias in the hours observed. This resulted in a total of 484 hours of data covering 14,528 documented activities. This is an extensive amount of data on which to base analysis and from which to argue that the activities should be reasonably typical within this setting.

iii) Method of data collection

The authors state in the discussion 'that it is always possible that being observed affected the behaviour of those in the study'. The extent to which it did influence the results is an unknown; however, the size of the sample and the numbers of activities

»

observed makes it difficult for those in the study to act unnaturally for such extended periods of time.

Reliability

The observation checklist used in the study to collect data had been developed in previous American research, and had already been adapted to suit the Australian context. This was argued to give the tool both validity and reliability.

The 10 minute observation samples were chosen over continuous sampling as there is evidence to support a greater level of accuracy and precision when the observation is carried out over short as opposed to long time periods.

To increase the accuracy in recording observations, research assistants received 16 hours of training on filling in the observation check list by a researcher experienced in using this method. Training was continued until the accuracy of observation between the research assistant and the experienced researcher reached a level of 90% agreement between the observations (inter-observer reliability also referred to as inter-rater reliability). Spot checks were carried out during data gathering to ensure that the accuracy in categorizing the type of activity was maintained. All the research assistants were also trained nurses so were able to accurately identify the type of activity.

Areas to note

The study fits the criteria of a descriptive study as it provides a picture of a pattern of behaviour in numbers. The tool of data collection and the rigour with which it is used appears very high in this study. The effort to gain consistency in recording between data gathers (inter-observer reliability) is very good. A large data set (amount of collected data) means that the statistical processing of the data should increase the likelihood of accuracy in the results.

Time sampling means that some activities may have been missed. The authors also identify that there are problems where nurses are carrying out more than one activity at the same time but only one of them is recorded in data gathering. Not all nurses in the clinical areas were observed, and there is no guarantee that nurses were working 'naturally' while being observed. It is therefore difficult to argue that the accuracy of such findings is 'high'.

Work patterns, abilities and organizational influences will vary from hospital to hospital and may even vary within the same hospital. This, combined with the Australian location of the hospital, means that the ability to generalize widely from this study would be difficult. However, the finding that there was little difference in the type of work carried out by lower qualified grades of staff and minimum qualified support worker was interesting and may highlight the problem of deciding who does what in the ward area, and at what cost to the organization.

This descriptive study provides some hard evidence on the kind of activities carried out in the study areas and provides a clear comparison of these staff. However, it does not provide a great deal of argument or evidence to say that this is a guide to optimal or 'best' skill-mix for this type of area. It provides the reader with a source of information on how nurses spend their time and a comparison between grades. Descriptive research is a relevant approach to answer the type of question posed here.

Surveys

Surveys are a form of descriptive research that can be used to determine the nature of a problem where evidence-based action needs to be introduced. It can determine what people know about a situation, or it can describe current practice in caring for certain patient or client groups. In this way it can help to identify practice in terms of what is most commonly carried out (this does not necessarily mean 'best'). This may be useful knowledge where it may be difficult to carry out an experimental design to answer the question of most effective outcomes. Such a survey of opinions or activities could be one solution to the problem of finding a better way of producing successful clinical outcomes. Although this may not be high up the hierarchy of evidence (see Chapter 2), at least it produces some basis for decision-making.

Surveys provide a snapshot of existing situations to provide a clear idea of how things are, for example the number of patients with difficulty swallowing, or the number of nurses who feel they would like to develop specialist skills in a particular clinical procedure. The researcher is not interested in manipulating or changing things, only in saying how things are. To achieve this, the emphasis is on including a large number of respondents so that they are likely to capture a range of diverse views, characteristics, or experiences.

One of the biggest problems in surveys is selection bias, that is, where the researcher cannot be sure that the people who have agreed to take part in a study are representative of the group required. Polit and Beck (2008) say that selection bias is one of the biggest problems and most frequently encountered threats to the internal validity of studies not using an experimental design (p. 295). This is particularly true where the researcher is dependent on individuals to return questionnaires, and there is a low response rate. It could be that those who have decided to take part in the survey are different in ways that will affect the results to those who have not taken part. The important point here is that although results can be impressive, the safety of the interpretation can be in doubt.

When reading survey results it is extremely important to consider the response rate and the characteristics of the sample included in the group. Sometimes the researcher will compare these characteristics to the larger group they represent in an attempt to demonstrate how typical the group is, and to increase the chances of being able to generalize from the results. If for example a study you read had a response rate of 80% of a group of 1000 questionnaires that is an excellent return rate, whilst a return rate of 10% would not be. When reading articles where surveys have been undertaken, it is expected that this is commented upon.

> **! Key points**
>
> A frequent method of collecting measurements in surveys and other types of research is the use of the Likert scale. This is named after the originator Renis Likert so is always spelt with a capital letter. The scale consists of a number of statements called 'items' and invites the respondent to respond to it using the alternatives 'Strongly agree', 'Agree', 'Undecided', 'Disagree', 'Strongly disagree'. Each point is given a value from 1 to 5 usually giving 'Strongly agree' a value of 5, but it can be reversed so that 'Strongly Agree' equals a value of 1. An example would be a statement such as 'When I think about my health I see myself as a very healthy person'. Someone who feels very healthy and choosing 'Strongly agree' would score a value of 5 for this response. All total scores can indicate an individual's belief on their health status. Different groups, for example age groups, or males and females, can be compared numerically using such forms of measurement.

Cross-sectional studies

A popular type of survey is the cross-sectional study. This looks at different sections or subgroups of a population at one point in time, rather than follow a single group over the course of their development. One example would be nursing students and their experience of mentorship during their training. It would be possible to follow one group through their training years in the form of a longitudinal study, where the researcher would go back at each year of training and remeasure. The alternative is to use a cross-sectional design where the researcher collects information from students in different year groups at one survey point in time.

The advantage of a cross-sectional study is one of cost and resources. The cost of repeatedly going back to the same group over time would be considerable. There would also be a long wait for the results. The disadvantage of a cross-sectional design is that we do not measure the same people at repeat points in time and so miss the consistency and control for personal variations across groups. It could be that the newest group of students is very different in their needs and relationships within mentorship than those in the 'oldest' group within the study. However, it would give us an indication of student experiences of mentorship at a given point in time over the different groups, an important issue if we had to consider making a change to student–mentor working within a given time span.

As so often happens in research, there is always a trade-off of advantages and disadvantages; however, we should feel that in the design of the study the researcher has been aware of disadvantages and compensated for this in the design as far as possible. So, for instance, data may be collected on characteristics that might make a difference to the study variable of interest so that comparisons between the groups concerned could be made. Example 5.2 provides a useful example of a cross-sectional study.

> **! Key points**
>
> The alternative to a cross-sectional study is a longitudinal study. This will typically fol-
> low one or more groups over time, instead of several groups at different points in their
> natural life, for example nursing students in different years. The advantage of cross-
> sectional studies is that they are cheaper to carry out and produce an answer in a
> shorter time compared to a longitudinal study.

Example 5.2 Example of a cross-sectional study

Title: Exploring knowledge and skills on HIV in student nurses and midwives

Authors: Veeramah *et al.* (2008)

Aim: The aim of the study was to describe the knowledge of, skills related
to, and attitudes of, a sample of final year student nurses and midwives
towards people who are infected with HIV or who develop AIDS.

Method

A cross-sectional survey of 42 final-year student nurses and 20 student midwives
registered on a preregistration nursing and midwifery programme at a university in
the south-east of England and agreeing to take part in the survey.

Data were collected using a self-administered questionnaire sent to those who agreed
to take part on their last day of their course. Postal questionnaires were sent to their
home addresses following receipt of willingness to participate. The questionnaire
contained 77 items (questions); these included socio-demographic information, e.g. age,
sex, marital status. The respondents' levels of knowledge on HIV/AIDS were tested using
a modified version of the State University of New York at Buffalo School of Nursing
AIDS Study Questionnaire. Attitudes towards patients with AIDS were measured
using the AIDS attitude scale (AAS). Further questions determined if respondents
had the necessary skills to meet the intense physical and psychological needs of patients
with AIDS and their relatives. They were also asked if they had sufficient information
and/or training to protect themselves against any infection while caring for this group
of patients and the skills to help prevent the spread of the HIV virus.

Methodological issues

There are a number of areas that can be highlighted in this study, these include:

i) Sample

Although the sample was based in only one education centre, the questionnaire had
a good response rate of 76%. This represented 47 out of 62 agreeing to take part in
the study. Where response rate falls below 50%, those not replying could have a very
different view from those who did take part. Here, 76% clearly represents a majority

»

view; however, this is not a percentage of the total student group as there were 116 in the cohort of students. This means that those returning a questionnaire represent 41% of the total group. The results may not necessarily be reflected in the knowledge and skills and attitudes of the whole group. Those who had a negative view of HIV/AIDS may have been more likely to not respond. It is also unclear how far the findings could be typical of other groups of students in different Schools of Nursing and Midwifery. Are those who volunteer to take part in a study by returning a questionnaire the same as those who do not? This is referred to the problem of the self-selected sample; there may be characteristics that prompted them to reply that make them different from those who do not take part, The issue is one of how representative is a self-selected sample?

Reliability

The questionnaire is made up of a number of scales that have been used in a number of studies. There is a clear attempt by the researchers to demonstrate reliability in the tool by looking statistically at its consistency in use through applying a statistical tool (Cronbach's alpha coefficient). This compares the extent to which individuals respond across the whole of the questionnaire in a consistent manner and so demonstrate the internal consistency of the measuring instrument (Burns and Grove 2009: 379).

Areas to note:

The study fits the criteria of a cross-sectional survey as it provides a picture of a reasonable number of respondents from different groups at one point in time.

One of the problems of all such studies is that we are dealing with a self-report method. This means that what people say is their level of skill or their attitude towards something may not be accurate. The results provide an indicator or a measure of 'perception', it lacks an objective measurement. Although a more reliable method may be difficult and costly, it should always be remembered that asking people what they do is not the same as what they may be observed to do in practice. This point is accepted as a limitation of the study by the researchers.

There is a good attempt to ensure the tool of data collection is to a high standard through the use of questions used in a number of previous studies on the same topic. This cross-sectional study provides some indication on the extent to which final year students may have developed knowledge, skills, and positive attitudes to working with this client group. The researchers are appropriately cautious in their claims to the generalizability of the results. The study does answer its aim and does provide some evidence on the need to ensure that key areas of nursing care are covered during the education of students.

Correlation studies

Surveys can be used to provide a numeric map of a number of variables within an identified group of respondents. It is possible to use survey data to look further for patterns between variables in the study to see if there is a clear connection or association

> **! Key points**
>
> You may have noticed under the 'Methods' section in Example 5.2 above the phrase 'Data were collected using a self-administered questionnaire'. A common mistake is for students to write 'data was collected'; however, this is incorrect as 'data' is a plural word, so needs a plural form of the verb. Similarly, we would write 'data are presented in the form of tables', rather than 'data is presented'.

that may help predict situations or better manage care. This is the role of a correlation study. It makes use of statistical calculations called '**correlation coefficients**'. Polit and Beck (2008: 272) define a correlation as:

> 66 *An interrelationship or association between two variables, that is, a tendency for variation in one variable to be related to variation in another (e.g. height and width).* 99

A further clear explanation is provided by Brown (2009: 91), who explains that correlation is where '**two variables are connected when they change in accord with one another'.** She explains that 'accord' relates to how strongly they are connected and in whether the direction of the relationship is positive, where they both increase with each other, or negative, where as the value of one variable goes up, such as amount of information about a condition, the 'linked' variable goes down, such as level of anxiety.

The statistics bit! Part 1: correlation

For quantitative research to have meaning, it requires some statistical analysis of the results. Without it, a reader would firstly have difficulty making sense of all the figures, and secondly would not know how much weight to place on the usefulness of the results. Statistical analysis is integral to quantitative research approaches. This section, and a similar one later, will provide you with some essential pointers to making sense of some of the statistical ideas you will commonly encounter.

Firstly, it is useful to know that statistical processes can be divided into two types:

i) Descriptive statistics

These summarize a host of figures produced by data collection in order to make them easier to understand. They often simplify the information in the form of an 'average' figure to allow the reader to grasp what may be a 'typical' numeric value within the group, such as typical age, or typical level of patient dependency. In statistics the word 'average' is not used, instead it is expressed as one of three measures that attempt to illustrate what is typical in the group. These are the mean, which is closest to our understanding of 'average' as it adds all the values together and divides by the number within the group, the median, which is the mid-point when all the values are put in order from the smallest value up to largest, and the mode, which is the most commonly occurring value.

Descriptive statistics also looks at how close each value in the set of results is to the typical value. It uses calculations of this such as the range, that is, the ones furthest away below and above the typical value. You will also see a measure called 'standard deviation' (abbreviated to s.d.), which is used to show how close to the typical figure most of the results lie. These last two calculations are called measures of dispersal.

ii) Inferential statistics

This is the second category of statistic. As the name implies, the purpose of this type of statistic is to make 'inferences' about a total group, based on the results of those in the study sample. They are used to establish if there is a difference between the groups, or sub-groups, in a study such as a RCT that is unlikely to be explained by chance variations. In other words, they confirm the extent to which a clear pattern in the results can support a hypothesis about the nature of relationships between the variables.

Correlation is one example of an inferential statistic. Its purpose is to test how closely two variables are similar. The strength of a relationship and its direction (explained below) are measured and expressed in a study through a numeric indicator called a correlation coefficient. This is produced by a calculation made by the researcher using the study data. The correlation coefficient is a figure between −1 and +1 that indicates how closely two variables change in relation to each other and if that change is in the same direction, a positive (+) relationship, or the opposite direction, a negative (−) relationship. A negative relationship is where as one variable increases, the other decreases to exactly the same degree. A perfect positive relationship would be indicated by a correlation coefficient of '1' where a change in one variable was proportionately identical to a change in another factor. If the correlation coefficient was estimated as zero (0), it would mean that there was no pattern between the variations in these two variables. This continuum of positive to negative correlation coefficient is shown in Fig. 5.2.

The correlation coefficient measures both the direction of the relationship, and its strength. Although +1 and −1 would be perfect relationships, in reality most relationships may be described as strong if they were below one with a decimal such as 0.6 or 0.7. A weak relationship may be 0.3 or 0.4 for positive relationships, and −0.6 or −0.7 and −0.3 or −0.4 for negative relationships.

Correlation studies are useful in that they confirm that two variables are linked in some way and have a predictable outcome. They increase our knowledge and allow us to predict events given the occurrence of certain situations. However, they do not

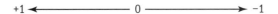

+1 ←————————— 0 —————————→ −1

Figure 5.2 Strength of correlation ranging from a perfect +1 to −1

mean that one causes the other, as they could both be linked to another variable that influences both of them in a causal way.

> **!**   **Key points**
>
> The important point about correlation studies is that they examine similarities in the behaviour of variables within the sample and indicate close patterns or associations. This is not the same as experimental studies that look for clear differences existing between the experimental and control group so it can be deduced that any differences are due to the experimental variable, or independent variable.

An example will clarify the points made so far. Example 5.3 presents an interesting clinical study examining whether we can predict the kind of people who are more likely to look after their health following the diagnosis of heart failure. In particular, the study wanted to establish if there was a pattern between men and women and the extent to which they were likely to take preventative action against further heart problems.

+ ....

EBP in action

Obtain a copy of this paper if possible and consider the issues noted in Example 5.3.

....

Example 5.3 Example of a correlation study

Title:	Gender differences in and factors related to self-care behaviors: A cross-sectional, correlational study of patients with heart failure
Authors:	Heo *et al.* (2008)
Aim:	The aim of the study was to identify correlates of self-care in patients with heart failure (HF) and to determine whether there are gender differences in the correlates.

Method

A cross-sectional, correlation study design was used. The study recruited 77 men and 45 women, a total of 122 patients with HF, who visited the outpatient clinics of one academic medical centre and two community hospitals in a Midwestern city in America for their routine cardiology follow-up. The sample size was estimated in the planning stage based on prior studies identified from the literature.

The data were collected by the authors, or the nurse research associates, using questionnaires, medical record reviews, and patient interviews at patients' homes, the clinics, or the general clinical research centre of a university-affiliated hospital.

»

A number of variables were measured using recognised scales. These included:

Self-care behaviours using the self-care maintenance subscale of the Self-Care of Heart Failure Index (SCHFI).

Depression using the Beck Depression Inventory (BDI)-II

Perceived control (patients' perception about their ability to control their heart, HF symptoms, and lives) measured by the Control Attitudes Scale-Revised

Patients' confidence in their ability to self-manage HF symptoms measured by the self-care confidence subscale of the Self-Care of Heart Failure Index (SCHFI).

Knowledge of HF management measured by the HF Knowledge and Barriers to Adherence Scale.

Functional status measured by the Duke Activity Status Index. This is a self-report measure that assesses functional status based on the individuals' assessment of their abilities to perform specific daily activities.

Social support (emotional support from others) measured by the Multidimensional Scale of Perceived Social Support.

Other demographic (age, educational level, marital status, and ethnicity) and clinical characteristics (New York Heart Association [NYHA] functional class, and Charlson Comorbidity Index score) collected by the Demographic and Clinical questionnaires, medical record reviews, and patient interviews.

This produced a large amount of numeric measures for each individual. The data were analysed using statistical techniques that establish the link or correlation between the factors that might influence the level of self-care. This allowed the aim to be achieved.

Methodological issues

There are a number of areas that can be highlighted in this study, these include:

i) Sample

Although there is an adequate sample size to allow the statistical processes to be reasonably accurate, it has to be remembered that they have been 'recruited' into the study and may not necessarily be similar to those who chose not to take part. They are a 'self-selected' group of individuals. There is also an imbalance in the number of male to female, which means that as it is shown there is a different pattern between male and female behaviour, care has to be taken when there is such a size difference between the two gender groups.

Reliability

The variables in this study are measured using a large number of well-known scales that provide numeric scores for the variables of interest. This gives the study a high level of rigour. Confidence in the accuracy of measurement of many of the scales is increased by details on the Cronbach's alpha coefficient (described in Example 5.2 above). The reasonable sample size also provides some assurance in the ability of the statistics to reflect a true reading.

Areas to note

The study fits the criteria of a correlation study as it concentrates on one outcome measure (taking self-care behaviour) and attempts to establish a pattern between it and other variables (such as level of knowledge about effective self-care behaviour, functional level, degree of depression, feeling of control, and gender). Such patterns or associations are determined statistically and interpreted according to the size or 'strength', and direction (positive or negative) of the statistical outcome (the correlation coefficient).

As with the research in Example 5.2, as some of the assessments were based on what patients said they did, there is the problem of self-report and the issue is that what people say they do is not the same as what they may be observed to do in practice. This point is accepted as a limitation to the possible accuracy of the study by the researchers.

There is a good attempt to ensure the tool of data collection is to a high standard through the use of questions that have been used in a number of previous studies on the same topic.

This correlation study demonstrates that for this sample, the level of self-help behaviours were low but did vary by gender. Studies like this make a small but important contribution to our knowledge about patients' reactions to illness and the steps they are likely to take in reducing another attack. The conclusion is that preventative behaviour is not as frequent or thorough as might be anticipated.

Retrospective studies

Retrospective studies are those where the researcher gathers descriptive data that relates to past situations or measurements. This can measure a variable such as high body mass index (BMI), and retrospectively collect information on eating patterns or BMIs at different ages through collecting information from past records or recollections of the past.

In terms of in-built limitations, you should be able to anticipate some of the problems, for example the accuracy of recall, or the accuracy or existence of records containing data crucial to building up a picture of the past. Missing data or values are often a problem with retrospective studies, as they do not allow any control over the accuracy or consistency of the data. This is why prospective studies (where data are collected from a particular point in time forward) are preferred because the researcher has the opportunity to influence the type and quality of information yet to be gathered. There is far more opportunity for quality control over data gathered prospectively that simply do not exist in relation to retrospective studies. However, prospective studies following a large group of people over time can be expensive to conduct.

> ❗ **Key points**
>
> The choice of a retrospective or prospective approach is often dependent on practical aspects of time, money, and staff. Where it is not possible to control or manipulate variables, the researcher may have no other choice than to 'backtrack' and look for trends in data or events that have already happened. Where possible, the researcher would usually choose a prospective study, as there is a greater chance of quality control over the data by building in safeguards on the accuracy of the information.

Experimental studies

This section highlights some of the essential features and variations in experimental designs. It will also highlight some of the things to look for when you read experimental studies. Although this section contains a large number of specialist terms and ideas that some people can find difficult, do persist with these as they will help you get the most from experimental studies. We have attempted to present information on a 'need to know' basis rather than cover all there is to know about the subject. The example of an experimental study in Example 5.4 will reinforce the information covered in the coming sections, but do be prepared to spend some time studying the key components and issues related to experimental designs.

EBP in action

If you had to explain to a friend in general terms how an experimental study is structured, how would you describe some of the processes used and principles applied in experimental studies?

There are clear differences between descriptive studies and experimental studies. A good question to start with then, is how do I recognize an experimental study when I see it? Polit and Beck (2008: 250) suggest there are three major attributes we would expect to see in a true experiment; these are: manipulation, control, and randomization.

Manipulation

Where the researcher does, or introduces, something to at least some of those in the study and so manipulates or makes a difference to the situation that existed. This is in contrast to descriptive studies, where the researcher does not introduce or change anything in a setting to examine what happens to one or more of the variables in the study. In an experiment, the researcher sets out to make a difference in relation to who gets what variable, or quantity of a variable. There is also an attempt to make sure that where the researcher introduces a treatment or drug, it is standardized between those who are meant to receive it. The ability of the researcher to alter aspects of the situation is fundamental to the concept of manipulation.

Control

Where the researcher must be able to influence or take into account the effect of some of the many things that happen to those in the study. This sounds similar to manipulation, but relates to the researcher's ability to convince the reader that they were able to control other variables that could influence the outcome of the study. In other words, the researcher is able to ensure that 'extraneous factors' (also referred to as 'confounding variables'), that is, variables that may also affect the outcome measures in study, are equally present in both groups or are excluded from the situation, so that they do not provide an alternative explanation for the results of the study.

Randomization

Where the researcher ensures that those within the study could have been allocated equally to either the control or experimental group by using a table of random numbers or, more usually, computer-generated random numbers. This is also called random allocation or random assignment and describes the ability of the researcher to ensure that there is no biasing influence on who is allocated to which group in the study.

Randamization is perhaps the most important of the three major attributes and has been described by Polit and Beck (2008: 256) as the 'signature of an experimental design', as without it a study cannot be classified as a true experimental design. However, the idea of randomization can be frequently misunderstood. This is because in everyday life we tend to talk about 'random', when there is no pattern or system to it, such as 'I picked a book from the shelf at random' meaning little thought was given to it. In fact such activities are far from random; there are subconscious factors that will make us select one object like this rather than another. In research, random is a very structured activity. The basic principle is that through this process any characteristics that might make a difference to the outcome are evenly spread between the two groups, or do not account for a large influence. The only major variable that should be different between the groups is the experimental variable, which the researcher controls. The process can be described as follows.

Random allocation

All those who could be included for selection in the study are listed in a sampling frame, which is a list of numbered names or identifiers. The sequence or order of names is not important. All names, or 'items' where the sample is not people, should receive a number. There are a number of ways to then select which individuals are chosen from the sampling frame. The main two options are, firstly, using tables of random numbers from a book of random tables. Such tables comprise blocks of numbers throughout the pages of the book. Illustrations of such tables can be found in many research texts books (e.g. Polit and Beck 2008: 256), so will not be illustrated here. The alternative is computer-generated numbers.

The total size of the sample to be extracted from the sampling frame is first agreed, for example, 80 with 40 in each group. The first 40 numbers selected with the help of the random numbers would then be matched against the names in the sampling frame and would form the 'experimental group', and the second 40 selected would form the control group.

In this way there is no possibility of the researcher influencing who will end up in which group, as there is no matching of individuals to numbers until after the allocation has been made.

Where the study is a prospective study, such as the first 80 patients entering the clinical area and agreeing to take part in the study from next Monday, the researcher would number 80 envelopes from 1 to 80. Inside the envelopes would be a note or card saying to which group the individual had been assigned, or which treatment or intervention they were to receive. Naturally, it would not say 'experimental' or 'control' as this would affect the masking of the allocation.

The examination of these three features of experiments illustrates the high level of planning and forethought built into the design of an experimental study. The complexity will also be reflected in its cost. Although some studies are still straightforward and can be done for a modest sum if they do not involve complicated measures and analysis of outcomes, on the whole experimental designs can be costly. For this reason, nursing has historically found it difficult to work consistently in this kind of research arena through lack of funding and sponsorship, and has found itself faced with little option than to adopt research approaches that do not require the same level of costs and staffing.

Experimental studies involve two variables; the independent variable is the one that the researcher introduces to at least one group of participants; it is the 'cause' part of the equation. The second variable is the dependent variable, which is the outcome measure, usually the factor the independent variable is designed to improve, such as pain level, or level of mobility or knowledge. Table 5.3 provides examples of dependent and independent variables in experimental studies.

Clear definitions must be given for both dependent and independent variables in order to achieve accuracy and consistency. Such a definition is called a concept definition as

Dependent variable	Independent variable
Pain levels	Level of pre-operative information
Anxiety levels	Daily structured relaxation session
Ability to concentrate in school children	Daily morning vitamin tablet
Cessation of smoking	Brief intervention by nurse

Table 5.3 Examples of dependent and independent variables in experimental studies

it provides a definition for the key concepts in the study to increase clarity. It is important in experimental designs that the researchers give precise details of the quantities of any variable introduced (such as information, vitamins, brief intervention session), and if factors such as duration or circumstances under which the variable is given are important, these must also be detailed as these could form a confounding variable, that is an additional influence on the outcome.

The need to have clear concept definitions and to be aware of any confounding variables is important when a particular study is compared with other studies, as it will influence the degree of comparison possible. So for example in two studies looking at the effect of pre-operative information given to patients, one group may have received a great deal more information at a different time before surgery, and that had a different effect on levels of pain experienced post-operatively. The standardization of the 'amount' of the intervention is clearly crucial to the outcome of a study, and to the ability to compare one study with another. The procedures followed in carrying out the experiment should therefore be described in detail by the researcher, so that it is possible to picture how the study unfolded. This should include clear detail on the control group and what they received so that the extent of the differences between the two groups can be assessed.

The hypothesis

One feature of experimental designs is the use of a hypothesis. These are more likely to be used in experimental studies than in descriptive studies, although they can be used in correlation studies. If we look at the definition of a hypothesis, you will be able to understand these variations in their use, although you will meet many experimental studies that do not have a stated hypothesis.

A hypothesis can be defined as a statement linking the dependent and independent variable or variables in a study, and indicates the researcher's anticipation of what the study may find. Polit and Beck (2008: 93) express this simply by saying a hypothesis is:

> 66 *a prediction about the relationship between two or more variables.* 99

It is, according to Parahoo (2006: 169), the researcher's 'hunch' of the relationship that they expect the study to demonstrate. This relationship between the variables is demonstrated statistically. Using this definition, studies that just look at one variable, or where no relationship between variables is being examined, do not require a hypothesis. In a correlation study a hypothesis predicting the relationship between variables may be used, but not in a 'cause and effect' way, only in terms of 'they will be related' or 'a pattern will be seen'. In an experiment that attempts to establish if one variable (the independent variable) has a direct causal effect on another (the dependent variable or variables) then a hypothesis is useful in testing whether that relationship can be clearly demonstrated by means of the results.

> ! **Key points**
>
> When talking about hypotheses, the researcher does not say that the hypothesis has been proved or disproved, as there are always problems in being 100% certain, instead they say the hypothesis was 'supported' or 'rejected' (not supported).

Types of hypotheses

There are three different ways of writing a hypothesis:

I) Directional or 'one-tailed' hypothesis

This predicts that one variable will result in an outcome that will be 'higher/greater' or 'lower/less' in size (whichever is advantageous) than the alternative (or usual) option.

2) Non-directional or 'two-tailed' hypothesis

This predicts that there will be a difference found between the outcome measurements of the two groups, but does not specify whether the difference will be greater or less in one group, only that a difference will be found.

3) Null hypotheses

This predicts that there will be no difference between the results for the options. This is also known as the 'statistical' hypotheses and is used as any difference found means that this hypothesis has to be rejected and the alternative, that there is a difference between them that could not have happened by chance, must be accepted.

These three alternatives can be illustrated with an example that you will find later in Example 5.4. This is an example of a RCT by Brodie *et al.* (2008), who looked at ways of encouraging patients with chronic heart failure to exercise. The purpose of this was to reduce the risk of future problems. The intervention was the use of motivational inter-views with patients. In this example, the independent variable would be the method of intervention (motivational interviews as opposed to usual encouragement to exercise by a specialist nurse) and the outcome measure was quality of life using a quality of life scale. The hypothesis for the study could have been written in any one of the options in Table 5.4 below.

You will notice that a hypothesis is written as a statement and not a question. You can also see that the way the hypothesis is written is slightly different in each example, so, for instance, in the second, non-directional hypothesis there is a possibility that their quality of life score could have gone down rather than up. For a non-directional hypothesis the researcher is not so much interested in the direction of the relationship between the dependent and independent variables, but only to indicate that a relation-ship can be shown to exist. The null hypothesis means that if the scores were not the same then the 'no-difference' prediction would have to be rejected and the alternative that the motivational interview does have an impact (either positive or negative depend-ing on the direction) would have to be accepted.

Type of hypothesis	Hypothesis statement
Directional (one-tailed)	There is a higher quality of life score at 5 months from baseline in patients with chronic heart failure receiving motivational intervention compared to those receiving standard care.
Non-directional (two-tailed)	There is a difference in quality of life score at 5 months from baseline, in patients with chronic heart failure receiving motivational intervention compared to those receiving standard care.
Null hypothesis	There is no difference in quality of life score at 5 months from baseline, in patients with chronic heart failure receiving motivational intervention compared to those receiving standard care.

Table 5.4 Alternative ways of structuring a hypothesis

The example above looks at just one dependent variable, if the researcher wanted to consider the effect of an independent variable such as relaxation therapy on pain and anxiety, two hypotheses would be stated, one linking relaxation therapy to pain, and a second linking relaxation therapy to anxiety, as a hypothesis can only relate to one dependent variable.

EBP in action

To practice constructing your own hypothesis, go back to Table 5.3 and the examples of dependent and independent variables. Try and construct a hypothesis from one or more of the options, then write it using an alternative format chosen from directional/non-directional/null hypothesis.

Blinding or 'masking' in experimental design

In assessing experimental designs one of the key criteria is blinding or 'masking' (Morris and Fraser 2007). It can also be defined as a method of 'allocation conceal-ment' (Polit and Beck 2008), where those involved in a study, including the subjects, do not know to which group individuals were allocated. This is an attempt to reduce the effect of conscious or unconscious bias in the way individuals are treated or outcomes interpreted. In many nursing studies, blinding can be difficult.

In the study by Robson et al. (2009) the wound healing property of antibacterial honey was tested against conventional wound treatments. In this situation it is difficult to 'blind' the patients in the honey group and those involved in data gathering may also be clear on which wounds have had honey applied. Although this does not invalidate the findings, it does put nursing research at a disadvantage when compared to the majority of medical research as the criteria of blinding cannot always be achieved because of the nature of the intervention. However, as the hierarchy of evidence (see Chapter 2) demonstrates, knowledge does exist at different levels and this provides us with the best available knowledge at the time. It is also a demonstration that research varies in its form. Robinson *et al.* (2009) did everything they could to produce a rigorous study, but reading their work you will see that many things can affect the outcome of a study that are not within the control of the researcher.

Why a control group?

If we are looking at the effect of a particular intervention on an outcome, it is difficult to know if it has been successful unless we compare it with a near identical situation where the same intervention did not take place. For example, if we are looking at the effect of relaxation exercise on patient anxiety then several individuals in a relaxation experimental group may have become more anxious anyway without the intervention and we would be mistaken in thinking there was a causal link between relaxation and anxiety if we just looked at a relaxation intervention group alone. The use of a comparison group who are as similar as reasonably possible who do not have the same intervention and are compared on the outcome variable then will help us decide if relaxation exercise does play a part in anxiety levels. Through such a design where individuals are allocated to either the experimental variable or the control we can see what might have happened without the intervention, and the statistical testing of the results will reinforce the ability to say that differences between groups are due to the independent variable and not other explanations such as chance.

In view of the information so far on RCTs it is little wonder they have such a high status in EBP and are constantly referred to as 'the gold standard' for research in this field. Their focus on accuracy and their ability to rule out other explanations for outcomes mean that they play a large part in deciding between alternative options for treatment and care. It is also on the basis of RCTs that most systematic reviews of the literature are carried out, which again influences their position within health care.

Threats to validity

Using an RCT design, however, is not an automatic guarantee of accuracy; in fact RCTs are perhaps one of the most demanding research designs to ensure that accuracy, or more correctly accuracy of interpretation of the results, has been achieved. The problems relating to interpreting the results, have been examined under a number of headings. These relate to factors that happened within a study and those that relate to applying the results outside of the specific study or study location. These are known as internal and external threats to validity. The problems were identified Cook and Campbell (1979) by (cited in Bryman 2008) and form a lengthy list of possible problems; some of the major ones are identified below in Table 5.5 and Box 5.1.

One of the big problems in experimental studies is the 'reactive effect', that is that people are influenced in their perceptions, behaviour, and actions because they are part of a study. The two terms frequently associated with this are the Hawthorne effect, and the placebo effect. These are outlined in Box 5. 1 below.

Problem	Detail	Reduction
Bias	Individuals are unrepresentative making generalizations difficult	Random allocation to ensure similar range of individuals are represented in each group
Groups are not comparable	Study mortality or 'attrition' where individuals drop out of the study leaving remainder who are not comparable, particularly where one group is affected more that the other	Large study size to account for attrition. Ensure characteristics of those dropping out are tracked and checked for trends
Individuals not acting normally	Hawthorne effect or placebo effect (see 'reactive effect' below).	Ensure masking as far as possible so those taking part are unaware of who is in which group.
Measurement inaccuracies	The tool of data collection varies in its ability to accurately and consistently measure key outcomes	Quality control over measurements. Use of recognized tools. Training of data gatherers to ensure consistency in how the data are collected
Independent variable is not wholly responsible for differences between the groups	Strong or confounding variables have an influence on the outcome and have not been 'controlled' or identified by the researcher	Control and power over the study needed to ensure that the independent variable applied as planned, and the influence of competing variables controlled as far as possible or at least recognized as influential
Inaccurate interpretation of results	Other explanations can viably account for differences between the groups Small difference in results between the groups means that statistical relationships cannot meaningfully be established Characteristics of the setting or those working there are unrepresentative of other areas and so form another variable that limits the generalizabily of the study	i) Consider possible competing explanations at design stage and build into selection of subjects ii) Ensure sample size adequate to establish real differences between the groups through the use of *power statistics*, which help to estimate sample size needed to show true effects iii) Statistical tests to ensure the possibility of chance playing a part in explaining differences between the two groups can be calculated and considered in the interpretation iv) Studies are carried out in more than one location or centre to ensure that a range of situations are representative and broaden out the idiosyncratic features of the setting
Ethical issues	Problems include fear that necessary treatments are being withheld from individuals or that appropriate care is not being given according to patient clinical need	It is important that individuals do not have appropriate treatment withheld through the study where that treatment is known to be beneficial. Researchers should avoid the problem when dealing with vulnerable groups of exploiting their ability to give true informed consent as a result of being unable to weigh up possible risks and benefits. Coercion of individuals and withholding the truth should similarly be avoided
Study environment produces additional variables	Lack of control over environment in which study takes place and inconsistencies in the way the research protocol was followed	Tight control over factors affecting an individual's outcomes and greater consistency between environmental factors and variables

Table 5.5 **Problems in experimental design and possible methods to reduce them**

Box 5.1 The reactive effects of experiments

Name	Description
Hawthorne effect	This comes from early work in America looking at motivation and output in industry. It is known as the 'Hawthorne effect' after the name of the factory in which the study was carried out. Researchers found that despite thinking that the dependent variable motivation was influenced by independent variables from the environment in the form of increased heating and lighting levels, the increases in productivity noted in their experiments could be explained by workers feeling special because attention was paid to them and their levels of productivity. In other words it was the effect of being in the study, not the experimental variables, that was having an effect on outcome measures.
Placebo effect	The placebo effect explains much the same thing. It comes from the realization that in drug trials even those receiving a placebo or false drug can report improvements to their condition that can be explained by being a part of a study where improvements were expected. Again it is the effect of being in a study that produces the outcome, not the experimental variable.

It is clear that experimental designs are amongst the most complex to plan and carry out. Although there are growing numbers of experimental designs in nursing now, for a long time they have been a small proportion of the total number of studies carried out by nurses.

The statistics bit part 2: Tests of significance and 'p values'

As we saw earlier, in order to be able to suggest there is a correlation between a number of variables in a study, statistical calculations have to be carried out using the numeric results. The same is true of experimental designs. Here the statistical principle underpinning the calculations are different, whereas correlation calculations search for *similarities* between the groups of numbers, in experimental designs they look for *differences* that cannot be explained by the element of chance. The researcher uses 'tests of significance' to establish if there is a statistically significant difference between the results of groups in the study. In this context 'significant' does not mean 'important' but a 'real' or 'meaningful' difference that can be demonstrated statistically. The reason for a variety of tests rather than a single test is due to the different properties that different types of numbers posses. Whatever the test used, they have in common the use of the 'p value', where 'p' stands for 'probability' that differences between the findings are due to chance not a cause and effect relationship. This is similar to the correlation coefficient, which is a figure that helps to interpret the element of chance.

There are three main p values to look out for:

i) $p < 0.05$. This means that the independent variable has been found to have a direct effect on the outcome, but there is a chance that for some of the time chance factors may have produced the difference between groups in the study (experimental and control groups). However, this is only likely to have been the case less than (the '<' sign means 'less than') 5 times in 100, the rest of the time we can be confident the difference in results was due to the independent variable. This is taken as the minimum value to suggest that a cause and effect situation exists between the dependent and independent variables. It rests on the assumption if the study was repeated to test the role of the independent variable on the dependent variable, in how many repeat cases the difference between the two groups in the study could be achieved by chance. Anything above 0.05 such as 0.08, the role of chance is taken as too large to make an assumption that the independent variable has been successful in having a direct effect on the independent variable.

ii) $p < 0.01$. This is a better result as the probability that chance is responsible for the difference in results is smaller. There is only a 1 in 100 chance that the results are not due to the independent variable.

iii) $p < 0.001$. This is the strongest indicator that chance, although still a possibility, is only likely to be an influence in 1 in 1000 times. This makes it pretty certain that a cause and effect relationship has been supported by the results.

In addition to these three main figures, you will see the abbreviation 'NS' to indicate 'non-significant'. In other words, the results did not achieve a p value of a minimum of 0.05.

Although a good understanding of the statistical principles is essential for those carrying out research, if you are mainly applying research findings to practise, an understanding of the interpretation of p values will be sufficient in many cases. Providing you are using research that has been published in 'peer-reviewed' journals, that is where the quality of the research has been assessed by experts, then the p value will be a good indicator of how far the researcher has been able to demonstrate that 'luck' or 'chance' has had little effect on the findings, and the difference between groups is largely due to the independent variable introduced by the researcher.

Example 5.4 provides an illustration of the elements of an experimental study covered so far in this section, and will reinforce the use of p values explained above.

Example 5.4 An experimental RCT study

Title: Motivational interviewing to change quality of life for people with chronic heart failure: A randomised controlled trial.

Authors: Brodie *et al.* (2008)

»

Aim: The aim of the study was to examine the effectiveness of (a) motivational interviewing, compared with (b) standard care, and (c) combined motivational interviews with standard care in a sample of elderly heart failure patients. The outcome measures were generic and disease-specific quality of life indicators measured by questionnaires.

Hypotheses

The researchers set out to test the following hypotheses:

There would be a higher quality of life score at 5 months from baseline in patients with chronic heart failure receiving motivational intervention compared to those receiving standard care. Additionally, it was hypothesized that motivational 'readiness to change' and self-efficacy for exercise would show significant increases in the motivational interviewing groups. It was hypothesized that Group 1 (standard care) would show non-significant changes.

Method

An experimental design was used with patients randomly assigned to one of three groups:

Group 1 (standard care) received the usual care package in which the heart failure specialist nurse advised patients to participate in a structured exercise programme.

Group 2 (motivational interviewing) received a behaviourally based, motivational interview programme from the researcher.

Group 3 (both) received both standard care and motivational interviewing.

Motivational interviewing is a method of facilitating decision-making about behaviour change. Rather than simply giving information, or telling the patient what to do, the role of the health professional is to stimulate thought and then support the patient through the process of decision-making and, perhaps, behaviour change (Brodie *et al.* 2008).

The motivational intervention comprised eight, 1 hour home-based sessions, delivered weekly by the researcher, who had no clinical qualifications. Three outcome measures were used. These were measured at the start of the study when the patient was in hospital, and again following the 5 months' treatment period. Two measures related to quality of life, one of these related to general health (the SF-36 which is one of the most commonly used general measure of health-related quality of life worldwide), and a second condition-specific measure (the Minnesota Living with Heart Failure Questionnaire or LHFQ), and the third measured motivational readiness for physical activity (the Readiness-to-Change-Ruler). All measuring tools were in regular use in other studies and all three combined only took 15–20 minutes to complete.

One of the researchers screened all patients 65 years or over admitted to the Care of the Elderly and the General Medical Wards with a primary diagnosis of chronic heart failure at two hospital sites. This resulted in 92 patients starting the study. Allocation to the three treatment groups was by 'block randomization'. This consisted of blocks of nine envelopes with three envelopes in the block each allocating individuals to one of the three treatments. The next consecutive envelope

»

was given to each patient entering the study in turn until the block of envelopes was exhausted, and then the process was repeated.

This produced a large amount of numeric measures for each individual. The data were analysed using statistical techniques that establish if there were clear differences between the three groups that were unlikely to have happened purely by chance. Following treatment there was a significant increase (p <0.05) for three of the dimensions of the health survey in the 'motivational interviewing' group. All groups improved their scores (p <0.05) on the heart failure questionnaire. Over the 5-month period there was a general trend towards improvements in self-efficacy and motivation scores. The aims of the study were therefore clearly achieved.

Methodological issues

There are a number of areas that can be highlighted in this study, these include:

Sample

Although power statistics were used to calculate how many patients were needed to form   good sized groups for accurate statistical analysis, the numbers completing both the pre-test and post-test was far less than the planned 30 per group despite adequate numbers at the start of the study. The numbers completing each group were respectively 18, 22, and 20. There was a high drop-out rate of 32 patients or 35% of the sample. The guidelines for pre- and post-test studies (where measures are taken at the beginning and end of an intervention) suggest that at least 80% of those starting should complete the final measurement to produce accurate results. Here the percentage was 65%, although the spread of demographic characteristics was similar for each of the three groups of patients at the end of the study.

Reliability

The questionnaires were piloted although they were well used in previous studies. This allows the researcher to become familiar with each data collection tool. It was at this pilot stage that it was decided to use the questionnaires in an interview situation rather than get individuals to fill them in. Given the age group and condition, this was a sound decision.

Areas to note

The study fits the criteria of an experimental RCT design as patients were randomly allocated to the groups fulfilling the criteria that everyone should have an equal or calculable chance of receiving any of the alternative interventions. The researcher then introduced the independent variable, which was the motivational interviewing to encourage people to consider exercise as part of their recovery. Data on the measurable outcomes were statistically analysed to establish if the variations in the findings could have happened by chance. This indicated that in this instance those in the motivational interviewing group did have outcomes that could be related to the motivational interviewing rather than chance factors.

Although experimental design often includes two groups, the experimental group and the control group, this kind of three-group design is not unusual. The extra group is used to compare not only one alternative against another but also one alternative compared to both alternatives to see if the second alternative still makes a difference when combined with the usual form of intervention, or whether any benefits are reduced through current practice.

The use of blocks of nine envelopes meant that there was equal distribution to the three groups as the study progressed. The decision to use the questionnaires in an interview situation would have improved the response rate. It may have also increased the accuracy of the results. In healthy patients there may have been an issue of 'social desirability', that is giving an answer that puts the individual in a good light and behaving responsibly, but here it is perhaps less of a problem.

The large number of those in the sample not completing the study is a problem for the study, as it weakens the accuracy of the statistical analysis, particularly as there was such a high study 'mortality' from one group. Although there are problems with the study because of this factor, the discussion makes an important point that nurses tend to talk 'at' patients in giving information, instead of working with the patient more collaboratively and asking what is their understanding of it all. This would result in working with the individual patient's information needs.

Quasi-experimental studies

For a variety of reasons, in some situations it will not be possible for the researcher to follow the strict principles of a randomized control group approach. However, it may be possible to carry out something similar to one in the form of a quasi-experimental study. As 'quasi' means 'almost' it is not difficult to work out the solution. In these situations the researcher still uses two groups, one where the experimental intervention is introduced and one to act as control, but there is no randomization to the groups. This design usually takes the form of two groups or locations where the intervention or change has already happened, or where it is possible to introduce the different intervention to everyone in a setting. A similar setting is then used as a control.

The study will measure if there is a positive change to the outcome measure, but this is where the difference comes, as there was not an equal or measurable chance for people to be in either group, we cannot be as certain that the only way of explaining the difference is through the independent variable, the intervention. There could be other explanations related to characteristics of those in each group, or differences in the two settings that could be responsible for the difference in outcomes. This is because unlike the experimental situation we are not starting with two comparable groups.

Quasi-experimental studies can be compared to a correlation study, in that there is a pattern here but we cannot say it is cause and effect. The statistic we would have to apply to demonstrate this is a correlation coefficient. This is taken as a weaker result compared to a RCT, but it may be the best that can be done under the circumstances.

+..

EBP in action

At the start of the section on experimental designs you were asked if you had to explain to a friend in general terms how an experimental study is structured, how would you describe some of the processes used and principles applied in experimental studies? Write another list based on what you know now, then go back and compare it to the list you made earlier to see if your understanding has changed.

....

Summary

- One of the hallmarks of a quantitative study is a strong study design and the researcher's ability to follow this design as closely as possible. In this way the emphasis on accuracy is assured through the researcher's control over the research design and implementation. Such quantitative studies can take a number of different forms depending on the purpose of the study.

- Descriptive studies will be carried out to numerically 'map-out' a situation. This may be followed by the attempt to establish a pattern between variables in the situation. For EBP, the most useful type of study to inform clinical decision-making is the RCT. This is performed under such careful conditions that it permits generalizations regarding cause and effect relationships to be made with some confidence. Where such studies cannot be carried out but where an intervention can be introduced, a quasi-experimental study will be used.

- The use of quantitative studies does demand some knowledge of statistical principles and some people can find the high level of statistical terminology and symbols off-putting. However, it is crucial for nursing that all nurses are prepared to make the effort to understand the basic principles underpinning the statistical procedures carried out. This is to ensure that nurses correctly adopt clinical practices that are sound and are founded on accurate and robust research.

■ Online resource centre

 To learn more about evidence produced using quantitative research, please now go online to **www.oxfordtextbooks.co.uk/orc/holland/** to find more resources.

■ References

Brodie, D., Inoue, A. & Shaw, D. (2008) Motivational interviewing to change quality of life for people with chronic heart failure: A randomized controlled trial. *International Journal of Nursing Studies* 45 (4) 489–500.

Brown, M. J. (2009) *Evidence-Based Nursing:* the research-practice connection. Boston: Jones and Bartlett.

Bryman, A. (2008) *Social Research Methods (3rd edn).* Oxford: Oxford University Press.

Burns, N. & Grove, S. (2009) *The Practice of Nursing Research: appraisal, synthesis, and generation of evidence (6th edn)* St. Louis: Saunders.

Chaboyer, W., Wallisa, M., Duffield, C., Courtney, M., Seatona, P., Holzhauserd, K., Schlutera, J. & Bost, N. (2008) A comparison of activities undertaken by enrolled and registered nurses on medical wards in Australia: An observational study. *International Journal of Nursing Studies* 45 1274–1284.

Heo S., Moser D., Terry A., Lennie T., Riegel B., Misook L. & Chung M. (2008) Gender differences in and factors related to self-care behaviors: a cross-sectional, correlational study of patients with heart failure. *International Journal of Nursing Studies* 45 1807–1815.

Macleod Clark (2009) Looking back, moving forword: pursuing the science of nursing interventions, Key Note presentation. RCN Nursing Research Conference, March 2009, Cardiff. London: RCN.

Morris, D. & Fraser, S. (2007) Personal views: masking is better than blinding. *British Medical Journal* 334 (7597) 799.

Polit, D. & Beck, C. (2008) *Nursing Research: generating and assessing evidence for nursing practice (8th edn).* Philadelphia: Lippincott Williams and Wilkins.

Parahoo, K. (2006) *Nursing Research: principles, process and issues (2nd edn).* Houndmills: Palgrave Macmillan.

Robson, V., Dodd, S. & Thomas, S. (2009) Standardized antibacterial honey (Medihoney™) with standard therapy in wound care: randomized clinical trial. *Journal of Advanced Nursing* 65 (3) 565–575.

Veeramah, V., Bruneau, B. & McNaught, A. (2008) Exploring knowledge and skills on HIV in student nurses and midwives. *British Journal of Nursing* 17 (3) 186–191.

■ Further reading

Brown, R. B. & Saunders, M. (2008) *Dealing with Statistics*. Oxford: Open University Press.

Franklin, B. L. (1974) *Patient Anxiety on Admission to Hospital*. London: RCN.

Newell, R. & Burnard, P. (2006) *Research for Evidence-based Practice.* Oxford: Blackwell Publishing.

Stockwell, F. (1972) *The Unpopular Patient.* London: RCN. (see RCN 50 year celebration of research series: www.rcn.org.uk and Chapter 1)

■ Useful websites

Quantitative research:

> http://www.nottingham.ac.uk/nursing/sonet/rlos/ebp/qvq/2.html/

Survey research:

> http://www.socialresearchmethods.net/kb/survey.php/

Survey systems:

> http://www.surveysystem.com/sdesign.htm/ What is a survey: http://www.whatisasurvey.info/

Randomized control trials:

> http://www.bmj.com/cgi/content/full/316/7126/201/

Understanding research:

> http://www.unm.edu/~lkravitz/Article%20folder/understandres.html/

Designs for nursing research:

> http://nursing.unc.edu/modules/nsg_research/research_design/topic2.html/

Searching and retrieving evidence to underpin nursing practice

Colin Rees

The aims of this chapter are:

➤ To identify why you need to search the literature for evidence.

➤ To consider ways of constructing a question to answer through the literature.

➤ To illustrate how to develop a plan of how to source (find) the literature.

➤ To outline successful methods of searching databases for relevant information.

Introduction

Throughout this book we identify a number of skills that are fundamental to the delivery of evidence-based practice (EBP). Although it is difficult to say that any one of these skills is more important than others, the ability to search the literature with ease and confidence is a necessary part of many activities. This is because the ability to search for and retrieve evidence is one of the major aspects of successful decision-making, and the better the clinical decision, the better the quality of care. The skill of searching and reviewing the literature then, makes a major contribution to both clinical outcomes and the quality of care.

The focus of this chapter is also essential for Chapters 8 & 9, where we examine how to process and organize information found as a result of a search of the literature and how it can then be applied to practice (Chapter 8) and how to use evidence in student assignments (Chapter 9). This chapter will cover the ground work for those chapters by focusing on the skill of finding, or 'sourcing' appropriate evidence, using databases, these are electronic sources of references of mainly published works such as journal articles.

One of the key stages of evidence-based practice (EBP) is finding a source for reliable evidence that can inform practice. However, this process takes planning, careful thought, time and above all patience. The aim of this chapter is to provide a clear understanding of this process, whether the purpose of finding information is for clinical decision-making, or for academic work, such as for a tutorial, essay, or project-based or problem-based assignment. The chapter will also consider some of the important issues that need to be tackled in relation to this process. We will tell you how to find the best quality nursing information quickly and efficiently so you can use your time reading the literature rather than endlessly searching for it.

Making a start

Searching and retrieving evidence requires skills not unlike those used in our daily life; for example, most of us have had the frustration of wasting hours looking for information on holidays, moving house, buying a car, etc. only to find that a friend or neighbour knows the best website, classified section, magazine, or car repair garage that we have missed. This does not mean the answer lies in a recommendation from someone, as they may not always know the best places to search, but that searching in a haphazard way may overlook other sources that may be better. It is no surprise, therefore, to find that Burns and Grove (2009:94) claim that:

> ❝ the most complex part of a literature review is identifying the material, not obtaining it. ❞

The key is to have a systematic and consistent approach to searching, and to develop some essential skills to apply to this activity. Your ability to search and retrieve information will be increased if you know:

- *How* to construct a clear question that can be answered through the literature.
- *Where* to look for information to answer your question.
- *How* to use the main sources of information such as databases, websites, journals, books effectively.

Before examining each of these activities in turn, it is worth clarifying a misuse of words sometimes applied to this activity.

> **! Key points**
>
> Collecting information from sources such as libraries and through computer sources is sometimes referred to as 'researching' a topic, or even doing 'research'. As you will find from reading this book, research as carried out by a researcher is a very different activity from the gathering of information described in this chapter. For this reason, it is better to avoid confusion and call gathering information from published material as 'searching the literature', and only use 'research' to describe the activities of researchers engaged in research projects.

Finding evidence

Finding evidence is a time-consuming task; however, this can be made easier by being clear on what kind of evidence you need, and where you might find or access it. In both clinical practice and as part of course work, your need for evidence may vary from the latest policies or guidelines on nursing activities, such as removing catheters, to gaining factual information or statistics such as how many people in the UK have a certain condition, to more specific information on, for example, the best nursing treatment for leg ulcers.

Such information may be available close at hand, and include such sources as local guidelines on procedures, local audits or surveys on nursing interventions in your or neighbouring clinical areas. This type of information may be searched through local or regional information departments or through local internet resources (Intranet).

Guidelines that affect practice, and policy documents such as National Service Frameworks or government White Papers, may be available through the internet using professional bodies such as the Royal College of Nursing (RCN), Department of Health (DH), or the National Institute for Clinical Excellence (NICE).

✦ ....

EBP in action

Use a search engine to locate information on the following:

- Guidelines on managing anxiety attacks in adults.
- Incidence of Crohn's disease in the UK.
- Recommended nursing treatment for pressure ulcer management in the community.

Once you have found the information consider how you would convince someone that this was sound information and could be used confidently to make decisions on the topic for clinical practice.

....

You may find that the type of information varies for each category of information in the activity above, and what you might use to judge whether the information is 'good quality' may also vary. For all of them, being clear on what you are looking for is the first consideration, and then considering where you found the information may influence your feelings about its possible quality. For example, voluntary groups or drug companies may use different arguments or types of information in comparison to sources and bodies such as the DH, or government sites, such as NICE. In addition the date the information was produced will affect how applicable it might be to current situations. Information does have a 'use-by' date, and can become quickly past its best as new situations in health care and social circumstances arise.

This chapter will focus mainly on evidence from health journal articles to answer clinical or nursing care questions, as this tends to be one of the most frequent sources of information used by nursing students when undertaking an assignment related to clinical practice.

Where is the evidence?

One positive aspect of searching for evidence is that probably at no other time in nursing's history has it been so easy to access information that can have a direct influence on the quality and effectiveness of care. The availability of databases on the internet has made information previously only available to a few clinical or scientific specialists accessible to many. However, this is not without its problems, as there are now so many sources of information available, and so much information to choose from, that we can suffer from 'information overload'. We can then be faced with the problem of making choices as to what to include, and of trying to work out the true quality or reliability of the information available. This is why Polit and Beck (2008) warn that when it comes to searching for information you need to be prepared for a lot of digging, sifting, and sorting of information. It will not simply emerge from the databases complete and useable.

It is important to distinguish however between some of the databases on the internet and the databases you can gain access to using your university information resources. Learning what is available as a student early on in your course of study will also help you to focus on key areas of literature, not only for nursing practice-related course work, but also those which focus on other subjects such as psychology and sociology which you will apply within a nursing context. It is also important to identify a wide range of evidence sources, for example books and reports.

+..

EBP in action

Identify a range of databases available in your university library information resource centre. What other sources of evidence are there in a library? Make a point of familiarizing yourself with the range of databases available and also linked resources such as an e-library, where whole books can be accessed for learning purposes.

....

Searching skills

The philosophy of evidence-based nursing care creates new demands on the essential skills of the nurse. The repertoire of skills now includes a high standard in both accessing information and also evaluating the quality of the information found. Certainly, nurses have increased their skills in obtaining information, and their ability to apply that information to creating guidelines and standards to inform practice. This has been undertaken sometimes purely as a nursing activity, and at other times as part of the multidisciplinary team.

It is inevitable that the skill of searching the literature will increase in importance as internet access increases in each clinical area, and health consumers becoming more knowledgeable through their increasing skills in accessing information on the internet too. It is important, then, to put a high value on your ability to access and use databases and do everything in your power to achieve a high degree of competence in this aspect of your work.

Finding information is not simply about its availability or quantity, but whether it is fit for the purpose intended. As with most things, **where** you buy something, whether it is goods, services or meals, will influence its quality. So with information; some places will provide more trustworthy and better quality evidence than others. However, it also depends on your ability to recognize and test the quality of the information that can make all the difference. Taking a quick snatch at information may not result in a complete or representative sample of the available information. What is easily available may not be of good quality or may be flawed. You need some kind of structure and strategy to follow. One of the best ways of

! Key points

The aim of searching the literature is to examine the body of work on a topic. This has to be made manageable, as for some topics it would take you most of your course time to go through the material. The advice is to keep the majority of information new and up-to-date by limiting how far you go back in time to search for articles. Remember that more recent articles will usually mention or draw on the most important previous authors in that topic area. Refer to Chapter 9 on this issue of what are often known as 'classic' texts or articles.

learning about searching and retrieving evidence is to follow the process of reviewing the literature outlined in this chapter using a specific topic so that you learn the skill first hand.

Reviewing the literature

A review of the literature can be defined as the careful and structured collection of published work that can help answer a specific question. The review should be based on good quality information and should include the writer's views on the information presented. So, although Burns and Grove (2009: 91) state that the:

> 66 *purpose of the review is to convey to the reader what is currently known regarding the topic of interest.* 99

Your interpretation of what you feel it says, and how well it says it, is crucial to the production of a sound review, as you will see in Chapter 9.

Why review the literature?

There are a number of reasons for reviewing the literature. The first is to establish what is known about a particular topic or problem. This is similar to a mapping exercise that will provide you with some insight into the extent to which a topic has been examined in the literature, and a quick idea of key points.

The second reason for reviewing the literature is to apply the findings to clinical decision-making, for example, where you need to decide between a number of assessment, or treatment options. A single research study may give a possible answer to a question, such as the best way to care for catheters; however, because there may be problems with the accuracy of one study (as will be seen in Chapter 7) it is far more reassuring if findings are repeated in several studies. We can then have more confidence in the evidence provided by a well produced review of the literature. As long as only good quality studies are included, a similar result across studies (particularly randomized control trials), suggests the findings are more likely to point to 'best practice' compared to a single study. For this reason a systematic review of the literature, that is a comprehensive review selecting only high quality research such as randomized control trials, and carried out following strict guidelines, is seen as the very top of the hierarchy of evidence (see Chapter 2).

A further reason for producing a review of the literature as part of the research process is to provide a justification for undertaking the study. Such reviews are included in a proposal that will be submitted to an ethics committee to gain approval for the study. It will also be used when the study is written up for publication to help people understand the context in which the study is placed. Any study should be placed within the context of current knowledge, and the review allows the researcher achieve that.

Skills for nursing practice

> **! Key points**
>
> A review is not an academic exercise or only something that is used in 'essay writing'. It is a clinical practice tool to help inform nursing decision-making. In other words, it is a mistake to see reviewing the literature as simply a 'student' skill it is a preparation for when you qualify as you will be expected to critically read reviews of the literature and maybe take part in producing them for the clinical area.

Developing the skill of searching the literature, then, is an important professional skill, just as important as learning a practical clinical skill. Although this might seem a surprising and somewhat exaggerated statement, it is worth considering this claim in the following reflection point.

> **? Thinking about**
>
> How far would you support the view that learning the skill of searching the literature is as important a professional skill as learning a clinical technique? In other words, would someone's health be disadvantaged or life put in danger because of a lack of skill in searching the literature?

Skills gained through education and course work are often seen as separate from those needed in the clinical area. It is not unusual to hear these referred to as 'academic' skills where it is felt that these are not really useful or are something not really relevant to practice. Although at first sight you may think that learning how to review the literature will not improve care or save a life, the reflection above should have helped you see that poor care can be the result of wrong decisions being made on the basis of drawing on single inappropriate studies, or on a poor analysis of information available. In the clinical area, you may need to question the quality of reviews of the literature produced by others to ensure that they are trustworthy and can inform your clinical practice. This depends on your knowledge of what makes a review of the literature sound.

From an educational point of view, where you are producing a review, it is important to be clear how your review will be judged, as this will influence how you go about searching for the literature based on your understanding of the purpose of carrying out a review. A useful insight into this is provided by Bryman, who says that (2008: 81):

> 66 *Your literature review is where you demonstrate that you are able to engage in scholarly review based on your reading and understanding of the work of those in the same field.* 99

This has to draw on the work of those who are the leading thinkers and researchers in a particular field. So, your literature search should provide you with the key works of writers who can be judged as producing sound work and ideas. The priority, then, should be on databases that draw on only good quality journals. However, this is not easy to know when you are starting out to learn how to search the literature and you also need to ensure that the journals you search publish articles which are themselves based on evidence and are also relevant to your field of practice (branch of nursing).

EBP in action

Access your University library through its website and identify the database list of journals in the following databases. You may need to use an additional password for this purpose, for example an Athens password that will enable you to access a database such as Internurse. Using the words 'communication skills' as a search term, which you will learn about later, identify the number of journals and their titles that show articles on the topic. Two examples are the *British Journal of Nursing* and *British Journal of Cardiac Nursing*. We will return to these journals and database again.

The next sections will provide some guidance on searching skills to produce your own reviews, but at the same time it will allow you to evaluate the search aspects of the reviews of the literature published by others.

Developing a clear question to be answered through the review

Searching the literature needs planning, and a clear starting point. A review of the literature is not a random event, but should provide an answer to a specific question related to a clear purpose, for instance an assignment question or clinical problem. Where the review is for an assignment, your reader (including your markers and academic supervisors) will expect to be told the question you set out to answer through the literature, and have an idea of why that question was seen as important. The question should be relatively specific and should avoid being too general or vague. For example:

> 66 *This review will look at literature on the elderly.* 99   ✕

The problem here, according to Cronin *et al.* (2008), is that the title is all encompassing, and will be too wide to be manageable for a review. The wording gives no hint of the kind of direction or purpose such a review will serve. For anyone undertaking such a review it is difficult to know what to leave out, as providing an article mentions the elderly potentially it would be relevant. The outcome, warns Cronin *et al.* (2008), is it will result in something that will be too long and superficial, and you may have problems with the word limit. Similarly, Timmins and McCabe (2005) advise that if the searcher does not have a clear focus and only poor keywords, it is easy to spend a whole afternoon surfing the web and find that you have achieved very little by the end of it. It is far better to have a specific question that you can return to in the conclusion of the review and answer. For example:

> 66 *The aim of the review is to identify common causes of falls in the elderly whilst in hospital, and to critically evaluate the possible solutions for reducing them.* 99   ✓

The results of this literature review would allow clinical areas dealing with this patient group to ensure that the environment they provide is safe and maintains high standards in preventing falls to older patients. It would also form the basis of a well structured student assignment. The wording would provide guidance on what to include in the review and would also give something specific to answer in the conclusion to the review. This wording also follows the advice of Cronin *et al.* (2008), who encourage the novice reviewer to ensure their reviews are narrower and more focused than the first example.

In EBP, one way of developing a good search question is to use the PICO format as this will help identify appropriate literature.

The PICO formula was developed by Sacket *et al.* (1997) and is cited in a number of texts such as Beecroft, Rees & Booth (2006: 95). They state that this approach 'works well for questions about health care interventions' but a different one might be needed for a broader topic.'

PICO is an acronym and stands for:

Population—those (patients/clients) who form the focus of the review.

Intervention—that is, the treatment.

Comparison—with an alternative treatment or no treatment.

Outcome—the measurable way that success is measured.

This structure for questions is used where the aim of the literature review is to establish what might be best practice and improve the kind of treatment provided for individuals. As the question is structured to identify what intervention might have a desired outcome, it needs evidence provided by randomized control trials as these compare different interventions (experimental variables against each other or placebo controls), and establish which has the best measureable clinical outcome. The following is an example of a review question using the PICO format:

> 66 *Will elective surgical patients (P) who are assessed using a pain scale prior to surgery (I) compared to those who are not assessed for pain (C) report lower levels of pain post-surgery (O)?* 99   ✓

Such wording gives direction to the search as each part can be used as a key word for searching the literature. It also gives clear purpose to the review by indentifying what to include in the search and what to reject. The conclusion to the study will also be easier than the previous example as it should clearly answer the question posed. The reviewer's success can therefore be assessed in terms of whether the question has been clearly answered.

✛···

EBP in action

Write a PICO format question for a review that looks at a comparison between counting calories as opposed to considering portion size in achieving effective weight loss in adult males attending an obesity clinic.

···

If your literature review is not 'intervention' focused, the use of PICO may not be relevant. The use of a carefully selected question, however, will always help you to identify key words for your review.

Where to look for evidence

The basic question we answer in this section is where can you find the good quality evidence you need to answer a review question? The main source of literature for reviews will be in the form of published research in a vast variety of international journals. Many of these will be available online; so one major method of locating them is through a search of databases that contain these journals. As mentioned above, such databases may be accessed through your university library or university website 'information online' page. A common alternative to using a database is to access databases using a web search engine.

Does it make any difference which method is used? The answer is that the system you use to search for sources of information can make a considerable difference to the outcome of your review. This is because in education, there is a need to demonstrate 'scholarly activity' and this means demonstrating that you are aware of the goals of scholarly activity, and the approved methods of achieving them. Scholarly activity can be defined as those actions that will lead to a well searched topic using logical, complete, and systematic methods, and an accurate interpretation of their findings.

Search engines

Accessing search engines such as 'Google Scholar' have the advantage of gaining a quick idea of how much information there is available on a topic and will allow you to quickly get some apparently relevant articles to download. Although this can give you a starting point and certainly allow you to make a decision on whether you have chosen a topic that will provide you with literature, there are disadvantages to its use. For example, unlike the more academic databases (Science Direct; CINAHL; SCOPUS), Google and Google Scholar do not list the 'hits' in time order, starting with the most recent. This means that important new literature may be well down the list of suggestions, and you may have given up searching all the hits before you arrive at the best references. It is possible to alter this by using 'advanced search' and specifying the timeframe you require. In addition saving those searches does not occur in the same way unless you save the sources for example in your *favourites list*.

One tip that is helpful to students is that, if your university has the journal cited when you have searched Google Scholar, there is often a direct link to that article in the university database. To give you an example:

1. Access Google Scholar. If you do not have this already as a favourite, you can access it through the Google site by clicking the pull down menu under the word 'more' on the top of the screen where it lists 'Images, Video, Maps, etc.

2. Once in Google Scholar, insert the author name Nicky Cullum, run the search and you will see many cited papers and books for this author.

3. To make the search more sensitive chose the option 'Advanced Scholar Search' at the top right of the screen. On that page you have the option to limit the search to more recent years. Look down the list of options and you will see 'Date–return articles published between', and then two boxes. In these put the year, say, 3 years ago from the present in the first box, and in the second box enter the current year. Click search and you will get a more recent search. For each article listed look underneath the reference for options such as 'cited by' followed by a number. Clicking this will give you more recent articles that have cited this article. Following this system is an example of 'Forward chaining', described later. There may also be the option 'Related Articles' and clicking this will allow you to find other relevant articles for your search.

4. Where you find a relevant looking article, you can click the link and if asked for a user name and password, and your university subscribes to this journal you will be taken to it once you have provided your user name and password.

Although this system seems to provide an adequate method of gaining some information, it does not allow you to track your search method and build up combinations of key words in the same way as other databases such as the British Nursing Index (BNI), PsycINFO or CINHAL. Do check with a member of teaching staff or library staff how your university prefers you to work in relation to databases.

Perhaps the most important disadvantage of using search engines is that they do not exercise any judgements on the quality of the information sources they list. In other words, unreliable and possibility misleading sources of information will be listed alongside dependable sources. So, the literature that could end up in your review may provide you with unknown or poor quality sources of knowledge. It is very important that you consider this in relation to the topics covered in Chapter 9 when using evidence in an academic assignment.

Nursing databases

Remember that part of the goal of academic activity, and particularly reviewing the literature, is to source good quality information. This is usually in peer-reviewed journals that filter the quality of the work before accepting it for publication by getting other experts to ensure that the information contained in articles has been assured. It is the editors of these journals who have the overall responsibility of ensuring that this is undertaken. These peer-reviewed journals are the ones included in many of the academically accepted databases. For reasons such as these, it is recommended that you choose to search the individual databases to ensure that you include the best quality information, and demonstrate you have high standards when reviewing the literature.

As databases will differ in the journals they include, it is always worth checking a number of the most popular ones (Table 6.1).

The use of a number of databases is important in any review. Most university websites allow their students to access a number of the key databases through their library or information web pages. A list of databases to which the university has a subscription will be offered on those pages.

Finally, under this heading, there are a number of websites that specialize in evidence-based practice searches for topics where there is literature to inform clinical

Databases	Websites
MEDLINE	Centre for Evidence-Based Nursing
CINAHL	Cochrane Collaboration (for randomized control trials)
SCOPUS	Joanna Briggs Institute (JBI) (Australian nursing site)
BNI (British Nursing Index—includes midwifery information)	
PsycINFO (Psychological information)	

Table 6.1 Popular databases and search websites

practice. One limitation is that many of these are very medically orientated as medicine has been using the concept of EBP a lot longer than nursing. These may still be useful if you add 'nursing' or similar word to the search.

Try for instance the Trip Database: **http://www.tripdatabase.com/**

In using such sites it is important to recognize the medical approach taken in articles and to consider the nursing implications.

EBP in action

Take time out now to search some of the common databases and use some key words connected to topics of interest or areas you are currently exploring in your work. Use this as an opportunity to develop searching skills and increase your awareness of some of the common sources of literature for topics.

Where to begin

Searching the literature effectively on any particular topic is a major task. This is because many databases require a good practical knowledge of how they work and how you can gain maximum control over the way in which a search of the database is conducted. Where you have limited time to complete an assignment, it can be difficult to know where to begin.

Key words

One of the first stages is to consider the search or key words you will need to trawl the databases. You are often given a choice of where you want the database to search for these words, such as in the title or in the abstract of an article, or even to search for an author's name. It is useful to think of these words as the keys to unlock the doors behind which the information you are looking for are stored. These will result in a 'stripped-down' version of the PICO statement structure we explored earlier. So, using the earlier example on the use of pain scales, the key words might include:

- Elective patients
- Pain scale
- Surgery
- Pain levels

This might provide a good starting point, but it will also bring up a large number of hits, including a number of references describing the construction of, or advantages and disadvantages of, pain scales, or different types of surgery. For this reason, it may also be useful to include the key words *'research'*, which will narrow the search to include mainly research articles, and *'nursing'*, to increase the inclusion of articles taking a nursing perspective.

If the search comes back as 'nothing found' or 'zero hits', then you may have to consider how you use the key words. Most of the ones in the bulleted list above were in the form of more than one word. Some databases require you to either put inverted commas around words that need to be seen as one phrase or 'field' so that they look like this:

> 66 'elective patients' 'pain scale' 'surgery' 'pain levels' 99

Alternatively, they may require them in brackets also called 'parentheses'. So they would look like this:

> 66 (elective patients) (pain scale) (surgery) (pain levels) 99

Databases usually have a 'help' section, where they will suggest how you can make the search easier for yourself. Reading these sections carefully, or asking advice from a librarian, will save you a lot of time and is well worth it to develop your skills for the future.

Record your progress

When writing up the results of your literature review, you will probably be encouraged to give a very clear description of how you went about your search process for information. Right from the start of conducting the search, you should carefully record each decision you make and the steps you take. In particular, Polit and Beck (2008) encourage anyone searching the literature to write down at the start their decisions and rules on what to include and exclude, and stick to them. These decisions and criteria may well be summarized in your assignment to demonstrate how thorough you have been in your work.

Carefully recording your way through the literature is an essential part of the process, according to Timmins and McCabe (2005), who go on to suggest that once the search has begun it is essential to manage the whole process in a logical, systematic, and retrievable way. It is recommended that you make a written or electronic note of important information such as the key words you used and how you screened or reduced the total number of 'hits' you had. Periodically printing a page summarizing your search is also worthwhile, or if you are offered the opportunity to 'save search' do so. The information should allow your reader to follow in your footsteps and repeat as close as possible the journey you took in arriving at your literature. You can record this information in a table such as the one shown below in Table 6.2. The column headings are just suggestions for you, as there may be alternative headings that you would find more useful for your particular search.

If you use a similar layout to this table, an electronic version can be developed as a 'landscape', rather than 'portrait' layout to give you more space under each heading (see the further reading list for a very useful practical book by Brettle & Grant 2003).

Database	Key words	Inclusions	Exclusions	Timeframe	Hits	Numbers reduced by:

Table 6.2 Record of search progress

+ ·

EBP in action

Consider starting an assignment to answer the question 'what are the major reasons for falls in the elderly in hospital, and what interventions have been found to reduce the number of such falls?' Write a list of the key words you might use to search the databases, and secondly use these to search at least two different databases. Note differences in the number of 'hits' and methods of searching the databases. Which would be your 'favourite' database?

· ·

Use several databases

Different databases work in different ways. Some will allow you to enter a string of search words into the same search 'window', and give you the ability to download articles located in the search, whereas others build up your search details using combinations of key words that must be added one at a time and then combined by ticking appropriate boxes (see Table 6.3). Although you might have entered your own key words into a search 'window', some databases will suggest ways of changing your search term to ones it knows already. This means you have to gain experience in using several databases so that you can maximize your chances of getting a good response to your search.

Using more than one database is a good search strategy as no one source will provide you with all you will need. Younger (2004) also points out using the same key words in different databases will produce different results. All databases are to some extent incomplete, and where your review is for a course assignment, you will be expected to explore a number of databases to ensure you capture as many high quality and relevant articles as possible.

This aspect of searching the databases is not necessarily completed before going on to reviewing the articles you have found. Timmins and McCabe (2005) point out that the reviewer may return to the databases several times to repeat the search process as they work their way through organizing the literature and considering what they have found.

Your experience of using more than one database may have raised the issue that some databases use a variety of words to mean the same thing, such as 'older person' and 'elderly', 'falls', and 'untoward events'. Similarly, some words are spelt differently in American databases and articles, compared to UK sources, for example, 'labour' and 'labor', 'tumour' and 'tumor'.

Some of the databases will allow you to perform an 'advanced search' where you can add certain conditions to the way the database searches for articles that will improve the search by limiting some of the criteria or allowing you to choose from certain criteria what is included in the search. In Table 6.3 below, the BNI database was searched for information on falls in the elderly and possible ways of reducing them. As with some other databases, this one only allows a limited number of keywords at a time. The searcher can, however, get the database to combine the results of the different searches. This has the effect of reducing the total number of articles found as it combines the searches and excludes those common to each search result. This combined method usually results in more appropriate titles and allows an initial large number of 'hits' to be drastically reduced.

This demonstrates the advantage of using a database such as BNI, or similar database that allows key words to be combined and so eliminate duplicates and some irrelevant articles. There may still be some articles that are irrelevant but this method cuts down many of the problems.

A number of databases allow the use of 'Advanced Search', which introduces 'filters' that also reduce the scope of the search into more relevant titles for your purposes. These often allow the searcher to control the span of years being searched, or the country in which journals are searched. The BNI was searched for 'falls', elderly, and hospital. By clicking on 'Advanced Search' it was possible to choose articles between 2000 and 2010, Journal subset 'UK and Ireland' and Age Groups 'Aged, 65+'. This took the total of hits down from 194 to 48, making it far more manageable. It is worth gaining experience of such methods through experimenting with the databases and clicking

Stage	Key words	Operation	No of hits
1	Falls		432
2	Elderly/elderly accidents	Thesaurus offers 'elderly accidents'	477
3	Hospital	Thesaurus offers many alternatives, keep to 'hospital'	7232
4		Combine results for 1 & 2 & 3	33
5	Accidents prevention/or elderly falls	Key word 'prevention'. Thesaurus offers 'accidents prevention/or elderly falls	770
6		Combine results for 4 & 5	33
7		'Show results'	

Table 6.3 Example of using British Nursing Index database

on 'help' where you are in any doubt or are unsure how to progress. Your university may also provide training in how to use the search engines. They may also provide online resources which you can use to learn how to undertake searching and then saving the links.

Once a final figure is produced, clicking 'display' will show the titles selected. If you have accessed the databases through your university, even off-campus from home, you will often find it possible to download a PDF version of the required articles.

Learning to use the university resources is one of the most important things to learn when you start your course, as it will in the long term save you much time and will also be an asset when it comes to writing assignments, working with others on a class presentation, and also most importantly enabling you to search for information which will help you in the practice learning environment.

Improving your search method

i) Boolean logic and database searching

Part of the system of a number of databases like the BNI is the ability to apply special terms that will either increase or decrease the amount of hits produced as a result of combining key words. This involves 'Boolean logic', which works by linking your key words together to cut down the number of hits to those that overlap the variety of words you used, accept alternative words, or exclude words by typing in the words *'and'*, *'or'* and *'not'*. Table 6.4 demonstrates how these three words work.

ii) The use of truncation and wildcard

There are other useful techniques used in this process, such as the use of truncation where an asterisk or star (*) or dollar sign ($) at the end of a word to find variations in

Inserted word	Effect
And	Using '**and**' between your key words will exclude all references to the words in titles and abstract unless the other word is also found, So 'falls and elderly' will exclude those references that only relate to 'falls' which could be related to other patient groups, and similarly will exclude papers on the elderly unless they concern falls.
Or	The use of '**or**' will allow you to include alternative terms in your search, 'elderly or older person' will include articles that use either term. Another example would be 'reduce or decrease'.
Not	This is used to rule out the inclusion of certain words such as '**not** medication' to rule our article that look at the use of medication to reduce falls. Similarly 'elderly not children' would exclude papers looking at falls in children.

Table 6.4 Key words in Boolean Logic

the ending of a word. An example would be nurs* to find either 'nurse' or 'nursing'. This needs to be used with care, as Burns and Grove (2008) advise that truncation to under four letters can lead to too many irrelevant hits.

The use of a 'wildcard' is similar, where a question mark is used at the point where alternative spellings may be possible such as 'lab?r' for 'labour' or 'labor', or, 'catheteri?ation' for 'catherterisation' or 'catheterization'. These examples emphasize the difficulties arising from the differences between UK and US spellings for health-related concepts and medical procedures.

iii) Increasing your relevant keywords

As you find relevant articles, check the list of key words under which the article is listed. This will usually be displayed somewhere on the first page. You may find some options missing from the key words you are currently using, and these may increase the success of your search. If they are helpful, remember to add them to your search strategy so that it can be complete.

iv) Backward chaining and forward chaining

A popular way to increase your stock of relevant articles is to start with one that will be part of your review, and then look at their reference section. This can be repeated through a process of backward chaining and working your way through reference sections until you run out of relevant possible articles. This method can be applied to hard copies of articles, or, similarly, many of the databases allow you to access the references section of an article title. There may also be a link to 'similar articles' that would increase the number of possibly relevant articles.

Instead of going back in time from a particular article, as in backward chaining, it is also possible in some databases to go forward when you display a particular title or abstract. You may find the option 'cited by', or 'find citing articles'. This is useful for an influential or important article as it will indicate authors work following this publication that mentioned or cited the author and will therefore probably be of value. This method is called *forward chaining*. The BNI has both options for 'Find Similar Results' and 'Find Citing Articles'.

v) Limiting the timeframe

Another important way to manage the amount of literature that has been briefly mentioned is by controlling the timeframe covered by your literature review. It is difficult to be precise about how extensive the timeframe should be. Where a topic has been the subject of a lot of research and investigation, a timeframe of 5 years may be adequate to get a good spread of information. Where little work has been carried out, a timeframe of 10 years may need to be covered.

It is always worth remembering that for any topic there may be certain key or 'seminal' work that will be expected to be included. These are the influential pieces of work that started the interest in a topic and form the 'seed' from which later work grows, thus 'seminal' meaning carrying the seed. These classic articles may lie outside your timeframe, but can also be included. Burns and Grove (2009) also suggest the inclusion of landmark studies. These are research projects that indicated a turning point in our understanding of a topic or marked an important point in the research on the topic. However, the older the work, the more usual it is to show that you are aware that the information is quite 'old' and the findings may not always be as relevant as they were in the past. The timeframe and the decision to include some seminal and landmark studies outside of that timeframe should also be covered in your search notes.

Accessing relevant articles

There are a number of options to physically get hold of an article once you have identified possible sources of information for your review. These can take the following forms:

- Downloading full text article (often as a **PDF** from the web)
- Hand-searching libraries

i) Downloading from the web

As a student you will have access to a large number of electronic journals subscribed to by your university library. Some databases will permit you to access journal articles, usually in PDF format, or allow you to print them from a computer. Whenever you do this, it is worth writing on them the name of the course, or assignment it relates to, or put it in a folder with the information on the front cover. It is also worth checking that all the information you will need for the full reference is on the copy and add any information you may need. These kinds of actions will help you keep track of material and remember why it has been collected. Another more practical use is to download them onto a 'data stick' in order to save time and paper. This latter point is very important as part of considering the issues of 'saving the planet and trees'. This also helps reduce costs to you as a student and also enables you to store information when you may have a lack of storage facilities.

ii) Hand-searching in libraries

When reviewing the literature for an assignment, it is important to illustrate you have tried to cover as many ways of finding work as possible. Traditionally, scholarly activity meant spending time in libraries searching indexes, or examining past copies of journals. It is always worth checking copies of more recent journals to see if new articles exist on your topic. It is also worth remembering that databases cannot be guaranteed to be complete and some articles may not have been included or your university may not have subscribed to journals at that time, nor indeed will some journals have included early issues in an online database.

If you use this method of hunting for articles, then mention 'hand searching' in your description of how you conducted your search.

Primary and secondary references

So far, we have only talked about full versions of articles that you read in their original form by the author whose name will go in your reference section. This is known as a primary reference. The alternative is a secondary reference, where you read one author talking about the work of another.

The problem with secondary sources is that they are basically someone's ideas of what someone else did or said. Such authors may have good reasons for being selective in how they report this information in their work, or simply may not have the space to present all the information you need. It is important, then, to avoid this source of information and concentrate on your own views of what authors have said or done by only using the original articles or textbooks.

It is advisable to avoid including secondary sources in your review as much as possible.

Similarly, a point that was made earlier is to keep to the full article and do not simply use the abstract taken from a database. This is because unless you are sure you are looking at the original work you may find the information from elsewhere inaccurate of biased, or if taken from an abstract incomplete or misleading.

Most of the articles in reviews of the literature used in EBP are research reports. If you sometimes find it difficult to be sure you have a research study, the format is well signposted and consists of the following:

- An introduction
- A review of the literature that puts the study in context and justifies why the study is needed
- An aim
- A comprehensive method section including:
  - Details of the sample and how they were chosen
  - An ethics section saying how individuals were safeguarded and made clear about the nature of the study. This will usually involve an ethics committee
  - Results
  - Discussion
  - Conclusion
  - Recommendations

If you can identify all those components then you can be reasonably confident you are looking at a piece of primary research (see Chapter 3 for more details regarding these headings). Part of showing your academic or scholarly ability is to demonstrate you are quite clear on the differences between opinion articles, audit, primary research, summaries of research, reviewers of the literature, audit, and practice development. If you feel unsure about the exact nature of any of these, it will be worth checking their definitions in this book.

> **! Key points**
>
> It is essential to keep track of your review processes when collecting literature. Using computer bibliographic software such as 'Endnote' and other alternatives will help you build up your references section not only for one assignment, but also provide the basis for other assignments that might draw on some referenced work that has been previously covered.
>
> Endnote is a computer program that lists articles in a format that fits the reference system of most courses. It also helps you to keep track of articles.

Including published reviews of the literature in your work

You might be concerned about the inclusion of reviews of the literature that have already been completed on topics you review, feeling that it may be cheating to include them or feel that the work has already been done. Both of these concerns are unfounded. Reviews of the literature can include reviews that have been completed by other people, but it is best to make it clear to the reader that you are talking about a review by using such phrases as 'in a comprehensive review of the literature, Hauxwell (2010) found that... etc.'

Knowing when to stop

Finally, one of the most frequently heard question from students is the request to know how many articles are needed for a review. This is difficult to answer as each type of assignment requires a different approach to how many articles are needed. Only general advice can be given. For example, Polit and Beck (2008) suggest that the searcher looks at their review in a similar way to carrying out a piece of qualitative research and just as the qualitative researcher will stop gathering data once 'saturation' is reached, that is, when the same information keeps coming up, so someone searching the literature should stop when the same authors names keep coming up and they have already been retrieved.

Although this may be good advice for those conducting reviews for higher degrees, it is perhaps more something to be aware of, or a case of understanding the principle.

Bryman (2008) has more practical advice and suggests that you should set yourself a timetable to conduct the review and then stop when you reach that cut-off point, hopefully after accessing the most important papers. He adds that you can check with your supervisor to see if they feel the references seem adequate. Do bear in mind that in many instances, once you start writing the review you will find that you may want to revisit certain themes that are included anyway.

There does come a point, however, when the searching has to stop and the writing and analysis has to start. Knowing when that point has been reached is yet another skill that comes with practice!

Summary

- Reviews of the literature are not just an academic activity but provide clear guidelines for best clinical practice.

- Searching the literature is a skilled activity.

- An effective search is the result of a very clear and systematic process so record how you carried out the search.

- The search should be conducted with a clear and specific question in mind, using the PICO formula if relevant.

- Clear criteria should be listed for what you will include and exclude from the search.

- Searches should be limited to good quality sources of information, resulting in peer-reviewed articles where possible.

- Search for as much material as is reasonable for the size of the assignment and the time available.

- Searching abstracts should help determine which articles need to be recovered as full text articles for the review.

- Abstracts only should not be included in the review.

- Keep a list of databases, key words, and the timeframe used in the review.

- Use a range of techniques to make the search as focussed as possible.

- Use backward and forward chaining to capture relevant articles.

- Use a variety of databases as no single one has all the articles you need.

- Finally, although you may go back and search further articles it is important to know when to stop searching when to start writing.

Online resource centre

 To learn more about searching the literature, please now go online to
www.oxfordtextbooks.co.uk/orc/holland/ to find more resources.

References

Beecroft, C., Rees, A. & Booth, A. (2006) Finding the evidence. In Gerrish, K.A. & Lacey, A. (eds) *The Research Process in Nursing* (5th edn). Oxford: Blackwell.

Brettle, A. & Grant, M. (2003) *Finding the Evidence for Practice: a workbook for health professionals.* Edinburgh: Churchill Livingstone.

Bryman, A. (2008) *Social Research Methods* (3rd edn) Oxford: Oxford University Press.

Burns, N. & Grove, S. (2009) *The Practice of Nursing Research: appraisal, synthesis, and generation of evidence* (6th edn) St. Louis: Saunders.

Cronin, P., Ryan, F. & Coughlin, M. (2008) Undertaking a literature review: a step-by-step approach. *British Journal of Nursing* 17 (1) 38–43.

Polit, D. & Beck, C. (2008) *Nursing Research: generating and assessing evidence for nursing practice* (8th edn). Philadelphia: Lippincott Williams and Wilkins.

Sackett, D. L., Richardson, W. S., Rosenberg, W. & Haynes, R. B. (1997) *Evidence-based medicine: how to practice and teach EBM.* New York: Churchill Livingstone.

Timmins, F. & McCabe, C. (2005) How to conduct an effective literature search. *Nursing Standard* 20 (11) 41–47.

Younger, P. (2004) Using the internet to conduct a literature search. *Nursing Standard* 19 (6) 45–51.

Further reading

Aveyard H. (2007) *Doing a literature review in health and social care.* Maidenhead: Open University Press.

Fink, A. (2005) *Conducting Research Literature Reviews: From the Internet to Paper* (2nd edn). Thousand Oaks: Sage.

Pearson, A., Field, J. & Jordan, Z. (2007) *Evidence-Based Clinical Practice in Nursing and Health Care: Assimilating Research, Experience and Expertise.* Oxford: Blackwell.

Useful websites

Evidence-Based Nursing users' guide:

http://ebn.bmj.com/cgi/content/extract/3/3/71/

How to conduct an effective and valid literature review:

> http://www.nursingtimes.net/nursing-practice-clinical-research/how-to-conduct-an-effective-and-valid-literature-search/217252.article/

Carrying out your literature search:

> http://edina.ac.uk/getref/background/research/page_5.html/

Advanced Literature searching: using databases:

> http://www.nottingham.ac.uk/nursing/sonet/rlos/studyskills/lit_search_advanced/

Using databases:

> https://www.kcl.ac.uk/iss/ir/subject/nursing/litsearching.html/

Trip database:

> http://www.tripdatabase.com/

Searching for evidence:

> http://www.southampton.ac.uk/library/subjects/sonm/pdfdissertation searchingevidence08.pdf/

Searching the literature for evidence-based medicine:

> http://missinglink.ucsf.edu/lm/EBM_litsearch/case1page.html/

7

Evaluating and appraising evidence to underpin nursing practice

Colin Rees

The aims of this chapter are:

➤ To outline the importance of evaluating and appraising evidence.

➤ To enable you to understand the importance of critiquing evidence for nursing practice.

➤ To develop the skill of critiquing evidence through the use of a framework.

➤ To understand some of the language of critiquing research.

Introduction

Previous chapters have introduced the idea of evidence-based practice (EBP) as a fundamental part of providing care. They have also emphasized that research is an ideal source of evidence and is a major part of the 'hierarchy of evidence' referred to in Chapter 2. Research evidence is highly regarded within EBP because of the careful way information is collected to answer important questions for practice through the research process.

Inevitably then, an essential part of evidence-based practice is using research articles to guide best nursing practice. Both students in nurse education and qualified practitioners must therefore develop the skill of assessing or 'critiquing' research articles to establish if they contain valuable information that might improve patient care.

This chapter will develop your understanding of the process and language of critiquing, and illustrate how this can be a straightforward and enjoyable activity. Although we agree with Parahoo (2006: 401) that:

> ❝ the task of critiquing is a challenging one, and can only be acquired through practice. ❞

We believe that you can easily learn how to recognize some of the common parts of research articles, and with a little help, begin to ask the right kind of questions about the quality of the studies you read.

What is critiquing?

Critiquing is perhaps one of the most important skills a nurse can develop, as it is an essential part of so many activities. As a student, it is a clear illustration of your ability to produce critical analysis, which demonstrates a high level of academic development. Little wonder, then, that critiquing is a familiar activity in assignments. Within this book it is one of the key skills we will help you develop, not only in this chapter, but also as a continuing theme throughout the book. Some of you will have to critique an article for an assignment and most of you will require critique skills for undertaking reviews of the literature and evidence for other assignments such as a research proposal or an in-depth review of evidence as part of a dissertation at higher levels of study.

! Key points

Critiquing can be defined as taking a balanced view of both the strengths and limitations of a study in order to evaluate the extent to which it provides a sound basis for decision-making. It involves the reader considering the way the research follows some of the basic principles of the research process. Parahoo (2006) points out that words such as 'evaluate' and 'appraise' can also be used as an alternative word to 'critique'.

It is easy to assume that critiquing means 'criticizing' a research study and that more marks will be gained the more negative you can be about it. However, all that you will demonstrate is what Greenhalgh (2006: 40) refers to as the 'science of trashing a paper'. This approach to critiquing is not only wrong, but leads to a negative approach to evaluation that does not benefit you or the researcher. A balanced view is an indicator of a higher-level skill, as it requires a more rounded and unbiased assessment of situations.

The purpose of critiquing, then, is to ensure that the evidence we use as the basis for practice is sound. This is clear from the way studies are conducted and presented. In education, critiquing allows you to demonstrate your knowledge and understanding by explaining what is to be admired in a study or where you can see limitations in the researcher's decisions or experiences.

As research is an unpredictable activity, there will usually be some things that the researcher was just not able to do, or do as they would have liked. They may even draw attention to these limitations themselves in the discussion part of the article. This idea of research rarely being perfect will help you if you find it hard to criticize someone who clearly has a lot of knowledge and has worked hard on their research project. However, constructive comments are part of good 'science' in that research-ers recognize that there may be weaknesses in their work and highlighting these helps others to avoid accepting the findings without question.

> **?** **Thinking about**
>
> How would you describe your attitude to published research? Do you believe what you read in research articles without question? Are you the kind of person who dismisses all research as likely to be untrue? Consider some of the skills you will already have gained in earlier chapters in determining your answers.

How you answer this reflection point is important, as you need to show that you hold neither a blind acceptance of all research, nor that you instantly dismiss it, but rather that you base your opinions on reasoned arguments. This means you should not quickly dismiss research, without good cause. Particularly in assignment work you need to show that you understand the principles of good practice in research and can apply them to the work that you read.

The importance of critiquing to the individual nurse

Nursing is committed to the philosophy of EBP (see Chapters 1 and 8), and so an understanding of research issues is part of being a competent reader of research papers. If you recall in Chapter 6, reading evidence is a skill in itself, without then determining its value and quality.

If we do not fully understand how a study has been conducted and particularly the limitations to a particular study, there is the danger of accepting published articles as 'the truth' when, in fact, they may be unreliable or only partially helpful. This is rarely because the results of a particular study are false, but more likely because research can only cover a small aspect of an area of knowledge at a time, and it may require several well conducted studies to build up our knowledge of a particular situation with different groups of individuals in different settings before a bigger 'answer' becomes clear. So, for instance if we are concerned with how we can help anxious patients facing surgery, we may find that the research on anxiety and surgery relates to different patient groups, and perhaps individuals of different age groups and genders.

It is only when several researchers come up with the same answer in different situations that we can be more sure that the answer can have a general application. This is why we consider the 'generalizability' of studies, that is, can the findings from one location be applied equally elsewhere? The limitations that are built into all studies is also why, in the hierarchy of evidence (see Chapter 2), there is an emphasis on systematic reviews of the literature, as these illustrate the similar findings of studies that have been selected because of the attention given to accuracy of the method and the size and representativeness of the sample. It is important to note however that research reported in a journal article is only a summary or part of the whole, and that we critique it based on what the author has chosen to share with us, and gives us the best précis of the actual full study. To gain a full appreciation of the whole research study often requires access to the report itself.

To achieve EBP, then, a nurse will need a number of skills relating to knowing what to look for when trying to answer evidence-based questions (the clinical question that has to be answered), where to look for specific questions, and how to search for appropriate evidence (searching skills), and how to evaluate the research once they have been able to get hold of it (critiquing skills).

+

EBP in action

One of the challenges when asked to find a research article to critique is that the article you choose may not be research. It could be a review of the literature, a practice development, or a summary of best practice drawing on research. If you were asked for advice, how would you help someone decide if an article was a research article or not? What could you then look for to confirm it was research? You may find revisiting Chapters 3, 4, and 5 helpful in answering this.

Recognizing research articles

At this point it is helpful to clarify what makes an article a research article, as it does not mean that if a journal page has the word 'Research' on the top, that it is a research article. There are some clues we can look for to help us decide if it is research. One helpful indicator is the headings or ingredients in the structure of research articles. These will reflect key elements in the research process covered in Chapter 3. For the majority of articles published in journals there is an abstract, which is meant to summarize the whole of the study as it is reported. The abstract is what you will often have access to when searching and retrieving evidence (Chapter 6).

We should find a description of the methods used to collect information to answer a specific question. This does not mean searching the literature for the answer as in the case of a review of the literature. These methods might include the use of questionnaires, observation, or measurement scales of some kind in an experimental study or randomized control trial (RCT). They will collect the information from people, events or objects, such as pieces of equipment, and these will form the sample or participants in the study. You will see the word 'empirical' as in 'empirical evidence', to describe this situation. The term 'empirical' means 'in the real world', where information is gathered through our senses such as observation, hearing, and so on.

! Key points

Research involves collecting data and so useful headings to look for to indicate an article is a research study will be 'Aim', Method' 'Sample' and 'Results'. Whilst many of these headings are also used in audit and reviews of the literature, only the heading, or reference to 'ethics', or ethical issues, will be normally be found in research articles.

This is an illustration of how important it is to recognize the 'signposts' that are found in published work. If we take an example from a research paper we can see how we can quickly spot the elements that together will confirm that this it is a research study.

Example of research 'signposts'

We can illustrate the points made in the last section with the help of a published example. Mitchell (2008) was concerned with patients receiving day surgery who were 'awake' throughout the procedure and received local or general anaesthesia. He wanted to establish what factors in the environment in which the surgery took place may influence the level of anxiety of patients and which, at least to some extent could be controlled by the nurse.

This could have been the subject of a review of the literature, a personal opinion article, or a case study of what happened in one unit to tackle the situation. These would not have been research. What were the indicators that this was a research study? Firstly, the opening page of the article had the subheading on the top of the page 'original research', which indicates it is not a summary of available research or a literature review. The abstract under the title quickly confirms that this is a research study as it includes the subheadings 'Method' and 'Findings'. In the article itself the reader finds the subheadings 'Design', 'Participants', data collection, 'Ethical considerations', 'Data analysis', and 'Results', all of which mirror the research process outlined in Chapter 3 and so confirm that this is a research study.

Note: We will return to this study throughout this chapter so you need to search and obtain this paper to use as a framework to refer to as we work our way through aspects of critiquing.

The 'how' of critiquing

According to Nieswiadomy (2008) every nurse should be involved in the evaluation of research findings. In other words, it is not possible to say 'I do not need to know about research, I am a clinical nurse, not a researcher', there is a professional obligation to base practice on the best available evidence. So, for instance the Nursing and Midwifery Council's (NMC 2008: 4) code of professional conduct states under the heading 'Use the best available evidence:

- You must deliver care based on the best available evidence or best practice.
- You must ensure any advice you give is evidence-based if you are suggesting healthcare products or services'.

This means that where evidence is in the form of research papers, the nurse needs to be able to understand it and be able to know the extent to which it can be safely related to practice. As a student you will also have seen in Chapter 1 how you have to develop competencies that enable you to:

66 *engage with and evaluate the evidence base that underpins safe nursing practice.* 99

(NMC 2004)

However, it is difficult to read a research paper without knowing something about the different forms that research takes. That is why we have already covered some of the basic principles of the research process in Chapter 3. The research process acts as a kind of 'road map' the researcher follows in completing research in order to achieve a successful outcome. The exact form of the map is influenced by the type of research chosen to answer the study aim. Knowledge of these variations will help to understand why different researchers make different decisions in undertaking their research, and how in turn different decisions will have different implications for the quality of the outcomes.

Similarly, there are principles the researcher is encouraged to follow when writing up their study for publication. This is because it helps a reader to anticipate what information should be available to check the quality of the study, and know where it should be found. Before going through the details of the critique framework, a simplified broad structure of a research article is presented in Table 7.1 below.

This format for published research papers is sometimes reduced even further and is referred to by the acronym IMRAD, which stands for:

Introduction

Method

Results

Discussion

This is very 'basic' key to what is expected in a research article, in particular that related to quantitative research papers.

EBP in action

Identify a research article from a journal that links to your own practice, e.g. children's nursing (or the one by Mitchell (2008) mentioned above which has an adult nursing focus).

Check that the researcher has followed the IMRAD structure and the individual sections outlined in Table 7.1. Is this structure visible? Once you can see this pattern you will feel more confident in finding your way around research articles.

Try this again with other papers from other journals that publish research studies.

Having considered the structure of any research article, we can now look at how to critique the various aspects of a study. That is, the principles of research that the researcher should demonstrate to have followed in their study. As a reader of research, you need to know what these are, so you can evaluate it.

Element	Purpose
Setting the scene	The title, abstract, introduction, and review of the literature all contribute to giving the reader an idea of what the study is about and why it was conducted.
Aim	This describes what the researcher set out to do, and should clearly include clues on what information will have to be gathered and from whom.
Method/methodology or research design	This provides the technical aspects, or important details of how the study was conducted.
Results or findings	This is what was found when the data were collected and summarized.
Discussion	This is the sense the researcher made of it all: the issues that were raised by the results.
Conclusions and recommendations	This forms the end part of the study, the conclusion first provides the 'answer' to the aim, and the recommendation tells us what the researcher feels should happen now: who should do what and how as a consequence of the results and discussion.

Table 7.1 The basic structure of a research article

Critiquing a research article

Looking for the clues the writer has given to convince us that the study was carried out to a high standard relates to the concept of **rigour**. This concept has been defined by Burns & Grove as follows (2009: 720):

> 66 *Striving for excellence in research through the use of discipline, scrupulous adherence to detail and strict accuracy.* 99

The more rigorous the researcher has carried out a study, the more we can feel we can trust in the findings and our ability to transfer the results to nursing practice. When writing an article, the researcher should be as transparent as possible in describing the key decisions that were made which influenced the design and conduct of the study, that is, how it was carried out. However, we should always remember with all research that we should handle it with care because of the difficulty of achieving absolute rigour. Similarly, rigorous research does not mean the content must be sound, it only means that the researcher has attempted to carry out the study to the best of their ability.

EBP in action

We need a way to make sense of articles so that we have an idea or plan of what we should be looking for. There are a number of useful frameworks and checklists to achieve this, some are very simple and concentrate on the structure of articles, and others are far more complicated and depend on an in-depth understanding of many aspects of research. A simple framework will be provided later in this chapter.

A framework to assess research

Cullum & Petherick (2008) point out that we need checklists to help us assess the quality of research so that we can critique articles systematically and efficiently. They suggest that if the research is assessing treatment and prevention methods there are three broad questions to ask (Cullum & Petherick 2008: 104):

- Are the results of the study valid?
- What are the results?
- Can I apply the results in practice?

The point to note here is that unless you can be satisfied that the study has been carried out in such a way as to make the results accurate, there is no point in looking at what they found. Put another way, the starting point for real assessment comes from looking at the methods section where the researcher describes what they did and how they did it.

Greenhalgh (2006) similarly suggests that if you are deciding whether it is worth reading a paper, you should make the decision on the basis of the design outlined in the methods section. Is it likely to produce results that are sufficiently sound to make a contribution to our knowledge or practice? However, your first action is to ask whether the paper fits in with what evidence you are attempting to find—i.e. does it relates to your research question or your own practice focus? To do this you need to search and retrieve the abstract which should give you an overview of whether the study is going to be useful or not. So we can rephrase the above as:

> **! Key points**
>
> It is important to note that different journals have different requirements of how research is presented and these need to be taken into consideration when critiquing a research paper. It is worth looking at the author guidelines for the chosen journal article to determine whether it is the journal requirements and not necessarily the author that has determined what is written and explained in the actual paper being critiqued.

- Is the study relevant to my research question?
- Are the results of the study valid?
- What are the results?
- Can I apply the results in practice?

The second point to note from the three questions from Cullum & Petherick (2008) is that the point of critiquing is not to admire an article like a photograph or painting, but to see it as a means to an end—will it make a contribution to practice? There should be a clear advantage to the patient, or at least indirectly for the patient by improving the nurse's ability to provide care and treatment, or by changing or restructuring the health care system so that it can deliver services in the best way. However, as a student, you may have chosen to critique a paper which explains and helps you to understand the student experience of caring for patients, for example those who may be anxious about going for surgery or caring for a patient with a mental illness. One kind of article will help you to use evidence as a nurse in practice and the other will help you to understand how students learn to give care through their different clinical placement experiences.

The challenge presented by Cullum & Petherick's (2008) questions is that to get started in critiquing you need to know a great deal about research to know if the method of carrying out the research will produce accurate results. This requires a lot of technical knowledge that is beyond the scope of this book. We will, however, cover some of the straightforward principles you need to be more informed about research.

Although the points made by Cullum & Petherick (2008) relate to research looking at treatment and prevention interventions, the three issues relate to almost all kinds of research, and provide a good starting point to think about critiquing. However, it is helpful to use a framework that will work on a broader level and provide some guidelines on what you might question. To achieve this you need to know some straightforward points that will help you write a critique in a language that your tutors will expect to see in your work.

When you are asked to critique research articles, you will be expected to do three things.

1. Describe some of the story line of the study—what they did and found.
2. Comment in a balanced way on how well they conducted the study.
3. Conclude whether these enable the researcher to arrive and valid findings.

The first part will demonstrate you have understood what they were doing and that you can summarize the key outcomes of the study (the clinical or educational aspects depending on the nature of the research). The second part will show your ability to have a view of your own, and make a balanced judgement on the researcher's ability to produce a sound study. The third part will enable you to determine if the first two led to their ability to make a sound judgement on their outcomes. When you write a critique, you do not cover these in order of first description, and then all the comments at the end; you combine these all the way through a critique by describing an aspect of the study and then providing your evaluation of it as part of that same section. For example see the extract of Mitchell's article below and the critique in Box 7.1

Ethical considerations

The study was approved by the appropriate ethics committee. Participants were given written information about the study and it was emphasized that a decision to withdraw at any time, or a decision not to take part, would not affect the care they received. All responses were anonymous.

From: Mitchell, M. (2008) Conscious surgery: influence of the environment on patient anxiety. *Journal of Advanced Nursing* 64 (3) 261–271.

Box 7.1 Describing, commenting, and critiquing

Although Mitchell (2008) has only a short section of three sentences on ethical considerations, he does cover the major elements expected in relation to ethical concerns in any study (**see Example box above**). For instance, he starts by saying the study was approved by an ethics committee. As their role is to protect those involved in research from harm through scrupulously examining a research proposal for any possible sources of harm, the fact that this study has passed that test provides the reader with confidence in the ethical rigour of the author. In addition, other elements such as informed consent and anonymity were also built into the study. Again this supports the view that the study was carried out following the principles associated with high ethical standards.

This example shows how critiquing is not just focussing on negative qualities, and that the writer should provide not just description but also analytical comment based on knowledge of the principles of research.

The frameworks in Tables 7.2 and 7.3 take the outline of a study framework suggested in Table 7.1, but this time highlights areas where you need to give analytical comment as well as description of what you see as important in a study and the types of issues about conducting the research the researcher should tell you about. The first framework Table 7.2, is for quantitative research articles that concentrate on measurement and numbers, and Table 7.3 is for qualitative research articles where the emphasis is on meaning, understanding, and experience. Revisit the section on research approaches in Chapter 3 if you want to refresh your memory of these two approaches.

What you have to do in both cases, is to confirm that they made good decisions or, identify that there were limitations or consequences as a result of their decisions when reasonable alternatives may have existed.

! Key points

Critiquing does not test your ability to summarize a research article. It tests your ability to critically assess the value of the study in terms of what was found, and how well it was conducted. This will demonstrate your understanding of research as well as your ability to make balanced judgements.

EBP in action

Take a photocopy (or print off a copy from the online resource centre of the frameworks in Boxes 7.2 and 7.3 so that you can keep them with you whenever you need to critique an article. Add any questions that are recommended to you as part of your course to the framework. Refer also to the student guidelines if undertaking a critique for an assignment (See Chapter 9).

Aspect	Questions
Focus	What topic is the concern of this article? Can you identify measurable 'variables' in the title or researcher's statement concerning their main interest? Is this an important topic?
Background	How does the researcher argue that the topic is worthwhile? How widespread or big a problem is it? Is the seriousness of the topic reinforced by the previous studies? Is there a thorough review of the literature outlining current knowledge on this topic? Are the key variables defined and an attempt made to consider how they can be measured? E.g. definitions of 'pain' or 'anxiety' and descriptions of scales frequently used to measure them.
Aim	What is the statement of the aim of the data collection? This usually begins with the word 'to', e.g. 'The aim of this study is 'to examine/determine/establish/compare/etc'. If it is a randomized control trial (RCT) there may be a hypothesis.
Methodology or broad approach	Within a quantitative approach, is it a survey, experimental (RCT),or correlation study? Does this match the statement of the aim?
Tool of data collection	What was the method used to collect the data? Had this been used in previous studies and so may be regarded as reliable or accurate? If not, was it piloted? Is there any mention of reliability or validity? Is there a rationale given for the choice of tool? Could an alternative tool have been considered?
Method of data analysis and presentation	Is the method of processing and analysing the results described in the methods section, such as statistical process through SPSS computer analysis, and are the results clearly presented in the results/findings section? Does the researcher clearly explain any statistical techniques or methods of presentation such as tables, graphs, pie charts?
Sample	On how many people, events, or things are the results based? If questionnaires, what was the response rate? If RCT, what was the dropout rate? Are either of these likely to have an impact on the results? Were there inclusion and exclusion criteria stated? Were these reasonable, given the research question and the nature of the sample? Do they limit to whom the results may apply? What method was used to select who got into the study (the sampling strategy)? Does the sample suffer from any kind of bias?
Ethical considerations	Did an ethics committee (LREC, or in US an Institutional Review Board 'IRB') approve the study? Was informed consent gained and mention made of confidentiality? Could the study be said to be ethically rigorous?
Main findings	What did they find in answer to their aim? What were the large results that relate to the aim of the study?
Conclusion and recommendations	Did they give a clear answer to their aim? If they stated a hypothesis, did they say if this was supported or rejected? Were clear recommendations made (who should do what, how, now)?
Overall strengths and limitations	What would you say were the aspects of the study they did well? What aspects were less successful? Did they acknowledge any limitations to the study?
Application to practice	How do the results relate to practice? Should any changes be considered?

Table 7.2 A framework for critiquing quantitative research articles

It is important to emphasize that qualitative research is so different from quantitative studies, that it is difficult to apply exactly the same criteria to judge both types of research. So, for instance, in qualitative research, the sample size will be small, and there will probably be no pilot study with the tool of data collection. These are not legitimate criticisms for qualitative research although they may be a limitation in quantitative research. For this reason, this chapter has one critique framework for each research approach and the framework for critiquing qualitative research articles can be found in Table 7.3.

Aspect	Questions
Focus	What topic is the concern of this article? Is this an important topic? The focus here will be broader than that of quantitative research and may emphasize experience of a condition or situation.
Background	How does the researcher argue that the topic is worthwhile? How widespread or big a problem is it? Is the seriousness of the topic reinforced by the previous studies? Is there a thorough review of the literature outlining current knowledge on this topic? The background may make the qualitative approach a logical choice.
Aim	What is the statement of the aim of data collection? This usually begins with the word 'to' and may concentrate on an exploration of a situation, e.g. 'The aim of this study is to explore the lived experience of chronic illness'.
Methodology or broad approach	Within a qualitative approach is it phenomenological, ethnographic, grounded theory, or broad qualitative design? Does this match the statement of the aim?
Tool of data collection	What was the method used to collect the data? Had this tool been used in previous studies of this type? A qualitative tool will not be piloted to check accuracy but may be used firstly on a small scale to give the researcher experience of its use in this situation. There may be mention of credibility where the researcher attempts to give clear details on the circumstances and environment in which data gathering took place. The descriptions of such things as individual interviews may be extensive to allow you to feel almost as though you were there. Do you feel this tool worked well or might an alternative have been more effective?
Method of data analysis and presentation	This is one of the most important steps in qualitative approach where the researcher's understanding emerges inductively from the data and their interpretation of what is going on with those involved. To make sense of large amounts of text the researcher may mention specific systems for analysing the data either in the form of computer programs such as NUDIST and NVivo, or systems designed by other qualitative analysts such as Colaizzi or Van Manon. There may be reference to immersion in the data where the researcher reads over and over the details of what people have said or done. Codes to categorized themes may be mentioned and illustrations of the way this was done may be presented to form an 'audit trail' to allow you to follow the way the researcher managed the data from transcript to coded themes. The data will be in the form of observed descriptions or verbal comments and statements from those involved. These may be quite powerful in their description of feelings and emotions where the researcher is attempting to provide evidence of 'credibility' so we can believe in the accuracy of the findings and the interpretation of them.
Sample	Here the numbers of participants will be low, perhaps under 10 and often not more than 20. Data collection may have stopped once 'saturation' was reached, that is, where no new categories emerged from the findings. Were there inclusion and exclusion criteria stated? Were these reasonable given the research question and the nature of the sample? Do the selection criteria limit to whom the results may apply? What method was used to select who got into the study (the sampling strategy)? Is this appropriate for this research question and approach? Does the sample suffer from any kind of bias?
Ethical considerations	Did an ethics committee (LREC, or in US an Institutional Review Board 'IRB') approve the study? Was informed consent gained and mention made of confidentiality? Could the study be said to be ethically rigorous?
Main findings	What themes or categories arose from the findings in answer to their aim? Was there an attempt to ensure that the accuracy of these themes was checked in some way, for example by peer checking with others not involved in the study, or more than one member of the team involved in interpretation of the findings?
Conclusion and recommendations	Did they give a clear answer to their aim? Is this well argued and supported? Were clear recommendations made (who should do what, how, now)? If grounded theory, is there an attempt to explain what might lie behind the findings?

Table 7.3 A framework for critiquing qualitative research articles (Continued)

Aspect	Questions
Overall strengths and limitations	What would you say were the aspects of the study they did well? What aspects were less successful? Did they acknowledge any limitations to the study?
Application to practice	How do the findings relate to practice? Should any changes be considered?

Table 7.3 (Continued)

This has many of the same aspects of Table 7.2, but you will notice some differences that relate to the principles of qualitative or interpretative research.

Using a framework can at first take you longer to read an article, as you have to consider each point. However, the advantage is that it ensures that you do not miss things you might otherwise not see. As you get familiar with using this approach, you should find that your speed in using the framework increases.

There is a language and style of critiquing. Learning to develop these will enhance your ability to demonstrate higher level of critiquing skills. The critique frameworks above contained some of the key words frequently seen as essential issues to comment on in a critique.

! Key points

The key words to use in a quantitative critique include 'reliability', 'validity', 'bias', and 'rigour', if it is a qualitative study, words such as 'credibility', and 'dependability', and 'fittingness' will be used'. These terms illustrate your understanding of the principles of good practice involved in assessing the standard of research reached by those responsible for it. You will find some of these terms defined below and in the Glossary of terms in this book.

How to work through a critique framework

A frequent form of assignment in both pre-registration and post-registration courses is a written critique of a research article. Critiques can also be used as a verbal activity

! Key points

If asked to produce a critique, choose your article very carefully. Choose one that allows you to illustrate what you have learnt about research. Avoid those that are too technical or overly statistical unless these aspects have been fully covered as part of your course. Find one that has both strengths and possible weaknesses so you can show a balanced approach. Where possible, choose one from a refereed journal. It will usually say 'this article has been submitted to a double-blind review' to indicate this.

in seminars. In this section we will look at the individual parts of the framework offered above and provide some advice on how to tackle each of the sections.

In choosing the article, remember that discussing the clinical aspects of the study in depth will not be your main concern in the assignment. This means that it is the research elements that should influence your choice of article, not simply the clinical aspect. If you are producing the assignment for a research or EBP module, it will probably be the understanding of the research issues that will be the focus of the work, and that is why a good starting point to look for a suitable research article is in the refereed journals. It is good practice to carefully check again the guidelines that accompany the assignment and ask for confirmation of your choice if you are concerned.

Each of the sections from the framework will now be considered to reveal the kind of aspects you need to examine when reading articles. Suggestions will also be made on what you can write about in producing a critique for an assignment. The main emphasis is on critical evaluation, which demonstrates knowledge of the research process and the issues involved in carrying out research.

EBP in action

Reading the section below with a copy of a quantitative article and a qualitative article to hand will help you to see how the points raised can make a big difference to your ability to critically assess an article. To help you, the quantitative article on patient anxiety by Mitchell (2008) will be used to illustrate a quantitative article. You might want to use your own quantitative and qualitative articles as well as using a copy of Mitchell's study as a guide.

Focus

The clue to the focus of an article is usually in the title. This will usually contain both the topic of interest, which will be the variable being examined, and the sample group from whom the researcher collects information. In Mitchell's (2008) article the focus is on 'patient anxiety' as one variable, and 'the environment' as another. (See Chapter 5 for explanation of a variable.) As these are joined by the word 'influence' this would seem to indicate a correlation study as it does not talk about a direct cause. In some qualitative research a quote from a respondent may be used and this may make the focus more difficult to identify. Check the abstract or the beginning of the introduction for clues if the title does not give a clear indication. See Table 7.3 for examples of titles along with the study aims.

Background

You need to consider how clearly and thoroughly the researcher makes the case for looking at this particular focus. This usually takes two forms. The first part will be the highlighting of a problem, the nature of the problem, how it originated, and an indication of the size of the problem. Although this part should be objective, it will play a persuasive part in convincing the reader that this was the right decision for the researcher to make; this topic really did need more research carried out on it. So for instance, Mitchell (2008) argues that the number of surgical operations is increasing, particularly those using local and regional anaesthesia when the patient is 'awake'. Whereas formerly, the patient was the concern of the anaesthetist, it is now the role of the nurse to look after the patient during the procedure.

The second aspect of the background will be a review of the literature. Articles vary in how they present this. Some have a separate heading where they explain how they carried out the review and under a number of headings present and discuss the research available on their topic. In some articles this aspect will be combined as part of the introduction and will look at both the problem and how it has been considered in the literature as a way of briefing the reader on the background to the study.

Critical analysis of this section should include whether you feel the researcher has convincingly presented a sound case for selecting the topic. Where there is a reasonably extensive review of the literature that considers the strength and nature of the studies, there will be an inevitability as to the method, or sample chosen for this study. Often the researcher will point to a gap in the literature that their study will fill. In producing your comments, you should not only say what they provided as a justification, but how well they justified the choice of topic.

Usually, little can go wrong in this section unless you feel that the researcher does not really present a strong case for selecting the topic, or little in the way of literature, which you feel was available, has been included. You can check the years over which the review of the literature is spread. There should be an emphasis on more recent research, but with earlier influential research being tracked for their contribution to the knowledge on the topic.

Interestingly, Mitchell (2008) presents the review of the literature under the heading '**Background**' and gives no information on how the literature was searched. It would have been more usual and helpful to the reader if the heading 'literature review had been used and search details given so that judgements could have been made on how thoroughly this had been accomplished. However, the actual article itself has to comply with word limits for that journal and the author may have decided for that paper to focus more words in other sections instead.

Aim

This is the most important section to locate in any research article. This is because you will judge the study by whether the researcher has successfully achieved their aim. There are two places to look for the aim. The first is in the abstract, usually under the title and before the article begins. It is often the first heading in an abstract. The second place to find it is at the end of the review of the literature, if there is one, and immediately before the subheading 'Method'. Sometimes it might have slipped just inside the subheading 'Method'. As indicated in Table 7.2, it will usually begin with the word 'to' followed by words such as identify/establish/determine. In some circumstances, because of the construction of the sentence, the word 'to' may be missing, and when you state the aim in any written or verbal work, you may have to insert it, to make sense.

Mitchell's aim is clearly presented in the abstract and is repeated immediately before the subheading 'Design' and is listed under the heading 'Aims' as (Mitchell 2008: 264):

> " (1) to investigate patient anxiety arising from the experience of the clinical environment during surgery under local/regional anaesthesia and (2) to uncover the specific aspects patients find anxiety provoking and possibly dissuade them form opting for local/regional anaesthesia. "

It is useful to see the different aspects of the study numbered by the author. If there are clearly more than one aspect and they are not numbered, do this yourself so that you can ensure the author does tackle all the aspects.

Qualitative research aims will often say '**to explore**, which indicates the exploratory nature of qualitative research, and so indicates a wide approach. Some phenomenological research will include the words '**lived experience**', again indicating the nature of the research. The main point is that there is a clear relationship between the title of the article, which provides the focus and the statement of the aim. This can be seen in Table 7.4 below.

✚ ⋯⋯⋯⋯⋯⋯⋯⋯⋯⋯⋯⋯⋯⋯⋯⋯⋯⋯⋯⋯⋯⋯⋯⋯⋯⋯⋯⋯⋯⋯⋯⋯⋯⋯⋯

EBP in action

Look at the publications outlined in Table 7.4 and in the titles, notice how the research approach and the sample form part of some titles. In the aim section, identify the aim starting with the word 'to' and notice where the aim is made up of more than one part. You should also be able to spot which studies take a qualitative approach.

⋯⋯⋯⋯⋯⋯⋯⋯⋯⋯⋯⋯⋯⋯⋯⋯⋯⋯⋯⋯⋯⋯⋯⋯⋯⋯⋯⋯⋯⋯⋯⋯⋯⋯⋯⋯⋯

If the study is a randomized control study, or a survey looking for correlations (patterns or similarities between variables) there may a hypothesis that will predict what the research expects to find at the end of the study. Unless the author says 'the hypothesis of this study was...' do not guess, or suggest that there was one, as it is easy to get this aspect wrong.

Author, title, source	Aim
STIRLING L, RAAB G, ALDER E & ROBERTSON F (2007) Randomized trial of essential oils to reduce perioperative patient anxiety: feasibility study. *Journal of Advanced Nursing* 60 (5) 494–501.	This paper is a report of a feasibility study to examine the effectiveness of essential oils in reducing anxiety in thoracic patients awaiting the results of investigative and staging surgery.
KUTASH M & NORTHROP L (2007) Family members' experiences of the intensive care unit waiting room. *Journal of Advanced Nursing* 60 (4) 384–388.	This paper is a report of a study to explore family members' perspectives and experiences of waiting rooms in adult intensive care units.
LAU LAU-WALKER M (2007) Importance of illness beliefs and self-efficacy for patients with coronary heart disease. *Journal of Advanced Nursing* 60 (2) 187–198.	This paper is a report of a study to assess the association between coronary heart disease patients' illness beliefs and their self-efficacy 3 years after hospital discharge.
MCCAUGHAN E & MCSORLEY O (2007) Consumers' and professionals' perceptions of a breast cancer review clinic. *Journal of Advanced Nursing* 60 (4) 419–426.	This paper is a report of a study to explore the health care needs of women attending consultant-led breast cancer review clinics from their own perspectives, how these health care needs were being met, and health care professionals' perceptions of ways in which the service could be delivered more efficiently and effectively.
BYRNE G, BRADY A, HORAN P, MACGREGOR C & BEGLEY C (2007) Assessment of dependency levels of older people in the community and measurement of nursing workload. *Journal of Advanced Nursing* 60 (1) 39–49.	This paper is a report of a study to explore the relationship between the dependency levels of older people who are part of the community nurse's caseload and the volume and nature of nursing input required.
MERRELL J, CARNWELL R, WILLIAMS A, ALLEN D & GRIFFITHS L, (2007) A survey of school nursing provision in the UK. *Journal of Advanced Nursing* 59 (5) 463–473.	This paper is a report of a study to map school nursing provision across the health and education sectors in Wales to identify the number, age, qualifications, terms of employment, location, functions, and access to continuing professional development and clinical supervision of school nurses.

Table 7.4 Relationship between research titles and aims

Warning:

The things that can go wrong in this section include a difference in the wording of the aim in the abstract compared with the statement of the aim in the part of the article. This can cause confusion in relation to the researcher's main intention in the study. Look very carefully at these wordings and assess how close they are in meaning, and which one is closest to describing what information the author did collect to answer their aim? This last question is always useful for determining if you have successfully identified the aim of the study as it should match the information they have collected.

When you present the aim, either verbally or in writing, keep to the author's own words. As you need to go back to this later on to see if the aim was achieved, the exact sense of what they set out to do is important. If you put it in your own words you may change the meaning.

Another very important point to consider if you are undertaking a critique of an article for a student assignment is that there may be an expectation that you support your critique with other evidence to explain your understanding, in other words go beyond the description of what is included or not. To use other examples such as: *'the author did not appear to have included evidence of a search strategy, which Rees (2010) states is an essential part of a critique.'*

Methodology or broad research approach

In critiquing research, you are looking for a logical relationship between all the elements in the research process carried out by the author. Following the link between the title and aim, the next major link is between the aim and the methodological approach. If the aim suggests measurement to provide an answer, then a quantitative approach will be a suitable approach. An assessment of the most appropriate or 'successful' intervention in treatment or care should use an experimental design, as this examines cause and effect relationships (See Chapter 5).

Where a study is 'exploring' a topic, especially in the form of an experience, then the more appropriate approach is a qualitative approach. If there is mention in the title or aim of 'the lived experience' of something such as chronic illness, then a phenomenological study would be most useful (see Chapter 4).

One area that can often confuse students relates to studies that refer to an 'attitude' towards something. These are often expected to be qualitative because they relate to subjective feelings; however, the usual method is to 'measure' attitude using a scale and so will take a quantitative approach. Similarly, some people see a study using a questionnaire with open comments as well as more structured ones and feel that this means it is using both a quantitative and qualitative design. However, all they have done is use a quantitative design and include some comments from individuals. The inclusion of some qualitative data does not make it a qualitative approach. This is often referred to as 'within method triangulation' where the researcher attempts to look at the situation from the point of view of collecting different forms of data within the same tool and which are intended to consider the same variable but in different ways (Burns & Grove 2009).

Looking at the tables and statistical analysis in Mitchell's (2008) study, this is clearly **quantitative**. Under the subheading 'Design' (Mitchell 2008: 264) states, 'this was a survey design' and goes on to say how he correlated the results to establish which factors related closely to high levels of patient anxiety.

Tool/method of data collection

There are so many aspects of the research process where a poor decision by the researcher can have a considerable effect on the quality of the study. This is true of the tool of data collection. The results of a study are only going to be as accurate, or as believable, as the tool the researcher has used to collect the information. We have seen in Chapters 3, 4, and 5 that the common tools of data collection included:

- Assessment scales
- Physiological measure in surveys and RCTs
- Questionnaires
- Interviews
- Observation
- Documentary methods

In quantitative research, the tool of data collection has to be as accurate as possible in the way in which it measures the variable highlighted in the aim. In experimental studies such as RCTs, both the dependent and independent variables have to be accurately defined (the concept definition) as well as accurately measured using a tool that is reliable (operational definition). Only then can the researcher hope to measure what they are setting out to measure (achieve validity).

In quantitative research, check that the tool of data collection has either been used in a previous study, and so is known to produce consistent and accurate results, or if it is a tool designed by the author that it has be piloted to ensure that the measurements are consistent.

> ## ! Key points
>
> Although the terms 'reliability' and 'validity' are often used together, almost as if talking about the same thing, they are very different. Reliability, relates to the tool of data collection, and its consistency and accuracy of measurement. Validity relates to the results and has the researcher measured what they believe they have measured. Chapter 3 explains these in more detail.

In qualitative research things are very different due to the flexible nature of the way the data are collected. Pilot studies are therefore difficult to carry out, as the researcher is not using a consistent tool, but one that is changing depending on the answers provided. It is important that you do not unjustly criticize the qualitative researcher for not carrying out a pilot study. You may find however that they did undertake some 'pilot' of their own experience in doing an interview, but not the actual interview schedule itself, especially if they were a novice researcher.

The problem that can arise with the tool of data collection is that it may not be a good choice for the type of information being gathered. An alternative may have been more suitable. If it is a quantitative study the researcher may not have used an appropriate tool that has been successfully used in other studies, or may have designed a tool and not piloted it prior to the study. This would leave the accuracy of the tool in question.

In tools such as questionnaires and interviews, the researcher is reliant on what is called *'self-report'*, that is, that people do what they say they do, or have had the experience identified. This may not always be accurate. It is important to accept these only as indicators or possibilities and not factual. Similarly, the researcher may lead the respondent by using 'loaded' words, such as 'would you agree that this is an unacceptable situation'. The results would therefore be biased as the researcher has influenced the responses.

If the research aim implies a qualitative approach, the researcher may have used a quantitative tool that really is not appropriate to the purpose of the study. For instance, using a list of alternatives from which an individual has to choose is not looking at the situation from their point of view, it is influenced by the researcher's preconceived ideas about a situation.

Mitchell (2008) gathered data on patient anxiety by means of a questionnaire that included the use of a Likert scale, which consisted of a number of statements to which respondents chose options ranging from 'strongly agree' to 'strongly disagree'. This had undergone a pilot study, and reference is made to the face validity of the questionnaire, which means that on the surface the questions appeared to measure surgical patients anxiety influenced by the environment (Polit & Beck 2008). The use of a questionnaire of this type is an appropriate tool for a survey approach such as that used here.

Method of data analysis and data presentation

The method of data analysis and presentation are areas that can prove difficult to assess for the novice in EBP. Both quantitative and qualitative research requires sophisticated methods of firstly grouping, and classifying the results or findings. Unless you have experience of these or are frequently evaluating such methods, this aspect of a study can seem daunting. In producing an assignment, it is important that you do not criticize an author for using something that may be quite commonly used, but with which you are not familiar, or do not fully understand. However, reading research approaches in Chapters 4 and 5 will help you develop this understanding, as will following suggestions for further reading.

> **! Key points**
>
> Every picture tells a story so it is important that you do not ignore tables and figures. There are ways of reading tables and graphs that reveal the story behind them. You need to gain experience of looking for these. Some of the research methods books will allow you to increase your skills in making sense of these key areas of the study.

Some of the problems you may encounter include researchers using an inappropriate or inadequate method of processing the data. In data presentation the headings for tables and charts can be misleading or missing. Similarly, the units of measurement may not be shown or be ambiguous. Do look at the author's comments on these presentations, particularly their interpretation of what the figures mean, and see if they correspond with your interpretation.

The data analysis and presentation in Mitchell's (2008) work is very strong. The findings are well laid out in tables and bar charts, and responses for some of the Likert scale questions are presented in a table. The relationship between variables is also appropriately presented using the strength of the correlation to indicate where the greatest relationships existed. These tables and figures are described by the author clearly.

Sample/participants

This aspect of research, like the tool of data collection, can have a considerable impact on the quality of the research. The big issue in quantitative research is getting a sample that 'stands for' or represents the type of population to which the researcher wants to generalize. In other words, it is an issue of bias. Bias is any distortion that affects the result, or the interpretation of the results (Burns & Grove 2009). Of course, a totally perfect sample is very difficult to achieve so it is important to recognize this in your comments in a written critique.

> **! Key points**
>
> You will get an idea of how representative the sample may be from the inclusion and exclusion criteria used to select the sample. The inclusion criteria cover those the researcher actively sought to include, and the exclusion criteria cover those who might have been unrepresentative, or may be put at risk by taking part.

A second major issue is the sample size. In RCTs, it is the difference anticipated in the outcome measurement that will suggest that the difference could not happen by chance that is important. The size of the sample is sometimes determined by a 'power statistic' that calculates the numbers needed to achieve confidence in the results. This number tends to be very large, so it is not always possible to achieve this goal. Unless a reasonable number are included in both groups, it may be difficult for the statistical tests to pick up real differences between the two groups in terms of the study outcomes with any degree of certainty. It is a design fault where this difficulty could have been anticipated from the start of the study and where steps were not taken to overcome this possibility.

Surveys can similarly run into problems where the numbers are too small to pick up differences between subgroups, or do not take the range of variation into account. This is why, as Polit & Beck (2008) suggest, quantitative researchers are advised to use as large a sample as possible. However, it is difficult to say what a reasonable number to include is; it will depend on the variations within the sample in regard to the issue or characteristics being studied.

There are a number of things that can go wrong with this stage of sampling. If the exclusion criteria are too strict or restricting, it may make the group untypical or limit the extent to which they can be applied to all in a population, such as only looking at a single sex group although both sexes would normally be expected to be included in the target group. This means the findings can only be related to those with the characteristics of the sample.

In RCTs, look at how many dropped out of the study, once it has started, or did not complete the 'post-test' or 'after' measurement. This is called experimental 'mortality'. This does not mean they died, although that can be one reason for people not completing the study, more usually it means they were lost to the follow-up, or 'post-test' measurement (Polit & Beck 2008). A large number dropping out from either the experimental or control group can make comparisons between the two groups difficult at the end of the study, as the researcher is now not comparing like with like.

Similarly in surveys, look at for the response rate in relation to the number's targeted. Where there is less than a 50% response rate to questionnaires, those not replying will outnumber those who did reply and could have very different experiences or views. A small response rate does not necessarily invalidate the whole study, but is certainly limits the extent to which we may confidently relate the findings elsewhere.

The method used to select the sample may also have produced an untypical sample, or one that did not allow the use of some beneficial statistical procedure. In other words, there may have been a better sampling method.

A frequent mistake made by those new to critiquing is to criticize qualitative research on the small sample size, or on the method of selecting the sample when small samples and more convenient or hand-picking methods are quite acceptable within the context of qualitative methods. Consider the issues discussed in Chapter 4 regarding qualitative evidence in research.

Attention should be given where the researcher claims they have undertaken a RCT, as for this to happen, everyone should have an equal chance of ending up in either the experimental or control group. If they have compared one clinical area with another without randomly allocating people, they have used a 'quasi-experimental' approach, that is they have introduced something to one group but not the other, but they cannot claim they have demonstrated a 'cause and effect' relationship from the results only a correlation, as there could have been something different between the two groups which led to them being in a particular group.

Finally, some studies omit vital information such as response rate, or how many were originally included so that response rate can be calculated. The sampling strategy may not be named, or inclusion and exclusion criteria may be omitted.

Mitchell (2008: 264) again produces a very well written section on his participants. This is what he says:

> 66 A convenience sample of patients scheduled for elective surgery in four public day surgery units (DSU) was invited to take part in the study. The inclusion criteria were those undergoing local or regional anaesthesia and having non-life-threatening day surgery, speaking English and being aged 18 years or more. The exclusion criteria were ophthalmic and dental surgery patients; as such patients may experience additional anxieties. Also excluded were patients with a history of chronic physical or mental health problems. 99

The study had a 41% response rate, which makes it a little difficult to be confident about how representative the replies are of the group as a whole. Neither this fact, nor the problem of this being a self-report study was acknowledged in the limitations of the study.

EBP in action

If you have not being doing so as we have been going through this structure, now is a good point for you to look at an example of a research study, and see if you can identify some of the strengths or limitations of your research study in relation to the sample. Are any problems inevitable, given the circumstances, or do you think the researcher could have avoided the problems with a little thought?

Ethical considerations

Throughout a study we are looking for the extent to which the researcher demonstrates 'rigour' by describing their thought process and actions in relation to the study. This allows the reader to form a clear opinion of the quality of the study. This process is related to the rigour demonstrated by the researcher to do the right things from the methods point of view. However, the researcher should also show ethical rigour in a study by recognizing, and addressing some of the ethical issues encountered or anticipated in their research.

> ## ! Key points
>
> Most studies should be approved by a local research ethics committee (LREC) or in the US, an Institutional Review Board (IRB). Other major issues include gaining informed consent from participants, and anonymity to protect the identity of those taking part. An assessment of possibility of harm should take place. This can include psychological harm such as anxiety, or distress in relation to the content or focus of the study. Although all research may involve some risk, this is usually minimal, and researchers should take steps to reduce risks and maximize possible benefits (Polit & Beck 2008).

The problems that can occur here include no mention of any ethical steps taken although it is clear there are a number of issues raised by the study. It is important to note that under research governance, even where health care staff are included in a research study, informed consent needs to be received and ethical approval gained.

One final point under this heading is to ensure that the study you are critiquing is a research study before criticizing a lack of ethical procedures. Audit and service evaluation can look very similar to research but do not have to gain ethical approval. However, the way these are conducted should safeguard the individual's safety and anonymity. The identity of the individual should be hidden from the reader; it does not mean that the person should be unknown or unrecognized by the researcher.

Main results/findings

These relate to the important information collected in the study and relate to the aim of the study and which in quantitative research, have a large number attached to them (at least in regard to what might have been anticipated). There may be only two or three main results for any study. These should be apparent if you look at key tables or figures, and be highlighted by the researcher in the paragraphs relating to the results.

If there is more than one part to the aim, each one should have a 'main finding' that answers that particular aim (see the 'Aim' section above). In qualitative research, the findings are often developed from the theme headings that have been used to group comments under relevant headings.

The main findings will be found in the 'Results' section if it is a quantitative study, and in the 'Findings' section, if it is a qualitative study. This distinction in names is one clue as to the type of research you are critiquing. However, one problem is the inconsistent use of these two terms by some nursing and health care journals.

The problems associated with this aspect of a study include the researcher claiming to have established a main finding when it has little to do with the aim of the study. This is another illustration of the importance of finding the aim of a study and referring to it as you work through the critique structure.

The overall sample size, or the size of the subgroups, can make it difficult to claim there is a clear pattern or finding, when there is little to chose between the results of groups or categories being examined. In qualitative research there can be little evidence that the main categories identified from the data have been systematically constructed and checked, either by those involved in the study (member's check) or by a peer researcher. In these cases, the author's claim that the themes are 'main findings' can be disputed by the reader.

In the study of patient anxiety, Mitchell (2008) found that 77% of those in the study experienced anxiety on the day of the surgery, although the degree of anxiety varied. The things that influenced the anxiety were grouped by Mitchell under three broad headings and these were intra-operative apprehension, anaesthetic information provision, and health control. These findings related to part one and two of the aim of the study.

Conclusion and recommendations

The conclusion to the study should give a clear answer to the aim, and use similar words to the aim. This forms the 'pay-off' or end point for the study and so is one of the most important aspects to consider. In other words, what was the answer to the question or aim posed at the beginning of the study? The conclusion also identifies the possible contribution the study can make to knowledge and understanding on the topic. In this respect you should find that the statement of the conclusion completes the study. The placing of the conclusion is at the end of the article and also in the abstract. Both should be worded in much the same way. This section is frequently followed by the researcher's recommendations, which should be based logically on the content of the conclusion.

You may be surprised to find that the section headed 'conclusion', particularly in UK nursing research, may not contain the conclusion to the study. Often it is used to present recommendations. This is easy to spot, as they will be written in the future tense and will indicate who should do what and how, from now on. If the conclusion contains the recommendations, then it is often the discussion section of the article where you may find the conclusion. It is worth checking if there is an 'implications for practice' box at the end of the article, as these can sometimes include the conclusion too.

The problem with this aspect of a study is that the conclusion can sometimes lead to the response 'so what?' where the usefulness of producing this knowledge can be challenged as either not being very enlightening, or that it is really no surprise, and hardly worth the effort of carrying out research to answer it. There is also a problem where there can be little done to change the situation.

The conclusion can also leave out some aspects of the aim and lead the reader to wonder what happened to an aspect that was part of the researcher's concerns at the beginning of the study. This demonstrates the importance of giving each aspect of the aim a letter to ensure that each part of the aim is answered at the close of the article.

The recommendations can also seem as though they have little to do with the main findings of the study, and were developed by the researcher before the study began. In other words, there is a feeling that the researcher did not need to have carried out the study, they could have just argued the case for what they would like to see happen in practice!

Mitchell's (2008) article is an example of where the conclusion to the study is placed in the discussion, and the heading 'conclusion' contains the recommendations including the suggestion that nurses should assess patients and if necessary dispel any myths associated with local and regional anaesthesia. It was also suggested they continue to develop a patient-friendly theatre environment, although he does not say what form this would take.

Overall strengths and limitations

Critiquing is concerned with the identification of what the researcher has done particularly well in the design and implementation of a study and where we can identify that there are shortfalls in the design. This section allows you to show your understanding of research in the way you demonstrate your knowledge of the principles of research, and your ability to be fair in your comments on any limitations.

> **! Key points**
>
> It is easy to be over-critical of an author and condemn the whole study because some aspects were not carried out perfectly. Research can be a complex activity. Clearly major flaws should be identified; however, it is important to recognize that perfection is rarely achieved, and compromises have to be made. The author will usually acknowledge these too. You should be seen as fair and understanding of this in your approach to this aspect of the critique.

The problems that can arise here relate to your misunderstanding of what was going on in the study, or unfairly criticizing authors when under the approach used, they were following convention. To avoid this, check your understanding of the point your feel you want to criticize or ask someone such as a tutor or supervisor for their opinion.

Mitchell (2008) produced a well-conducted study and revealed some appropriate information on what made patients anxious in day surgery. The paper was clear and the evidence supported the recommendations; however, there were some aspects of structure that could have been improved, such as heading the background 'review of the literature', recognizing the limitations of the study, and making the heading 'Conclusion' fit the content.

Application to practice

The most important aspect of research is that it benefits patients, nursing, nurse education, or health or social care generally. At this point you should ask yourself the question 'so what?' How would you see the results of this study being applied to practice? Will it provide a clear pointer for action and allow practice to be based on sound evidence?

EBP in action

No matter what limitations you have identified in the way the study has been conducted, look at this point for any ways in which the study may have stimulated thought over this topic, or might trigger others to launch a better study. Give thought to the broader principles that the study highlights that might be wider than just the clinical area or patient group they have included.

The problem you might encounter here is not recognizing the bigger picture that the study may highlight. It is worth at this point to be creative and think around the topic by considering who might benefit in what way from the results of this study. Do try and be positive and think, despite any methodological limitations, how can we argue the study was worth carrying out?

The study by Mitchell (2008) made a number of suggestions for improvement to how we consider patients' psychological needs and anxieties when faced by treatment. Many of these could be applied to other clinical areas. In achieving this, the study was successful in adding to our nursing knowledge over this important and growing issue within health care.

EBP in action

As a final activity in this chapter return to the examples of research that you have been asked to use at several points. Now look at them in terms of what understanding you have gained from this chapter. How do you feel your skill of critiquing has improved?

Summary

- Critiquing is a key skill in nursing, and a familiar feature of nurse education. It is not just criticizing a published report, it is taking a balanced view of the quality of the processes used by the researcher to complete the study. In this respect it is an assessment of the researcher's skill in carrying out research. It should identify both the things they have done well, in addition to any limitations of the study.

- Critiquing requires a systematic approach and so a framework, like the one presented in this chapter should be used. We need to ensure that the different approaches to research in quantitative and qualitative approaches are acknowledged and we do not dismiss a study, or part of it, when it may be quite legitimate within a different research approach.

- EBP requires all nurses to be skilled at critiquing and so we need to have a basic understanding of research processes so that we can correctly assess how well a study has been undertaken. The end point of critiquing, however, is the extent to which we can apply it to practice to improve care.

- Practice should not be based on the results of one study, as it is rarely possible to conduct the perfect study. For this reason, reviews of the literature, particularly 'systematic reviews of the literature' are needed, and these will be the focus of the next chapter.

◼ Online resource centre

 You may now like to visit the accompanying website for this book and explore the additional resources you will find there. **www.oxfordtextbooks.co.uk/orc/holland/**

◼ References

Burns, N. & Grove, S. (2009) *The Practice of Nursing Research: appraisal, synthesis, and generation of evidence (6th edn)* St. Louis: Saunders.

Cullum, N. & Petherick, E. (2008) Evaluation of studies of treatment or prevention interventions. In: Cullum, N., Ciliska, D. Haynes, R. B. & Marks, S. (eds) *Evidence-Based Nursing*: an introduction. Oxford: Blackwell.

Greenhalgh, T. (2006) *How to Read a Paper*: the basics of evidence-based medicine (*3rd edn*). Oxford: Blackwell.

Mitchell, M. (2008) Conscious surgery: influences of the environment on patient anxiety. *Journal of Advanced Nursing* 64 (3) 261–271.

Nieswiadomy, R. M. (2008) *Foundations of Nursing Research (5th edn)*. New Jersey: Pearson Prentice Hall.

Nursing & Midwifery Council (2004) *Standards of proticiency for pre-registration Nursing Education*. London: Nursing & Midwifery Council.

Nursing & Midwifery Council (2008) *The Code: standards of conduct, performance and ethics for nurses and midwives*. London: NMC.

Parahoo, K. (2006) *Nursing Research: principles, process and issues. (2nd edn)*. Houndmills: Palgrave Macmillan.

Polit, D. & Beck, C. (2008) *Nursing Research: generating and assessing evidence for nursing practice (8th edn)*. Philadelphia: Lippincott Williams and Wilkins.

■ Further reading

Coughlan, M., Cronin, P. & Ryan, F. (2007) Step-by-step guide to critiquing research. Part 1: quantitative research. *British Journal of Nursing* 16 (11) 658–663.

Cutcliffe, J. & Ward, M. (2007) *Critiquing Nursing Research* London: Quay Books.

Ryan, F., Coughlan, M., & Cronin, P. (2007) Step-by-step guide to critiquing research. Part 2: qualitative research. *British Journal of Nursing* 16 (12) 738–744.

■ Useful websites

NHS Public Health Resource Unit

http://www.phru.nhs.uk/Pages/PHD/resources.htm

Ontario Critical Appraisal of research evidence 101 publication

http://www.health.gov.on.ca/ (has links to CASP critical appraisal tools UK)

8

Evidence-based practice and its implementation in nursing

Karen Holland

The aims of this chapter are:

➤ To explore why it is important to use an evidence-based approach to nursing care and nursing practice.

➤ To examine examples of nursing practice where an evidence base has been used.

➤ To explore how different kinds of evidence can be used in nursing practice.

➤ To explore how evidence can be used in implementing nursing care plans.

Introduction

Patients require their care to be based on the best evidence possible. As we have seen in other chapters this requires a set of skills to be learnt, which include understanding what evidence is and being able to determine its quality. Student nurses are expected to gain these skills during their studies to become qualified nurses as well as being able to deliver the care that is evidence based as part of the required Nursing and Midwifery Standards of Proficiency (NMC 2004). This chapter will focus on developing the knowledge and skills required to help you implement evidence-based care.

Clinical governance and clinical effectiveness

Before we can examine how evidence can be utilized in practice it is important to consider how evidence-based practice (EBP) relates to the delivery and management of nursing and health care generally. Two phrases that you will come across frequently in relation to EBP, and each other, are: clinical effectiveness and clinical governance. It is important to define these in order to examine their relationship to EBP and nursing practice.

One definition which is used frequently in many articles and Clinical Governance reports is:

> 66 A system through which NHS organisations are accountable for improving the quality of their services and safeguarding high standards of care by creating an environment in which excellence in clinical care will flourish. 99
>
> (Scally & Donaldson 1998)

It is an overarching framework which, according to McSherry & Haddock (1999: 114), incorporates the elements of: clinical risk, clinical audit, quality and practice development, and research and development. Others include clinical effectiveness as one of the key components (Cox & Ahluwalia 2000). However they are expressed, it is clear that there is a clear relationship between them and, in turn, EBP. Clinical effectiveness is defined as:

> 66 The extent to which specific clinical interventions when deployed in the field for a particular patient or population do what they are intended to do i.e. maintain and improve health and secure the greatest possible health gain from the available resources. 99
>
> (NHSE 1996)

One can see from these definitions that it would be essential that ensuring health improvement and excellence of clinical care is underpinned by the best possible evidence. We have seen already how to evaluate the quality and relevance of various forms of evidence but need to know how to use these to inform practice and deliver the best care possible. The literature tells us that there are barriers to the implementation of EBP (Newman et al. 1998; McKenna et al. 2004) but that nursing needs to move away from this negative debate which focuses on these barriers 'towards seizing it as an opportunity', particularly in collaborating with other professions in order to implement evidence-based change (Tod et al. 2004: 211).

Let us first consider however what the perceived barriers are to implementing EBP. Issues such as access to resources and lack of knowledge and skills to search for evidence (McKenna et al. 2004) and also evaluate it (Nagy et al. 2001) are much noted, as is lack of time (Palfreyman et al. 2003). Lack of time in fact was the significant factor reported by participants in a recent study by Koehn & Lehman (2008). A study by Gerrish et al. (2008: 71) examining the experiences of junior and senior nurses in implementing EBP found that the junior staff felt less confident in doing so and also that nursing culture 'seems to disempower junior nurses so that they are unable to develop autonomy in implementing EBP'. This use of junior and senior is possibly misleading, as the reader may assume that this relates to length of time qualified, e.g. newly qualified (as junior).

> **? Thinking about**
>
> Consider one of your placement experiences.
>
> Who helped you to achieve your outcomes with regard to EBP? For example who helped you to learn how to use evidence in a planned nursing intervention? What resources were available in the practice placement to help you to achieve this? What barriers, if any, did you come across that hindered your finding that evidence?

However this is not the case. It is in fact related to their position in the organization, regardless of age or length of qualification in terms of registration. This lack of confidence in implementing EBP can of course also be seen in newly qualified nurses, but it is a general issue and not just limited to EBP (Ferguson & Day 2007).

It could be argued that given these two perspectives, developing the knowledge and skills of individuals in relation to implementing EBP (who seemingly, as outlined in Gerrish et al. 2008, lacked confidence) is essential if the newly qualified nurse is to develop confidence and be exposed to role models who use EBP in their work.

Utilizing evidence of any kind in practice and using it to implement any change, if necessary, does not however rely on using one piece of evidence but normally a body of evidence, that is a number of research studies which support the need for change in how care is delivered. As a qualified nurse you will be expected to develop an understanding of the body of evidence which underpins the care of the patients in your area of work, to ensure that the best and most appropriate care is delivered. This could be a body of evidence in relation to the need for good nutrition during ill health or something with a more clinical focus such as pressure ulcer prevention.

As a student nurse you will be expected to learn to use evidence in practice and there are specific learning outcomes in relation to this from nursing professional bodies, including the Nursing and Midwifery Council (NMC) in the UK (NMC 2004; NMC 2007). It is important to note here that the NMC is undertaking a review of these but that it is very clear that understanding the research process, current nursing research, and the application of this in evidence-based care remains central to the development of the new competencies which will become available this year (see NMC website for further details: http://www.nmc-uk.org/)

Utilizing evidence in practice: meeting the professional body requirements

As noted in Chapter 1 there are a number of Standards of Proficiency linked to EBP (NMC 2004) that a student has to attain in order to become a registered nurse. It is important that a student gains experience in practice in order to be able to do this.

We shall now consider some ways of achieving the following two current competencies (NMC 2004):

1. Identify relevant changes in practice or new information and disseminate to colleagues
2. Ensure that current research findings and other evidence are incorporated into practice

You may be asked to demonstrate these in a theoretical assignment which draws on practice experience as well (see Chapter 9), but for the purpose of this chapter we are focusing on how you would demonstrate achievement in practice. Examples from all four branches of nursing will be explored. It is important to note that the following example is just *one way* in which you could demonstrate use of evidence in practice, and that you should work with your tutors and mentors to identify other ways in which you could illustrate your developing understanding and use of evidence in practice.

✛

EBP in action

You are a final year student nurse and have to achieve the outcome in Point 1 above. You and your mentor have agreed that you will develop an evidence based information package for your placement and that you will also disseminate the evidence to a small number of staff and students. At this stage you only need to determine the evidence base and disseminate your findings.

Developing an evidence-based information package

What are the first things to consider in order to achieve this?

The first issue to consider is obviously the *choice of topic*. The second is **how to find and possibly obtain some of this evidence**; Thirdly **how you will organize this evidence in an information package**. Fourthly **how you will disseminate the findings**.

Many of the other chapters in this book will help you with these steps.

Choosing a topic

Depending on your placement, and whether you have specific topics to consider for a practice-based assessment, some possible topic examples for the information packages are provided below for you to consider:

1. Pain management in adults following surgery (adult nursing).
2. Parental involvement in caring for children in hospital (children's nursing).

3. Use of cognitive behaviour therapy with older people experiencing anxiety and depression (mental health nursing).

4. The role of the learning disability nurse in caring for young adults with learning disability (learning disability nursing).

Using these as examples for 'identifying relevant changes in practice or new information' we consider each in turn. The examples relate to each of the four fields of practice (NMC 2008a) or branches of mental health nursing, adult nursing, children's nursing, and learning disability nursing. However all pre-registration students need to experience exposure to all these. Later we will return to these same examples and examine how the findings could be incorporated into practice. To learn more about **finding** the evidence you can refer to Chapter 6 and Chapter 7 for **evaluating** this evidence.

Developing the information package

All of the four evidence-based information packages will require a structure, which will depend in part on the focus of the topic. This is unlike a learning package where there is an expectation that there are specific learning outcomes to be undertaken with regards the content. For example, you could be expected to demonstrate your knowledge of the theory of learning underpinning your learning package or you could build in test questions in the form of a quiz which tests knowledge on the content.

To convert the kind of information package we are discussing into one where learning can also occur, you could design questions and answers or quizzes and similar exercises which can engage the learner. Consider some of the ones in this book for example. You could also use a patient case study to illustrate how all the evidence can be used. Developing an information package for use by other students and mentors in practice is an excellent way to develop your knowledge and understanding of all the evidence required to care for a patient. (On a practical note you can use an A4 file with dividers for each section and possibly some plastic wallets if you need to include leaflets or to keep the information you are provided relatively clean etc. You may also want to include information already available in the placement to give to patients/clients.)

Converting the information package into a learning package where there is a 'testing' or checking of that knowledge and understanding could be easily achieved with the support of your academic supervisor or colleagues in practice. If you do decide to do this please remember to provide the answers or refer the person undertaking the exercises to further reading which will give them the answers. Examples of these can be found on the online website.

Often patient-related care studies which require the student to determine evidence-based practice and possible outcomes can be included. Let us consider this in the context of one of the topics identified.

Information package 1: Pain management in adults following surgery

Any information package on pain management will require an introduction to pain and how and why it occurs post-operatively. This will require some evidence from physiology books and articles relating to the physiological manifestation of pain. As the focus is on pain management post-operatively there will be a need to include a section on what is involved in caring for a patient who has had surgery. The content list could therefore look like this:

1. Title of information package: Pain management in adults following surgery
2. Contents page
3. Introduction to surgery and the kinds of surgery you might come across in this clinical placement
4. Caring for patients in the pre- and post-operative period
5. Post-operative pain and the causes
6. The physiology of pain
7. Nursing management of post-operative pain
8. The evidence base for managing post-operative pain
9. Reference list
10. List of related resources and websites

For example, consider the care of a patient who has undergone surgery for removal of a bowel tumour.

Case study Mrs Glenda Williams

Mrs Glenda Williams aged 58 years has undergone major surgery for removal a tumour in the large colon and has had to have a permanent colostomy.

As well as experiencing varying degrees of pain post-operatively as a result of the surgery she will also have other needs which may impact on how she perceives and experiences this pain. To help this patient you should demonstrate your knowledge of the surgery she has had, why it has had to be undertaken and the long-term implications for her with regards to managing the **colostomy**. (Definition: where there is a surgically created and fashioned opening directly into the bowel from the surface of the abdomen and through which faeces can pass into an appropriate bag.)

We can use this case study to focus on key issues (points 7 & 8) in this information package outline and also help you to understand how using different kinds of evidence helps you to care for patients experiencing pain:

a. Nursing management of post-operative pain
b. The evidence base for managing post-operative pain

To determine her needs both pre-and post-operatively you will have had to assess and plan her care, taking account of the evidence base to ensuring that a safe environment is maintained for her (both internally and externally). A nursing model that could be used to help you to do this is the Roper, Logan and Tierney Model of Nursing (Holland *et al.* 2008), as the activity of living: maintaining a safe environment, is an essential aspect of Mrs Williams's care. Pain will be an actual problem experienced in the post-operative period, and how patients experience this will differ. Carr & Thomas (1997: 194) identified that 'nine out of ten patients, when asked if they had experienced pain since their operation, said they had'. However there was 'a significant difference between patients' expected and experienced worst pain'.

During your clinical placement you will be talking to many patients who have undergone an operation. Consider how they have expressed their needs with regards to pain and pain control. How different were they? How did the nurses assess their level of pain? They may well have used an evidence-based pain assessment tool such as the Wong–Baker Faces Pain Rating Scale (Wong & Whalley 1986) or a 0–10 Numeric Rating Scale (McCaffery & Beebe 1983). You can include an example of this in your information package. A useful website for many topics on pain management is http://pain-topics.org/clinical_concepts/assess.php/. This is a particularly useful site for accessing pain assessment tools for children and older adults. A very useful paper on assessing pain in patients who are unable to verbalize or self-report their pain is the study by Herr *et al.* (2006).

It is essential however that in order to understand the evidence for managing pain by the patient and by the nurse you have an underpinning knowledge of the physiology of pain. For example in managing pain by the nurse there will be a need to offer medication post-operatively and the evidence for how this works will link directly to your understanding of the physiology. (See Allen 2005: 140–145; Davies & Taylor 2003: 111–131; Duke 2006: 735–761.).

+··

EBP in action

Imagine that Mrs Williams' husband asks you to explain to him and his wife why she is having pain relief via the 'pain pump'. What is the evidence base for choosing to give patient-controlled analgesia (PCA)?

··

You can discuss this with your mentor and agree what you are going to say. You will not of course be quoting references to them in your explanation of the reasons why the PCA is the preferred choice for providing pain relief but you can include these in your information pack. What you tell them will be based on this evidence. For example one of the major benefits of PCA is that patient has control of the pain relief, which has psychological benefits and also allows for immediate delivery of pain medication without having to wait for the nurse to come. Because the pain relief is given over a period of time this is also helpful given that a larger dose given at once has a shorter impact and the possible side-effects such as nausea are more easily managed. Some patients worry about overdose or addiction to pain medication but reassurance can be given that this will not occur (see NHS Quality Improvement Scotland (2004) Post-operative Pain Management—Best Practice statement for an EBP approach; **www.nhshealthquality.org/**).

Some additional references for including in your information package which may be of value as evidence for pain assessment and pain relief in general:

Carr, E. C. J. & Thomas, V. J. (1997) Anticipating and experiencing post-operative pain: the patient's perspective. *Journal of Clinical Nursing* 6 191–201.

Manias, E., Botti, M. & Bucknall, (2002) Observation of pain assessment and management—the complexities of clinical practice. *Journal of Clinical Nursing* 11 724–733.

Nash, R. *et al.* (1999) Pain and the administration of analgesia: what nurses say. *Journal of Clinical Nursing* 8 180–189.

Royal College of Physicians of London (2007) *The assessment of pain in older people:* National Guidelines, no.8, **www.rcplondon.ac.uk/**.

Information Package 2: Parental involvement in caring for children in hospital

For those of you who are undertaking a programme to becoming a registered children's nurse, communicating with parents and carers of children will be a major part of your clinical practice experience, whether in a hospital or home/community environment. Helping others to understand all the issues involved and ensuring that you know what the evidence base is for parental involvement in care of children in hospital is therefore a very appropriate area for you to consider either in developing an information package or in writing an assignment (see Chapter 9). This information package concerns the topic of parental involvement in the care of the child in hospital.

For the structure we can consider the following:

1. Title of information package: Parental involvement in caring for children in hospital.

2. Contents page.

3. Introduction to parental involvement in caring for children in hospital.

4. Needs of parents who are caring for children in hospital.

5. Nurses responsibilities and parents in hospital.

6. Communication between nurses and parents in hospital.

7. The evidence base for parental involvement in care of the child in hospital.

8. Reference list.

9. List of related resources and websites.

You can see here, as with Information Package 1, a basic framework that you could use, ensuring however that you add your own interpretation and additional sections as necessary.

Again a case study scenario could be used to explain the evidence base for parental involvement in care. Consideration of all kinds of evidence would ensure in this package that consideration is given, in particular to the National Service Framework (NSF) for Children, Young People and Maternity Services (DH 2003a). The NSF 'sets out clear standards that the NHS and other agencies like Social Services should aim to meet' (DH 2003b), including treating children and their families with respect.

+..

Case study Emma

Emma, a 6 year old child has undergone a tonsillectomy (removal of tonsils) and the nurses are trying to get her to eat and drink post-operatively without much success. They need to know she can do this before they send her home. Her mother wanted to help with this but was unsure whether she should. She felt however that she knew her child and how to get her to do things.

What does the research evidence tell us about this scenario and how the nurses could be made aware of the issues involving parental involvement in caring for children in hospital?

....

The NSF for children (discussed above) includes considering parents as 'partners in care' and the guide for parents and carers (DH 2003b) provides an excellent summary regarding this, which could be added to the package as key references. Use the skills developed in Chapter 6 to help you to search the literature.

+..

EBP in action

Consider the following statement (from Standards for Children in Hospital: A Guide for parents and carers (DH 2003b) and find the evidence to support some of the statements identified (we have indicated in **bold** where references to evidence are needed):

*In the past parents were discouraged from being around a child staying in hospital (**find reference**). In recent years, it has been recognized that a parent or carer being with the child can usually be helpful from everyone's point of view and help provide much-needed reassurance (**find reference**). It can also speed recovery (**find reference**).*

If you are a parent you are most likely to know about any special needs your child has and how best to meet them. It also means that when your child goes home, you are more likely to know what to do to continue any treatment that might be needed. You should therefore be able to stay with your child if you want to throughout the stay in hospital and should be given somewhere on the ward or nearby to sleep (**find reference**).

*You should not feel 'in the way' as you have an important role in helping to look after your child (**find reference**) (DH 2003b).*

....

Examples of possible references which may help you with this exercise are:

Coyne, I. & Conlon, J. (2007) Children's and young people's views of hospitalization: 'It's a scary place.' *Journal of Children's and Young People's Nursing* 1 (1) 16–21.

Espezel, H. J. E. & Canam, C. J. (2003) Parent-nurse interactions: care of hospitalized children. *Journal of Advanced Nursing* 44 (1) 34–41.

Kawik, L. (1996) Nurses' and parents perceptions of participation and partnership in caring for a hospitalized child. *British Journal of Nursing* 5 (7) 430–434.

Turner, P. (1997) Establishing a protocol for parental presence in recovery. *British Journal of Nursing* 6 (14) 794–799.

Information Package 3: Use of cognitive behaviour therapy with older people experiencing anxiety and depression

Depression in older people is a major health problem, as is anxiety. Both can cause a significant impact on the life of an older person, in particular where other illnesses are also present (Bird & Parslow 2002). Managing these issues have implications for health care professionals and health care services, in terms of both human and financial costs. An understanding of how a particular treatment can be of value in helping older people will therefore be an excellent information package to develop for your learning and also for use by other students in one of your clinical placements.

For our third information package we can consider the following:

1. Title of information package: Use of cognitive behaviour therapy with older people experiencing anxiety and depression.

2. Contents page.

3. Introduction to cognitive behaviour therapy.

4. Anxiety and depression in older people.

5. Cognitive behaviour therapy and the older person.

6. Nursing role and cognitive behaviour therapy.

7. The evidence base for cognitive behaviour therapy.

8. Reference list.

9. List of related resources and websites.

An understanding of why older people become depressed and anxious will be essential. The National Association for Mental Health (MIND) has some excellent information and fact sheets on aspects of mental illness and health, including some that focus on a number of different cultural groups such as South Asian and Chinese and Vietnamese communities in Britain (see **www.mind.org.uk/**). Many can be used by students and are evidence based, including links to additional websites and resources which will be invaluable for including in your information package. Some students are told by their tutors that information obtained via searching the web is not appropriate for use in assignments and not valid evidence. This of course is dependent on *where* on the internet information is found—care needs to be taken in what material is used and development of effective searching skills will enable you to identify what is good or not so good evidence. Sites by leading specialist charities such as this one by MIND is a very valuable resource and such organizations often have their own evidence-based papers available.

+··

Case study Mr John Underhill

Mr John Underhill is a 70 year old man with a 2 year history of anxiety and depression since the death of his wife. He has been referred to a nurse behavioural therapist at a primary care practice where you are undertaking a placement. He has been told by a friend who had himself used it, about something called 'Beating the Blues' which can be used via a computer. He has access to a computer at home as he likes to email his daughter and family in Australia, more so since his wife died and he wishes they lived closer.

Learning more about the **Beating the Blues** programme and other computer-based resources, will be essential for developing this information package.

··

Your other clients as well as Mr Underhill may also have access to the World Wide Web and a computer, and this medium is also being used to deliver cognitive behaviour therapy (NICE 2006) which in a study reported by Van Den Berg *et al*. (2004) showed positive results. This paper offers some case histories of the use of the CCBT computer system package called *Beating the Blues* which Mr Underhill has been told about. An introductory session video can be found at **www.beatingtheblues.co.uk/** and it provides an introduction to depression, anxiety, and CBT through actual narratives. However as Mr Underhill has already been referred to a nurse behavioural therapist, he needs to discuss this with her/him. It is not unexpected in such situations for patients to turn up with a print out of information they have found on the world wide web, and is part of the growing trend of patients' own 'evidence-based' searching.

You may know of someone who has had experience of this programme. If possible talk to them about their experience and how useful they found it. As this programme has been through rigorous randomized control trials the NICE guidelines indicate that *Beating the Blues* is 'recommended as an option for delivering CBT in the management of mild to moderate depression'. It can be available through a general practitioner.

Some additional references which may be of help to you in planning out the rest of the information package:

Boote, J., Lewin, V., Beverley, C. & Bates, J. (2006) Psychosocial interventions for people with moderate to severe dementia: a systematic review. *Clinical Effectiveness in Nursing* 951 e1–e15.

Curran, J. & Brooker, C. (2007) Systematic review of interventions delivered by UK mental health nurses. *International Journal of Nursing Studies* 44 479–509.

Frazer, C. J., Christensen, H. & Griffths, K. M. (2005) Effectiveness of treatments for depression in older people: a systematic review. *Medical Journal of Australia* 182 (12) 627–632.

Williams, C. & Garland, A. (2002) A cognitive behavioural therapy assessment model for use in everyday clinical practice. *Advances in Psychiatric Treatment* 8 172–179.

Information package 4: The role of the learning disability nurse in caring for young adults with learning disability

Pre-registration nursing can be undertaken in four 'branches' or fields of practice of which learning disability nursing is one. In some UK universities this is combined with social work to give a dual registration. It is therefore appropriate to ask: What is the role of the learning disability nurse and how can it be best illustrated? This question is also important to all health care profession students, given that working together in a multi disciplinary and inter-professional way is important to the delivery of integrated services. You may choose to develop this evidence-based information package for an acute surgical ward or a community health care practice.

Northway *et al.* (2006) edited a report called *Shaping the Future: a vision for learning disability nursing* published by the UK Learning Disability Consultant Nurse Network. This Network believes that:

> " *in order for the learning disability nursing profession to progress into the 21st Century, that it needs a shared vision to promote, articulate and drive the distinct identity and unique expertise of the learning disability nurse.* "
>
> (Northway *et al.* 2006: 3)

The report describes the changing role of the learning disability nurse, parallel with the changes that have taken place in moving from the more 'closed institutional settings' to community-based practice (Northway *et al.* 2006: 6). It is clear that caring for people with learning disabilities involves meeting both physical and mental health needs (Brown 2005). Let us consider these health needs in the context of young adults:

1. Title of information package: The role of the learning disability nurse and health education needs of young adults with learning disability.

2. Contents page.

3. The role of the learning disability nurse.

4. The health needs of young adults with learning disability.

5. Health education and young adults with learning disability.

6. Caring for young people with learning disabilities in the community: the key issues.

7. The evidence base for learning disability nursing and health education role.

8. Reference list.

9. List of related resources and websites.

Developing this package would ensure that you learn not only about the role of learning disability nurses but also how to approach health education with people who have learning difficulties—based on the evidence of how to meet their needs generally. Talking to qualified learning disability nurses about their role is another excellent way to understand what your future role will be (if you are a learning disability nursing student) as is talking to your future client group.

Case study Michael

Michael aged 24 years, a young man with a learning disability, has started to attend a local College. He has made friends with two young men in his group both of whom smoke and as a result he has also started to do the same. Unfortunately he has mild asthma and smoking is making it worse.

He has agreed after talking to his parents to attend the Stop Smoking group at his local health centre.

The searching and retrieving of evidence for this information package may also help you if you are a smoker trying to give up cigarettes! Northway *et al*. (2006: 29) state that:

> 66 *all learning disability nurses, regardless of the setting in which they work, have a health promotion element within their role* 99

As part of your package you can obtain copies of support materials from the NHS Go Smokefree campaign: Easy read leaflets see **http://gosmokefree.nhs.uk/quit-tools/for further details/**. The one appropriate for Michael would be Easy Read Leaflet—Go Smokefree Guide—aimed specifically at people with learning difficulties. This website can be included in your information package. Another excellent website is the Trip database for evidence-based medicine—which you can use to access evidence-based material at a large number of other World Wide Websites: **http://www.tripdatabase.com/**. Accessing this site enabled me to find another resource: Meeting the health needs of people with learning disabilities: Guidance for nursing staff (RCN 2006).

A small study by Whitaker & Hughes (2003: 92) was carried out 'to find the prevalence of smoking in people with learning disabilities who attended the local Social Education Centres and the local Technical College' as well as what their knowledge about the effects of smoking and whether there was a relationship between those who smoked and with their carers smoking behaviour. They found only a small number of people with learning disabilities who smoked in those two environments. There was an influence on those who smoked with who they lived with who smoked—which is something to be considered for Michael. The researchers recognized that their study was limited but that further research needed to be undertaken on the smoking behaviour of people with learning disabilities.

Two other studies which you might find of value in understanding smoking behaviour in people with learning disabilities are:

McGuire, Daly & Smyth (2007) Lifestyle and health behaviours of adults with an intellectual disability. *Journal of Intellectual Disability Research*, 51 (7) 497–510.

Taylor *et al*. (2004) Smoking prevalence and knowledge of associated risks in adult attenders at day centres for people with learning disabilities. *Journal of Intellectual Disability Research*, 48 (3) 239–244.

And two articles related to nursing disability nursing are:

Barr, O. (2004) Nurses for people with learning disabilities within the United Kingdom: Some challenges for the future. *International Journal of Nursing in Intellectual and Developmental Disabilities* 1 (1) 5. **http://journal.hsmc.org/ijnidd/**

Mitchell, D. (2000) Parallel Stigma? Nurses and people with learning disabilities. *British Journal of Learning Disabilities*, 28 (2) 78–81.

Dissemination of evidence

Dissemination of the evidence you have gathered in the course of this exercise in developing an information package could be undertaken in a number of ways. Only a brief overview is given here of one example of a dissemination activity. More detailed explanations and learning exercises can be found in Chapter 10.

Once you have developed the packages or even as part of these, you can consider how you need to share with others in the practice area what you have found. You may have had to develop the package as well for an assignment and it is hoped that the exploration in this chapter of some of the key issues to include will be of value.

Dissemination of evidence is essential in order to develop nursing practice and also to enable others to use this evidence in their own work. It is assumed that you will disseminate your findings to colleagues in practice, and this can take place as part of your goals for learning, or even if you are in the final year of the programme as part of a teaching session to other students.

Let us consider that in each of these case studies you will have 30 minutes in which to share part of the information package findings. You have decided to talk to a small group of other students on the ward and are going to use the package to disseminate what you have found and will also use it as a teaching opportunity. Teaching students is an essential skill required of a qualified nurse and as such an essential part of role development for a student nurse in the final year of their programme. There are some important points to consider when you are teaching students and these are identified below:

Here are some key steps for you to consider:

Dissemination of evidence to student nurses: a teaching session

A. Decide what you are going to disseminate (the topic).

B. What the aims of the session are (what you want the other students to learn).

C. Decide on how you are going to disseminate (you may not be able to use an overhead projector in the practice area nor use a computer for a PowerPoint presentation) so you may need to use a handout, and especially if it is part of your assessment in the placement.

D. Whatever means you are going to use make sure you have all the key points of the session clearly identified.

E. Provide some key references or refer the students to your information package— you can also show them this and tell them where to find it.

F. Leave enough time to enable the students to ask you questions—especially about the information package and how you developed it.

G. Consider how you can find out if and what they have learnt from the session. You could consider asking no more than five questions on the chosen topic.

Consider this framework in relation to the case study in Information Package 1: Pain management in adults following surgery. Please remember that this is only an example for the purpose of illustrating what kind of dissemination activity you as a student nurse can undertake. It can also help you to demonstrate your understanding of research studies and how theory and practice work together to inform others and influence how they undertake their care of patients/clients.

Dissemination example

1. The topic I have chosen to talk to you about is: Managing the pain of patients post-operatively.

2. The aims of my session are:
   a. to explain why patients have pain post- operatively
   b. what kind of medication is available for relieving pain post-operatively
   c. describe three research studies which have looked at the use of pain assessment tools
   d. offer some conclusions about which pain tool might be used on this ward
   e. to determine what you (the audience) have learnt from the session.

As the presenter you would then use these three aims as the basis of your presentation—remembering you only have 30 minutes in total. You could consider the information in 5 minute sections, thus allowing 5 minutes for discussion at the end. The main consideration is for you to have an opportunity to show what you have learnt through your searching for information to include in your package.

You can discuss your plan with your mentor. A mentor is the person who is named as your main supervisor, teacher, and assessor in a clinical placement. Mentors support students and help them to achieve their learning outcomes through enabling them to access varied learning experiences in a practice placement (see *Nursing Study and Placement Skills* by Hart 2010).

Utilizing evidence in practice: delivery of nursing care

As well as needing to meet the NMC Standard outcomes as seen in Chapter 1, there are also those specific outcomes related to the *Essential Skills Clusters* (NMC 2007). These are skills-based outcomes which nevertheless are supported by an evidence and knowledge base.

As with all nursing practice it is an opportunity to consider both the theory and the evidence behind why we carry out care skills. Some examples of Essential Skills, along with statements of how the student nurse can demonstrate these through being 'tested on their knowledge' and their 'performance' of the actual essential skill itself can be seen below in Box 8.1. These can be considered in terms of what evidence you can use to help you to achieve these and will be discussed in turn. (Please note the numbering applies to the original numbering used in NMC documents.)

Let us consider these in relation to the evidence required.

Essential skills 1: Organizational aspects of care

Assessment and planning of care and application of evidence to practice

You are expected to be able to demonstrate how you undertake an assessment of the needs of a patient/client, both holistically and systematically. You are then expected to develop a plan of care for the patient/client taking into account what will promote their health and well-being and minimizes risk of harm. Underpinned by this is your ability to apply evidence to practice.

Obviously this will be achieved as part of your 'fitness for practice' as a qualified nurse and all these Essential Skills will be built into your practice assessment documents.

To achieve this Essential Skill will require you to know why assessment and planning care are important and that these are different stages of the nursing process.

> **Box 8.1** Examples of essential skills (NMC 2007)
>
> 1. For entry to the register: Essential Skill: Organisational Aspects of Care:
>
> Patients can trust a newly registered nurse to:
>
> **9. Make a holistic and systematic assessment of their needs and develop a comprehensive plan of nursing care that is in their best interests and which promotes their health and well-being and minimizes the risk of harm.**
>
> > Demonstrated by: Applies evidence to practice.
>
> **16. Safely lead and manage care**
>
> > Demonstrated by: Bases decisions on evidence and uses experience to guide decision-making.
>
> **20. Select and manage medical devices safely**
>
> > Demonstrated by: Works within legal frameworks and applies evidence-based practice in the safe selection and use of medical devices.
>
> 2. For entry to the register: Essential Skills: Medicines Management:
>
> **41: Use and evaluate up to date information on medicines management and work within national and local policies.**
>
> > Demonstrated by: Accesses commonly used evidence-based sources relating to the safe and effective management of medicines.

You may also use a nursing model or framework which will enable you to do this in order to ensure a holistic and systematic approach.

To assess patient/client needs in any given practice placement you will be expected to know what the reason is behind your assessment, for example if your placement was in a surgical ward you would be expected to know that before patients have their surgery you would need to undertake baseline observations such as taking a blood pressure. However if during the assessment you find out that the patient is in fact a smoker what evidence would determine your plan of care to minimize the risk of potential problems post-operatively ? There is 'a body of evidence describing increased perioperative complications in smokers' (Stechman *et al.* 2004) and smoking clearly has a potential negative effect on wound healing (Pudner 2002). As part of your care plan for any patient who has not given up cigarettes it will be essential that you identify this and plan to help them to give it up post operatively.

Safely lead and manage care: basing decisions on evidence

Making decisions based on evidence implies that you will have been taught to do this in both the university and practice settings. Garret (2005: 38) undertook a study to explore

> 66 *what were final year graduate nursing students expectations and perceptions and their views of the value of clinical decision-making skills in their role as qualified nurses'. He found that they 'were aware of the requirements for professional practice but lacked the confidence in their own ability to make decisions'.* 99

? **Thinking about**

Consider a situation in practice where you have observed your mentor making a decision about patient/client care. What did he/she base that decision on? Was it clearly based on research evidence or on some other form of evidence?

Thompson (2003) for example found that nurses relied on experiential knowledge and intuition in clinical decision-making rather than systematic evidence-based knowledge for most of their 'day to day clinical decisions'. Welsh & Lyons (2001: 299) however stressed that:

> 66 *it is not always appropriate to disregard the tacit knowledge and intuition of experienced practitioners when making assessment decisions in mental health nursing practice.* 99

Unlike a student nurse however an experienced practitioner has a wealth of varied experiences to draw upon in any decision-making situation and consequently engages in expert practice (Benner 1984). As a student nurse however expert practice is something you will not as yet be able to provide. In certain situations there will not be research-based evidence on which to base your decisions; however, it is important that as a qualified nurse you make every attempt to do so.

Consider the example used by Thompson (2003) in Box 8.2 to illustrate how a nurse's confidence in what she was doing in terms of an 'evidence base' affected her practice. In this case 'evidence' was sought which altered the staff nurse's decision-making.

In this example however the 'research' evidence has been pursued through a 'decision audit', or in this case a small patient survey of effectiveness of an established pain control protocol.

As a student nurse you will not however be in a position to instigate this kind or level of decision-making. However you can learn from it in terms of not accepting current or established practice without questioning the evidence. It is important to ask questions if you are not sure of why a certain practice is undertaken and very often student nurses can bring to their clinical placements examples of recent evidence which their

Box 8.2 Clinical experience as evidence

Imagine that you are a staff nurse working on a day surgery unit. You have an informal analgesia protocol that you apply to most of your patients with hernia repairs because you are fairly confident (based on a couple of years' experience) that it works and that patients get a few hours relatively pain free at home after they have left the unit. However you have not really stopped to consider whether there are better alternatives, and you realize that you receive no feedback on whether the pain relief carries on working in the hours after discharge. You decide that if the pain relief was not effective after discharge that you would—in all probability—try and devise something better. You decide to 'test' whether your confidence is justified. You arrange for one of your colleagues or yourself to administer a pain measurement scale to each patient before leaving the ward and then phone them within 6 hours of discharge and simply ask them to complete it again and send it back. The findings surprise you, and you realize that in fact a large proportion of patients' pain is not well managed by the protocol after discharge. Obviously you would not have received this information if you had not sought feedback on your initial decision choice. Clearly you now have a solid footing for a more evidence-based approach to revision of the pain relief protocol, and repeat the 'decision audit' at a later date to see if this has worked.

(From: Thompson, C. (2003) Clinical experience as evidence in evidence-based practice. *Journal of Advanced Nursing* 43 (3) 230–237.)

tutors will have given them. It is important to note that evidence-based teaching is as important as EBP.

In considering the example by Thompson (2003) what kind of decision-making would you be involved with in relation to a patient or client and what would be based on evidence or experience?

Consider for example a patient who arrived at the Accident and Emergency Department, very agitated, talked about being depressed, and thinking about committing suicide.

There is evidence to suggest that there is a link between suicide and depression and one decision that could be made in the Accident and Emergency Department is to assess the risk of suicide during triage (Sands 2007). This is a decision which is clearly based on a substantive body of evidence, that has been translated into a nursing assessment tool.

Select and manage medical devices safely: applies evidence-based practice in the safe selection and use of medical devices

The increased use of medical devices by nurses has meant that it is essential for students to learn not only how to use them safely but also how to participate in evaluating and choosing appropriate ones. In a study by McDonnell *et al.* (2007) nurses, patients, and medical staff evaluated a disposable device for patient-controlled intravenous analgesia and found 'high levels of staff and patient satisfaction with the device'. One of the advantages was:

> *❝ compared with an electronic pump is that siphoning under gravity or excessive drug delivery cannot occur, so patient safety cannot be compromised in this way. ❞*
>
> (McDonnell 2007: 75)

A study undertaken in 1993 by McConnell & Fletcher focused on how registered nurses learn about device use. They stressed that 'nurses must be knowledgeable about the devices they use on behalf of the patients and that 'health care organisations in which nurses work as well as schools of nursing from which they graduate, are accountable and responsible for educating them about device use' (McConnell & Fletcher 1993: 1593).

A possible definition of a medical device which you can use to consider these questions is any piece of equipment used in the treatment or care of patients; this could also relate to that used in diagnosis as well.

❓ Thinking about

Consider your own experience to date.

How many devices have you seen used in clinical practice? How did you learn to use these and how did you know that this was evidence based?

You should not use any medical device unless you have received both written and verbal instructions on its use and then only under the guidance and supervision of a qualified nurse. The NHS Trust in which you will work on qualifying will have policies on the management and use of medical devices. These usually outline who can use different kinds of devices, what training is required and provided, as well as a list of those used in different areas. Examples of devices are: infusion devices, defibrillators, tympanic thermometers, blood pressure/vital signs monitoring equipment, glucose monitoring equipment. You may have come across all or few of these depending on your placements.

Essential Skills 2: Medicines management

Note: (The student) accesses commonly used evidence-based sources relating to the safe and effective management of medicines.

Medicines and the giving of them will be a core element of your practice learning, and you may also have experienced learning in the clinical skills laboratories in your university in addition to learning how drugs work (pharmacology). The NMC (2008b) has now published their Standards for Medicines Management for Qualified Nurses, which covers everything from dispensing, storing, transporting, and disposal of medicines to the standards for practice of administration of medicines (it would be advisable to access this document for your own reference as it contains a summary of the Standards published).

+ ··
  ### EBP in action

  Obtain a copy of the NMC Standards in the UK or those in your own country and consider the implications for you as a qualified nurse.
  ··

These are some articles which will help you to consider the evidence base to some of the Standards.

Banning, M. (2003) Pharmacology education: a theoretical framework of applied pharmacology and therapeutics, *Nurse Education Today* 23 459–466.

Banning, M. (2003) The use of structured assessments, practical skills and performance indicators to assess the ability of pre-registration nursing students' to apply the principles of pharmacology and therapeutics to the medication management needs of patients, *Nurse Education in Practice* 4 100–106.

Cowan, D. *et al.* (2002) Medicine Management in care homes for older people: the nurse's role. *British Journal of Community Nursing* 7 (12) 634–638.

Preston, R. M. (2004) Drug errors and patient safety: the need for a change in practice, *British Journal of Nursing* 13 (2) 72–78.

Summary

In this chapter we have seen the importance of using evidence in nursing care and how you as a student nurse can develop the skills to consider EBP in your learning to be a nurse.

- It is essential in order to ensure that all patients/clients receive the best possible care and that nurses base their practice on the best evidence.
- Developing the skills to determine this best evidence is a priority as are the skills to be confident in deciding which evidence to use.
- Implementing evidence-based practice however is not without its challenges, including finding out what the evidence is and sharing this with your colleagues to begin with and then having the support to change practice based on that evidence.
- As a student you will learn other skills which will enable you to do this and develop your confidence to be able to challenge practice which is not based on a sound evidence base.
- We recognize that not all nursing practice is based on evidence from research findings.
- Nursing is and possibly will always be a complex rich activity where valid decisions are made on evidence not easily explained.

- Learning to be a nurse is learning how to balance decisions which can clearly be based on research evidence from that which is based on intuition and experiential knowledge.

■ Online resource centre

 To find out more about the dissemination of evidences into learning packages and other resources, please go online to: **www.oxfordtextbooks.co.uk/orc/holland/**

■ References

Allen, D. (2005) The central nervous system. In: Montague. S., Watson, R. & Herbert, R. A. (eds) *Physiology for Nursing Practice (3rd edn)*. Edinburgh: Elsevier.

Benner, P. (2004) *From Novice to Expert*. California: Addison-Wesley Publishing Co.

Bird, M. J. & Parslow, R. A. (2002) Potential for community programs to prevent depression in older people, *eMedical Journal of Australia* 177, S107–110 http://www.mja.com.au/

Brown, M. (2005) Promoting Health, Supporting Inclusion: Developments in the nursing and midwifery contributions to improving the health of people with intellectual disabilities in Scotland. *International Journal of Nursing in Intellectual and development Disabilities* 2, (1).

Carr, E. C. J. & Thomas, V. J. (1997) Anticipating and experiencing post-operative pain: the patient's perspective. *Journal of Clinical Nursing* 6 191–201.

Cox, C. L. & Ahluwalia, S. (2000) Enhancing clinical effectiveness among clinical nursing specialists. *British Journal of Nursing* 9 (16) 1064–1073.

Davies, K. & Taylor, A. (2003) Pain. In: Brooker, C. & Nichol, M (eds), *Nursing Adults—the practice of caring*. Edinburgh: Mosby, Elsevier.

Department of Health (2003a) *National Service Framework for Children, Young People and Maternity Services*. London: DH.

Department of Health (2003b) *Standards for Children in Hospital: a guide for parents and carers*. London: DH.

Duke, S. (2006) Pain. In: Alexander, M. F., Tonks, J., Fawcett, N. & Runciman, P. J. (eds) *Nursing Practice Hospital and Home—the adult, (3rd edn)*. Edinburgh: Churchill Livingstone, Elsevier.

Ferguson, L. M. & Day, R. A. (2007) Challenges for new nurses in evidence-based practice. *Journal of Nursing Management* 15, 107–113.

Garrret, B. (2005) Student nurses' perceptions of clinical decision-making in the final year of adult nursing studies. *Nurse Education in Practice* 5, 30–39.

Gerrish, K., Ashworth, P., Lacey, A. & Bailey, J. (2008) Developing evidence-basedpractice: experiences of senior and junior clinical nurses. *Journal of Advanced Nursing* 62 (1) 62–73.

Hart, S. (2010) *Nursing Study and Placement Skills*. Oxford: Oxford University Press.

Herr, K., Coyne, P. J., Key, T., Manworren, R., McCaffrey, M., Merkel, S., Pelosi-Kelly, J. & Wild, L. (2006) Pain assessment in the nonverbal patient; position statement with clinical practice recommendations. *Pain Management Nursing* 7 (2) 44–52.

Holland, K., Jenkins, J., Solomon, J. & Whittam, S. (2008) *Applying the Roper, Logan & Tierney Model in Practice* (*2nd edn*). Edinburgh: Elsevier.

Koehn, M. L. & Lehman, (2008) Nurses' perceptions of evidence-based nursing practice. *Journal of Advanced Nursing* 62 (2) 209–215.

McCaffery, M. & Beebe, A. (1983) Pain: *Clinical Manual for Nursing Practice*, V V Mosby Co, Baltimore (cited by National Institutes of Health–Warren Grant Magnuson Clinical Centre **painconsortium.nih.gov/pain_scales/NumericRatingScale.pdf**).

McConnell, E. A. & Fletcher, J. (1993) Australian Registered nurse medical device education: a comparison of life-sustaining and non-life sustaining devices. *Journal of Advanced Nursing* 18 (10) 1586–1594.

McDonnell, N., Kwei, P. & Paech, M. (2007) A disposable device for patient-controlled intravenous analgesia: Evaluation by patients, nursing and medical staff. *Acute Pain* 9, 71–75.

McKenna, H. P., Ashton, S. & Keeney, S. (2004) Barriers to evidence-based practice in primary care. *Journal of Advanced Nursing* 45 (2) 178–189.

McSherry, R. & Haddock, J. (1999) Evidence-based health care: its place within clinical governance. *British Journal of Nursing* 8 (2) 113–117.

Nagy, S., Lumby, J., McKinley, S. & Macfarlane, C. (2001) Nurses' beliefs about the conditions that hinder or support evidenc-based nursing. *International Journal of Nursing Practice* 7 314–321.

Newman, M., Papadopoulos, I. & Sigworth, J. (1998) Barriers to evidence-based practice. *Clinical Effectiveness in Nursing* 2, 11–20.

NHS Executive (1996) Promiting Clinical Effectiveness: a framework for action in and through the NHS: In NHS Executive (1998) *Achieving Effective Practice* - a clinical effectiveness and research information pack for nurses, midwives and health visitors. Leeds: NHS (accessed on DH website).

NHS Quality Improvement Scotland (2004) *Postoperative Pain Management. NHS Quality Improvement Scotland, Edinburgh.*

National Institute for Health and Clinical Excellence (2006) *Computerized Cognitive Behaviour Therapy for Depression and Anxiety.* London: NICE.

Northway, R. Hutchinson, C. & Kingdon, A. (2006) *Shaping the Future: a vision for learning disability nursing.* UK Learning Disability Consultant Nurse Network.

Nursing and Midwifery Council (2004) *Standards of Proficiency for Pre-registration Nursing Education.* London: NMC.

Nursing and Midwifery Council (2007) *Essential Skills Clusters for Pre-registration Nursing Programmes.* London, NMC, Annexe 2 to NMC circular 07/2007.

Nursing and Midwifery Council (2008a) *Confirmed Principles to Support a New Framework for Pre-Registration Nursing Education.* London: NMC.

Nursing and Midwifery Council (2008b) *Standards for Medicine Management.* London: NMC.

Palfreyman, S., Tod, A. & Doyle, J. (2003) Comparing evidence-based practice of nurses and physiotherapists. *British Journal of Nursing* 12 (4) 246–253.

Pudner, R. (2002) Cigarette smoking and its effect on wound healing. *Journal of Community Nursing Online* 16 (8) 19–24.

Royal College of Nursing (2006) *Meeting the Health Needs of People with Learning Disabilities: guidance for nursing staff*. London: RCN.

Sands, N. (2007) Assessing the risk of suicide at triage. *Australasian Emergency Nursing Journal* 10, 161–163.

Scally, G. & Donaldson, L. J. (1998) The NHS's 50 anniversary. Clinical governance and the drive for quality improvement in the new NHS in England. *British Medical Journal* 317, 61–65.

Stechman, M. J., Healy, J., McMillan, R. & McWhinnie, D. (2004) Is current advice on smoking prior to day surgery in the United Kingdom appropriate? *Journal of One-Day Surgery* 14 (1) 5–8.

Thompson, C. (2003) Clinical experience as evidence in evidence-based practice. *Journal of Advanced Nursing* 43 (3) 230–237.

Tod, A., Palfreyman, S. & Burke, L. (2004) Evidence-based practice is a time of opportunity for nursing. *British Journal of Nursing* 13 (4) 211–216.

Van den Berg, S., Shapiro, D. A., Bickerstaffe, D. & Cavanagh, K. (2004) Computerized cognitive-behaviour therapy for anxiety and depression: a practical solution to the shortage of trained therapists. *Journal of Psychiatric and Mental Health Nursing* 11 508–513.

Welsh, I. & Lyons, C. M. (2001) Evidence-based care and the case for intuition and tacit knowledge in clinical assessment and decision making in mental health nursing practice: an empirical contribution to the debate. *Journal of Psychiatric and Mental Health Nursing* 8 299–305.

Whitaker, S. & Hughes, M. (2003) Prevalence and influences on smoking in people with learning disabilities. *British Journal of Developmental Disabilities* 49 Part 2 (97) 91–97.

Wong, D. & Whalley, L. (eds) (1986) *Clinical Handbook of Paediatric Nursing*, C V Mosby Company, St Louis (cited by National Institutes of Health–Warren Grant Magnuson Clinical Centre. **painconsortium.nih.gov/pain_scales/Wong-Baker_Faces.pdf** /).

■ Further reading

Craig, J. V. & Smyth, R. L. (2007) *The Evidence-based Practice Manual for Nurses*. Edinburgh: Churchill Livingstone.

■ Useful websites

Pain treatment topics:

http://pain-topics.org/clinical_concepts/assess.php/

Mental health needs of different cultural groups

http://www.mind.org.uk/Information/Factsheets/Diversity/

NHS Scotland Clinical Governance Resources and websites

http://www.clinicalgovernance.scot.nhs.uk/section6/Resources.asp/

9

Utilizing research and evidence-based practice in assignment work

Karen Holland

The aims of the chapter are:

➤ To explore how research and evidence-based practice can be used in the following student assignments:

➤ A literature review as an assignment

➤ A nursing practice-related essay or care study

➤ An broad topic essay

➤ A dissertation

➤ A research proposal

➤ To enable students to reference the evidence using the Harvard and Vancouver reference systems.

➤ To offer guidance on good practice in writing assignments.

Introduction

As a student undertaking a programme of study leading to both a professional and academic award you will be required to undertake a variety of assignments, usually as part of a module or unit of learning. Most of the academic-related assignments will require an evidence base or supporting literature. This chapter will focus on these assignments, although we recognize that your practice assessments may well include you having to demonstrate gathering information on topics within the clinical placements. This may require that you use your searching skills as seen in Chapter 6.

Some modules may also require that you present the evidence you have gathered to colleagues and this activity will be considered in Chapter 10.

It is not possible to consider all assignments that you may be asked to undertake as each university will have its own curriculum and assessment strategy. However some key types of assignments have been identified as the focus to the chapter. In addition it is essential that we revisit the use of two different reference systems and how to create reference lists and a bibliography. It is not a chapter however that will teach you how to write, but the basic principles of writing will be looked at.

A literature review

As we have seen in Chapter 6 searching and retrieving evidence is usually undertaken for various reasons. One of them is to enable a researcher to determine which research articles or other documents such as Department of Health policies would be important to support the evidence base of their research studies. Researchers would then critically review that evidence (see Chapter 7) and either include or exclude it from their work. This is called reviewing the literature and you will often see in either a research article or research study a section called: A literature review (see Chapter 3). Here the researcher presents the written evidence of the work they have undertaken, ensuring that it clearly demonstrates evidence of critiquing the literature identified (this is discussed in Chapter 7). Depending on the level of study you are pursuing you may well see another term which is also used with regards to reviewing the literature: critical analysis. This means that you need to be able to consider all the different opinions or evidence available in an objective way and then present a well reasoned and constructed point of view. It is not just describing what you have read but is about having your own views about what is being said, and then justifying this with supporting evidence: that is a well constructed argument. We will be returning to this later in the chapter.

Students also have to undertake a similar activity to a research study literature review as part of an assignment or an essay, in order to support the points they are making. Many such assignments will have credit and marks awarded for how well this is undertaken. Some assignments however ask students to undertake a literature review on its own and it is this kind of assignment that will be discussed here.

Writing a literature review

An broad example of this kind of assignment would be as follows in Box 9.1:

Obviously this is not exactly how your assignment guidelines would be written as they would have very specific issues related to your programme, module, or university. There may also be marking guidelines and information on what reference system to use. Further more general information is usually found in either a module handbook or programme handbook. For the purpose of this chapter however we will use the general principles outlined in the following example.

> ### Box 9.1 Assignment example
>
> You are required to identify a topic that is related to your specific area of practice or a more general health-related focus. You may have already had questions about why certain practices are undertaken and what the evidence base was in relation to care decisions. You are then required to undertake a review of the literature on the topic.
>
> Areas to include in the presentation of the literature review would be: search and retrieving strategy and databases used, rationale for choosing this topic, how it relates to practice and how the findings of your literature review could be used to support either a change in practice or the evidence base to current practice.

Let us consider the above assignment, which asks that you choose a topic you may be interested in. Here are some examples of practice specific ones related to the four fields (branches) of practice:

1. Pain management and children.
2. Death and bereavement in hospital and how nurses manage this.
3. Self-harm in women.
4. The needs of people with learning difficulties who are diabetic.

Here are some examples of broader topic areas, which you could choose in other modules where the focus could be on social policy, health promotion, sociology, or psychology:

1. Poverty and homelessness in young people.
2. Health promotion and smoking.
3. Stress and health professionals.
4. Nursing and medicine: development as professions.

All these broad topic areas however at this stage do not have a clear focus but do give an indication of the literature you will be required to search. With a literature review there will be a clear structure, and some of the expectations of this structure are clearly noted in the assignment expectations. These are: search and retrieving strategy and databases used; rationale for choosing this topic; how it relates to practice and how the findings of your literature review could be used to support either a change in practice or the evidence base to current practice.

We will now look at one of these topic areas and follow through the steps required to write the literature review underpinned by an evidence base: '**Death and bereavement in hospital and how nurses manage this**'.

You may have chosen this topic because of an experience as a student during a clinical placement or you may wish to prepare yourself by learning more about the evidence base to this before going out to a placement and you think choosing this as an assignment topic will broaden your knowledge base as well as learning how to manage this situation yourself. You may have asked yourself: I wonder how nurses manage the death experience for the patient and their relatives in hospital, especially if they have different cultural or religious needs. It is possibly an area where you have only minimal knowledge.

Your main area of interest in the topic is not just in nurses' management of death and bereavement but in how this is managed within the context of cultural and religious needs. Prior to starting to review the literature it would be useful to devise a question for yourself which can help you to focus. For example: *'How do nurses take account of the cultural and religious needs of patients who are dying in hospital*?

Steps to help you to focus:

Step 1: Develop a clear question to review the literature (as above).

Step 2: Identify all key words related to the topic area: death, hospital, nurses, managing death, culture, religion, and death. As the broad topic area includes bereavement as part of the death experience then this may also be a word you may need to consider.

Step 3: Undertake a search for evidence.

Step 4: Decide on which evidence fits in with your topic area (see Chapter 6 for how to undertake Steps 1, 2 & 3).

It is Step 4 we are concerned with here. Some of the same steps will also apply in the other assignments, especially a dissertation. What then should be considered in writing the literature review? We are focusing on what Cronin, Ryan & Coughlan (2008: 38) call:

> 66 a traditional or narrative literature review' which is a 'type of review that critiques and summarizes a body of literature and draws conclusions about the topic in question. 99

What then should be considered when writing the literature review:

1. The title of the literature review: You may have decided on something like this: *The cultural and religious needs of the dying patient in hospital: the nurses role.*

2. You may need to provide an abstract of the literature review (see example) especially if you considered publishing it. (The example of an abstract provided below is from a published review of the literature but it clearly illustrates the evidence found and the author's summary of that evidence which is clearly based on a critique of the literature.)

3. Immediately after the title you will need to 'set the scene' of the literature review, and it is here that you will need to offer some background to the topic being reviewed, its importance and also the rationale for choosing it. This can either be titled the Introduction or background to the review. You can see from Dingwall's (2008)

abstract that she has clearly set out the background context of her review by referring to guidelines for integrated continence services. In her full paper this is expanded on.

Abstract

Recent United Kingdom guidelines have identified the need for integrated continence services within health regions. While there is evidence of improvements in community services there is little evidence that the quality of nursing care offered for older people with urinary incontinence in care settings has improved. This literature review identifies some of the underpinning issues that impact on continence promotion for older people. Despite evidence that older people suffer physical, social and psychological distress as a result of mismanaged urinary incontinence, costs of promoting continence are higher in financial terms that containing incontinence. The extent of the problem is difficult to identify in terms of how many older people are affected by different types of urinary incontinence. Nurses' attitudes are found to affect the quality of continence care delivered, and there continues to be a lack of evidence around sustainable strategies for continence promotion in care settings.

Dingwall, L. (2008) Promoting effective continence care for older people: a literature review. *British Journal of Nursing* 1 (3) 166–172.

In relation to our choice of topic on cultural and religious needs of dying people and the nurses' role, you could refer to the Professional Code in relation to preserving dignity and not discriminating against those in your care (NMC 2007) and if you are a student nurse, to the Standards of Proficiency for entry to the register (NMC 2004). The standard for professional and ethical practice includes 'provide care which demonstrates sensitivity to the diversity of patients and clients'. Depending on which specialty of nursing you are pursuing as a student nurse, the focus to your literature review could either be and adult patient or a child. The adult patient may also have a mental illness or someone with a learning disability. All student nurses need to have some understanding of death and bereavement and caring for patients from different cultural backgrounds. The background to your review may also include specific policy documents such as the Department of Health *End of Life Care Strategy* (DH 2008a).

4. Review and search methods. Here you will need to explain how you searched the literature and what key words you used as well as the databases such as MEDLINE or CINAHL. You will also need to indicate which kind of papers you excluded from the review.

5. The next section will in effect be your findings section and the main body of the review. It is very important to show how you have grouped together the various

papers. In a literature review however it would not only be research papers used as supporting evidence. You may also need to use material from textbooks or theoretical focused papers.

Example of using subheadings to present evidence:

The nurse's role in caring for the dying patient.

The needs of the dying in hospital.

Cultural and religious needs of a dying patient (or the dying child).

These kinds of headings imply that there were some clear themes arising from the evidence, which focused very much on the title of the review and the original question posed. The papers in this section could also be organized as per the methodologies used in the studies reviewed, although this is more likely in a systematic review. It is important when presenting evidence in sub headings to ensure that there is clear link between one section and the next. One question often asked by students is: can I use the word I in an essay? (i.e. to write in the first person). In the case of this assignment it would be perfectly acceptable in the first section where you outline your choice of topic to do so. For example: **'My rationale for choosing this topic in which to review the literature . . .'** but in later sections of the review writing it would still be acceptable to refer to your views on what you read or what you are going to write about but not writing the word I. For example:

> ❝ *it could be considered that this is an example of ....***or**
>
> *From personal experience it is clear that ......***or**
>
> *This literature review will focus on the following ......* ❞

Gimenez (2007) has some excellent advice on all these issues for the student nurse and it is also important to refer to your university guidance on essay writing (see also the nursing care study essay later in this chapter).

6. Then you would need to have a conclusion which would summarize the findings. It is important here to refer to any gaps you may have found in the evidence, such as very little research found on some aspect of the review.

7. Referring back to the assignment guidance, you were also asked to show how the evidence you have gathered could be used to either create change in practice or to provide evidence of what was already happening. You could also in your conclusion or in a separate section make recommendations, either for future research or how practice could be changed in a specific area.

If this had been a systematic review, which according to Cronin et al. (2008: 39) uses a 'more rigorous and well-defined approach to reviewing the literature in a specific subject' and are 'used to answer well-focused questions about clinical practice', then this section would use a very focused framework to illustrate the key evidence. Coates (2004) offers a comprehensive definition of what a systematic review is:

> 66 *A systematic review is a process of reviewing all papers that can be located on a particular topic, which uses a specified approach that has been designed to minimise bias and errors that may have influenced the results published in individual papers. This process should result in a single paper or report to which a reader can refer, rather than many individual articles. Each paper is evaluated and those that are considered flawed according to the criteria applied, are identified ... by drawing together the results from a range of studies it is possible to check whether they are consistent across the investigations or whether they are contradictory. If different teams in different localities have investigated a topic, possibly using different methods, yet the research yields consistent results, then they can be used as a robust form of evidence.* 99

A systematic review is also considered by some to be secondary research (Beverley *et al*. 2006). Some examples of systematic reviews are:

Power, N. & Franck, L. (2008) Parent participation in the care of hospitalized children: a systematic review. *Journal of Advanced Nursing* 62 (6) 622–641.

Fernandez, R. S., Evans, V., Griffiths, R. D. & Mostacchi, M. S. (2006) Education interventions for mental health consumers receiving psychotropic medication: a review of the evidence. *International Journal of Mental Health Nursing* 15 70–80.

Smith, D. R. (2007) A systematic review of tobacco smoking among nursing students. *Nurse Education in Practice* 7 293–302.

Consider the above definition by Coates (2004) when reading these papers and determine whether there is a clear systematic approach taken in the review and decide whether there is sufficient evidence for it to be useful in changing practice.

In summary, a literature review is helpful in setting out the current evidence base of a specific topic area. It can also be very systematic, using a more structured approach to managing both the evidence and the findings (see Chapter 6 for further information).

+···

EBP in action

Now choose one of the other topic areas and undertake a similar exercise, focusing on identifying a specific question from the topic area in order to begin the literature search, then searching the literature yourself just to explore the evidence base and then making some key notes around the stages of the written literature review. You may find this useful as well in relation to other assignments, when the same principle can be applied.

···

A nursing practice-related essay or care study

Most students will have to undertake an assignment where they are required to consider a patient they have cared for in practice, review certain aspects of care, and support this with an evidence base. There is normally very clear university guidelines regarding confidentiality and anonymity, which may also include gaining permission from the patient to undertake a care study. Please refer to your university handbooks for this information. Giminez (2007: 77) calls this a 'care critique'. An example might be (Box 9.2):

> **Box 9.2** Example of care study/nursing practice essay title
>
> The focus to this assignment is the evidence base to an aspect of care you have been involved in delivering to a patient during one clinical placement. You are required to choose a patient, remembering to ensure that you do not identify him/her in any way nor the clinical area specifically. Describe the patient/client's history in brief, including the nature of what their health problem(s) is and choose one aspect of his/her care that has been identified during the assessment. You are then required to discuss the care delivered, the rationale behind that care, and any underpinning evidence base.

In this essay, unlike the broad literature review above, there are very specific instructions for you to follow as to what is required. After describing the patient and their health problem, which could also include evidence that you understand from using the literature what this means and the likely symptoms or behaviour, you will then choose an aspect of care on which to focus your evidence-based practice (EBP). It is important to remember that in this type of assignment that the patient remains central to what you write in terms of the evidence base and also the rationale for looking at the specific aspect of care. You can link what you find back to the care given and that way you ensure that you individualize what you are writing about. For example, if I was looking after the needs of a Muslim patient (Mr Mohamed Kalhid Quereshi) and I wanted to know how nurses were educated to look after patients from a minority ethnic background:

> 66 *It would appear that despite the need for health professionals to be prepared to meet the needs of patients from minority ethnic groups that the majority of qualified nurses in Chevannes' (2002) study did not have any education during their initial education programmes. Knowing the needs of patients such as Mr Quereshi, in particular their need to pray even whilst in hospital, would have helped us give him much better care than I believed we were doing. This lack of knowledge was also identified by Hamilton & Essat (2008: 104) when they interviewed service users from different cultural groups to 'determine their experiences of nursing care and in particular how they felt their specific cultural needs were by met by nurses ...* 99

You will also note in the above that I have also used the word I, the use of which is always a question I get asked by students. Although there are certain protocols to be used in academic writing and your tutors may have their own ideas, it is my view that much depends on the type of assignment it is. If it is a reflective essay (where it is your personal experience that is being written about), or where, as in the examples below, you are required to consider your care of the patient, then it would be perfectly acceptable for you to do so. Of course writing in the 'first person' does not require you to use I, me, or myself in every sentence and it is wise to avoid this. This is a skill that needs to be learnt and as you gain confidence in what you are writing about and how to say it, this balance will develop over time. Your university may have resources or individuals who can help you with this skill development.

Consider some of the following examples (drawn from student practice experiences) in relation to your evidence based care choices:

Example 1: A 78 year old lady who is being cared for in the community. She has a large leg ulcer which is taking a long time to heal. You have been visiting her every day with your mentor. You have decided to look at this aspect of her care, in particular the evidence base of different treatments and why the ulcer is taking such a long time to heal.

Example 2: A young child of 7 has suffered a serious fracture to his leg requiring a stay in hospital. This is causing him some pain. You have been caring for him for 3 days and have begun to consider his pain relief and pain in children generally. This is an aspect of his care you have decided to consider.

Example 3: A 45 year old man who has been diagnosed as suffering from serious depression has been visited by the community psychiatric nurse for the past 3 weeks and as your mentor you have been going with him. The man has suddenly decided he does not want to take his medication any longer and as a result his previous symptoms have been returning. You have decided to look at this non-compliance with medication as your topic, in particular as you wish to understand the reasons why people do not comply in order to help him and understand all the possible reasons why he will not take his tablets.

Example 4: A young girl of 18 with a learning disability who has been attending a centre for young people has recently developed a friendship with a young man of the same age at the same centre. You know that there is a possibility that they could develop their relationship further and want to be able to talk to them both about this. However you do not know the best way of doing this and have decided to find out what the evidence base of sex education and young people with learning disabilities in order to be able to talk to them and provide some guidance should they wish to discuss it.

In considering these examples you may have arrived at the following ideas:

Example 1: The literature you may have chosen to review would focus on the fact that she is elderly and what happens normally to the skin of an elderly person due to the ageing process. The leg ulcer she has is taking a long time to heal, and during your assessment of her needs you may have found out that she was on steroid medication, which also causes skin changes. The causes of leg ulcers not healing would need to pursued as would the treatment she is having for the leg ulcer. Wound healing generally would be considered and this can also lead you to considering aspects of her care such as diet, rest, and mobility.

Example 2: The young child has suffered a serious leg fracture, so your background literature would need to include evidence of your understanding of what this is and what has caused the stay in hospital. Depending on the position of the fracture and the severity of it there will be a need for either an internal or external fixing, so evidence would be needed of your understanding of this and how it could be linked to the pain the child is experiencing. You might choose to focus on evidence of studies that have looked at the experience of pain in children, possibly linked to phenomenological studies. You might have decided however that an aspect of pain management that you wish to look at would be how to assess pain in children and focus on different pain assessment tools.

Example 3: This man has serious depression and you would need to know something about this health problem and what causes it and how it is treated. The client is clearly taking medication but has decided to stop. Your focus is around what leads to non-compliance of people in taking medication. There is a need to look at the general evidence for all patients initially and then look at similar health problems to your client with depression. Their health beliefs may influence decisions as they may not believe they have a problem. In understanding the reasons for non-compliance you will be able to determine what kind of nursing actions may be required as well as the involvement of other professionals and, if he has members close by, the client's family.

Example 4: The young girl and her friend are in that age group where sexual relationships are clearly possible. Sex education is an important aspect of life for all young people but Doyle (2008) for example found that provision of sex and sexual relationship education for young people with learning disabilities was inadequate. Your review of the literature would need to focus on this education for all young people initially and then focus on such papers as Doyle's.

All I have highlighted in these examples are the kind of issues you may have considered in mapping out your area of review. Each of you will do that in your own way.

Regardless of the very different topic areas, there will still be key steps to take in order to find and review essential papers, and then discuss them in the context of the care of the patient/client you have chosen as per the brief example of Mr Quereshi. Following a description of the person chosen, their health problem and the topic chosen with a clear rationale, it is essential then that you focus your search of the literature (see Chapter 6), decide which evidence is relevant or not, and then review the literature found. You will then need to decide on how to group the evidence into appropriate sections and discuss it in the context of the care of your chosen patient. In conclusion you will decide how this evidence has a) helped you to understand the patient's/client's situation better and b) how this evidence can help you deliver future care. The findings can also help you to apply it in similar situations in the future, and if you are actually out in practice at the time of doing your assignment you may well be able to share what you are finding with your mentor and others with a view to possibly changing the current care being given. This kind of assignment is an excellent way of learning about nursing practice and most importantly the value of basing that practice on an evidence base. This is often called 'bridging the theory and practice divide'. Fig. 9.1 on the following page outlines the steps involved in writing this kind of assignment. For more advice, a useful paper to read in relation to essay writing and structure is by Hatchett (2006).

A broad topic essay

A broad topic essay is one which is on similar topics to those in the literature review section. An example is: '**Discuss the impact of poverty on families and their health**'.

Sometimes you may be given a quote and then be asked to discuss it. For example:

'**From a transcultural point of view, (Leininger 1978) argues that an understanding of cultural diversities is essential to the provision of effective and safe care for clients**' (Chevannes 2002). Discuss.

Reference Chevannes, M. (2002) Issues in educating health professionals to meet the diverse needs of patients and other service users from ethnic minority groups. *Journal of Advanced Nursing*, 39 (3) 290–298.

When answering the assignment requirements, again it is important to consider what is being asked in terms of finding the evidence. In any 'discuss' question, it is clear that you are being asked to provide evidence which can either support or disprove the points you are making yourself (personal view) or find evidence that does the same, but different views from the literature itself.

Let us consider this in the context of the essay topic: '**Discuss the impact of poverty on families and their health**'.

What is the question actually asking you to do? It is asking you to discuss what the impact of poverty is on families and their health. You may think '*I can answer that in one paragraph not a whole essay!*'. However the purpose of this essay will be linked to your module or course outcomes and there will clearly be expectations that you will need to demonstrate your knowledge and understanding across a wide literature and evidence base. As in all essays you will need: an Introduction, the main body, and a conclusion.

In your introduction as with other types of assignments you will need to demonstrate a broad understanding of the issue to be discussed, linking poverty, families, and health. The evidence for this may come from books, and may include a clear definition of how they are linked together. You will also need to define what poverty is as well. As this is a very broad question it does not single out any specific age groups, so you will need to be clear about what the main aim of your paper is going to be, together with at least three key areas that you will discuss in the paper.

A. Read the assignment guidelines carefully.

↓

B. Decide on the patient/client and draft out a plan focusing on all the assignment requirements. You may wish to discuss with your mentor your choice of patient/client.

↓

C. Discuss the plan with your assignment tutor and agree an action plan, including how you
are to communicate and meet with regards to the assignment.

↓

D. Your plan could include: make notes regarding patient/client ensuring confidentiality and
anonymity; choose aspect of care to be searched and reviewed; search for evidence; read
and review evidence after deciding which papers and reports were relevant; write notes on
each of the papers and keep an accurate record of all references as you go along. This stops
you hunting around for the reference you are unable to find at the last minute.

↓

E. Draft out the structure of your written work and use this
as a template for building up your assignment content.

↓

F. Write the first draft and discuss with your tutor. This may involve
sending it by e-mail rather than direct contact.

↓

G. Keep checking that you are following the guidelines of the assignment
and tick off the sections as you complete them.

↓

H. Be mindful of word limits as most universities have penalties for not meeting this.
Tip From my experience I do not count the exact words on the first draft nor as I go along
because it detracts from my writing. Once complete, I read the essay and take out sections
that I can see are not necessary for the assignment. This does of course depend on each
individual's way of working and each of you will develop the best way that works for you.

↓

I. Ensure that you are using quotes and paraphrasing read material and evidence
appropriately in order to avoid plagiarism.

↓

J. The tutor will normally read one complete draft of your work only. NB. Each university will
have its own student guidelines on this however.

Figure 9.1 Steps to writing an assignment

! **Key points**

Being clear about the main aim of your essay is important as it not only shows how you can focus on the topic but will also be an indication for you of the areas of literature and evidence you will need to obtain and summarize. Remember how in Chapter 5 we said identifying your research question is key to finding the right evidence—it applies to essays just as it applies to research.

For example, the question does not focus on the UK but after your introduction where you would need to make a possible statement about world wide poverty and causes and impact on families then you could state that your paper will only focus on the UK. You will however have clearly demonstrated that you have read material outside the UK and have made a link to your paper. For example whilst searching for material for this book I came across a paper: The impact of poverty on health—a scan of research literature by Phipps (2003). The focus to it was Canada (http://www.dsp-psd.pwgsc.gc.ca/—A Canadian Government publication). Despite this it had some very useful material with regards to definitions of poverty, measuring poverty, and most importantly evidence on the links between poverty and health and families. Another interesting piece of evidence was by Salway *et al.* (2007) which offered a different perspective, focusing on how ethnicity was seen in relation to long-term ill health and poverty. This was a large research study that offered evidence for national policy change.

The point in highlighting these two kinds of evidence examples is that when answering essays, demonstrating wide reading outside the standard literature found in research papers is very important. It demonstrates that you have made an attempt to not only widen your own knowledge base but also that of your searching skills.

In relation to a quotation question, the discuss part follows a quote. What is the first task to consider? You need to look at the actual quote, read it, and consider what it is telling you. First you will have noted that the quote is from an article by Chevannes (2002) and you should have been given the full reference as part of the assignment guidelines. You will need to access that article as it is your first piece of evidence. She is in fact making a point from her understanding of what Leininger said in 1978 in another paper. You will be able to obtain this paper (or in this case a book) in order for you determine yourself if that is clearly what Leininger said or meant. In order to discuss Chevannes point of view and that of Leininger you will need to look at the evidence around the statement for yourself. Consider what it is saying and break it down into smaller parts, for example:

From a transcultural point of view (Leininger argues that)

An understanding of cultural diversities

Is essential to the provision of effective and safe care for clients.

You do not know at this point whether Chevannes actually agrees with this view or not, and this is what you will need to consider for yourself in this essay. Is Leininger right and what is the evidence for you agreeing or disagreeing with this statement? You will need to understand Leininger's point of view and the evidence around transcultural nursing

---

Box 9.3 Assignment preparation

1) Make sure you understand the title of the assignment topic or assignment focus.
2) Underline key words.
3) Decide how many parts are there to the question or assignment.
4) Read widely, think and make some notes.
5) Prepare a plan.
6) Do at least one rough draft.
7) If a broad essay topic, have no more than three lines of argument or areas that you can develop through the essay.
8) **Support your claims with evidence.**
9) Indicate in your opening paragraph what your main issues are going to be.
10) Avoid sweeping generalizations or statements you cannot support (this is not the same as putting your view across based on the evidence).
11) Only write what you understand yourself.
12) If you are disagreeing with an author or position, offer an alternative.
13) Stick to the point and do not waffle or repeat yourself ! Be precise.
14) Answer the question—ensuring that you keep checking the guidelines.
15) Write in plain English.
16) Make good use of paragraphs and sub headings in longer assignments.
17) Keep to the word limit or the per cent extra allowed.
18) Have a dictionary handy—possibly one related to research methodologies or nursing.
19) Summarize the points raised or the argument taken in a final conclusion section or concluding paragraph.
20) Ensure your reference list is accurate and that all cited evidence is referenced in the reference list.
21) Check the final draft.
22) You may at various points in this check list also meet with your tutor to discuss your work.
23) In some seen examinations (which we have not discussed here) you are allowed to take textbooks into the exam room with you. Referencing your sources correctly are just as important.

and what it is. You will then need to look at the literature on provision of effective and safe care for clients/patients from different cultures. What is the evidence that care providers can offer this? Do they understand cultural diversity and therefore cultural needs in order to deliver safe and effective care? These questions immediately lead you to the evidence base which may also include (because I am familiar with the literature on this topic) literature and research on the topic of cultural competency. You may also be able to offer exemplars from practice to illustrate your point of view, and allowance for this should be indicated in your assignment guidelines.

The main point of this type of essay as with the other one is that you need to provide both sides of the 'argument'. You may say something like:

> 66 *In conclusion, having considered all the issues that even though it is clear that Leininger's (1978) argument is valid in relation to the need for nurses and other health care professionals to have an understanding and awareness of different cultures to provide safe and effective care, I do not believe that a transcultural approach or model as she advocates is necessary.* 99

These kinds of essays help you to learn to offer balanced views, to search wide and focused evidence and to develop your critical thinking and analysis skills.

A dissertation

A dissertation is often required to be undertaken as part of an Honours Degree programme. This is usually between 8,000 and 10,000 words (sometimes 15,000) and although on some programmes it can involve undertaking a piece of research, for the majority of student nurses this will not be the case. Hannigan & Burnard (2001) offer some useful guidance on 'preparing and writing an undergraduate dissertation', particularly in relation to: getting started, defining a topic, planning the work, and the literature review, which is the main body of the work. This is similar in structure to the literature review discussed earlier in the chapter and also the same process of defining the topic area and focusing on one aspects or question. It is however a much longer piece of writing and will require much more depth and evidence. The structure of the dissertation will also be different and there will be clear guidelines on how to set it out. One of the key differences will be that the different sections of the evidence and the other sections may be provided in chapters (see your own university guidelines for this).

The structure will include: a title, an **abstract**, an introduction, the literature review which could cover more than one chapter if not undertaking actual research, when a chapter outlining the research design would be required. This would include methodology, methods, ethical considerations, data analysis, validity and reliability or trustworthiness, sampling. In a literature-based dissertation you could still have a general discussion chapter where all the evidence from the literature chapters is pulled together and considered. A recommendations chapter may also be necessary, in order to be able to provide a link between the theoretical discussion and relevance for practice.

Your university library may keep previous student's undergraduate dissertations but this is not usual. Libraries normally keep Masters level studies and you may be able to have an opportunity to read some of these, especially if you are undertaking your pre-registration programme at Masters level study. It is important to remember however that all of these dissertations will have gained different grades and are therefore going to varied in the quality of the work.

+ ···

EBP in action

If you are having to complete a dissertation read Hannigan & Burnard's paper to obtain a general idea of what is expected from that kind of assignment, in terms of the evidence base and the level of academic study.

···

A research proposal

Some of you will be required to write a research proposal, either as part of a research methods module or a literature-based dissertation. This may also require preparing and writing a proposal form for an ethics committee. In relation to the former this will have specific guidelines and the proposal is a good way for your module tutors to see what you have learnt from their classes on different aspects of the research process. There will also be a word limit attached to writing a research proposal, and if you do not have guidance on how many words are appropriate for each section you will need to determine this early on. If you were allocated no more than 4,000 words and you had to ensure that there was enough evidence to support your proposal, then a large part of this would be attributed to the background literature and the justification of the various aspects of the research design.

A research proposal will usually follow the same structure as the research process found in Chapter 3 but, in addition, will possibly also require the student to consider outlining the time it will take to undertake the proposed research and for each stage of the research, and may also require a consideration of the possible cost in terms of researcher time and other non-staff costs such as administration or travel to undertake the research. In terms of evidence, there will be a need to provide evidence on all aspects of the research proposal to support topic area choice, methodology, method, need for ethical approval or ethical considerations etc. In particular will be the need to justify the choice of methodology and method and have a clear research question (Chapters 4 and 5 will be able to support this section).

Let us consider the elements of a research proposal. Read Chapter 3 on the research process as a reminder of everything that needs to be considered. Most research, unless you are preparing a proposal for specific funding or research bid, arises out of a need to answer a question or a problem. The following is a shortened version of a piece of research I undertook in 1991, and is used only to illustrate the use of evidence at various stages of developing a research proposal. I had to provide a proposal outlining my study for gaining access to the study area and submit to the local research ethics committee.

Title of the study

This will give the reader of the proposal an indication of not only what the study being proposed is about but also the methodology. I shall use my own experience to illustrate aspects of the proposal. For example: *'An ethnographic study of nursing culture as an exploration for determining the existence of a system of ritual'* (Holland 1993).

Introduction and background

Here you will need to outline the background information for the research being proposed and link it to some literature, as well as a rationale. For example in the above study I had developed an interest in anthropology and how nurses could learn from it, as well as how we could apply anthropology to nursing practice. I started to read the literature around linking them both and in particular whether nursing could be considered a culture and if yes were there aspects of that culture that I could study. During my reading of the literature to explore my ideas I had come across a paper by Chapman (1983) which reported on a study to explore rituals in hospital. I decided then that this is what I wanted to explore further.

Once I had found this paper by Chapman and established that this would be a different view of nursing practice, I undertook to widen my literature base, but at this stage all that was required was to provide enough evidence to demonstrate that I understood the topic area, the concepts from anthropology that I wished to use, and some evidence from the nursing literature which related to it. I made a summary of the key literature I had discovered. From this I was then able to narrow my area of research and define a clear research question. It was clear from my initial search that there was not a great deal of evidence on this topic and only Chapman's study in the UK.

I decided on the research question provided in the next section.

Research question

'Was there a system of ritual in nursing practice?'
To answer the question I developed a set of aims to be able to answer it.

Research aims

My overall research aim was to explore nursing as a culture in a specific environment to determine if a system of ritual existed. I would undertake this through:

1. Observing a group of nurses in their work environment.

2. Asking nurses about what they did as part of their everyday work.

Research design

This is another term which covers all aspects of the research that you will undertake up to the actual data analysis and findings.

As you will have seen in Chapter 3, if you have a clear research question and research aims you should be able to define your research methodology and methods quite easily.

Methodology

As this was an exploratory study, it was clearly a qualitative methodology choice. I chose ethnography as this was also related to anthropology and culture. It is important to provide evidence here on the choice of methodology and why you have chosen to use it. For me at the time it was Field & Morse (1985) from nursing and Spradley (1979) in relation to ethnographic methodologies. Spradley had undertaken a number of ethnographic studies and his experience of all aspects of the research was easy to understand and read. An ethnography if you recall can be both the methodology and the actual description of the research findings itself.

Methods

The research aims directed me to consider specific research methods and the researcher in qualitative research is the main data collecting tool, i.e by undertaking observation or doing interviews.

The research methods chosen:

Participant and non-participant observation

Interviews with key informants

In a research proposal it is important to justify this choice, so evidence as outlined in Chapter 4 was used to support the choice of methods. If you have to complete an ethics committee approval form as part of your proposal assignment then justification of methods is particularly relevant.

Ethical issues

The main ethical issues I had to consider in my research proposal were informed consent and how I was going to conduct the observation, in particular in relation to patients on the ward. It is important to provide evidence related to your professional code as a nurse and also the requirements of an ethical committee regarding, in this case, NHS staff. I made it clear that at no time were patients being interviewed nor directly observed but I would explain to patients that I was on the ward conducting research. It is important here to make clear the links between the research methodology, methods, and the ethical issues.

Data protection issues

Here you need to refer to the evidence of the Data Protection Act 1998 and what it is there for in relation to research data and processes involved in undertaking the research.

Time and budget costs

In a research proposal this is not necessarily based on evidence but you can include references from the research books on why it is important to ensure that enough time is built into any research project and for all possible events. Bond & Gerrish (2006) provide a very informative overview of preparing a research proposal for funding, including information on budget.

Dissemination

An area that requires inclusion in any research proposal is how the findings of your proposed study will be disseminated. It could be through a conference or publication. This is important as any research participant will need to be informed that the findings from the study will be published and do they agree to that within the boundaries set by the anonymity and confidentiality issues.

Assignments: summary points

All assignments have elements in common with regards to providing a clear evidence-based rationale for choice and evidence to support either key arguments in an essay or key justification points in relation to choice of methodology.

How this evidence is to be referenced and summarized will now be discussed. Referencing is an integral part of the writing throughout an assignment and it is the process by which you will identify where you have either read and summarized someone else's views or actually quoted them. It is an integral part of evidence-based practice (EBP).

Reference list, systems, and bibliography: the basics

All evidence used in any assignment must be acknowledged in the correct way. This includes material found on the World Wide Web.

It is important initially to differentiate between a reference list and a bibliography. A reference list is a list of referenced or cited authors/resources which you have used in your assignment. A bibliography is the list of resources that you have read during the course of preparing your assignment but have chosen not to reference. In some universities both of these are called bibliography, but for the purpose of this book we will differentiate between them as indicated. Please refer to your own university guidance on all matters concerning references and a bibliography.

References are usually cited in one of two ways.

1. Through referring to the author's work that you have read and summarized but not quoted, for example:

   Holland (1999) suggested that:

   In a recent editorial Holland (2008) describes her initial observations on the Darzi report (DH 2008b) ...

2. Or as a direct quote:

   When assessing older people using the Roper–Logan–Tierney model it is important to determine the cultural or religious factors that can influence each AL before commencing the assessment. (Rawlings-Anderson 2004: 31)

Referencing is important as it shows that you recognize other people's work and that you have clearly undertaken to both search and use the evidence for your assignment. It also allows your tutors to check out some of the references to see if you have used the evidence cited, and also used it correctly, and to read the original material for themselves. We shall be looking at this wrongful use of evidence in the next section on plagiarism.

There are two main reference systems that are used in assignments. It is important that you do not mix them in the same assignment. Your university will have guidance on referencing and how to use the different systems. One is known as the Harvard System and the other the Vancouver System. The Harvard System is often known as the author/date or in-text referencing and the Vancouver as the numeric system or end-notes/footnotes. It is not the intention of this section to go into great detail about the two systems other than to offer brief examples of each.

Harvard system

In this system all references are cited in the reference list in alphabetical order. If quoted material is also included, then the actual page number of the quote is also cited in the reference, after the data. All references in the text are identified by both name of author (s) and the date of publication, as well as the publisher, city of publication. The title of the book can either be underlined or placed in italics. If it is an article however it is the title of the journal that is either underlined or placed in italics. Whatever system is used it is essential to have conformity throughout. You will also note in the reference list for this chapter that references by the same author are listed in order of date of publication (see Holland in the reference list) and an author who publishes different papers or reports in the same year has to have the references differentiated both in the text and in the list with an alphabetical sequence (see Department of Health in the reference list). Here are some examples of Harvard references:

In the text referencing

Gimenez (2007: 3) in Chapter 1 of his book, offers 'an introduction to academic writing', where he discusses not only key words such as what does discuss mean but also offers a checklist for an academic essay.

If there are more than two authors of a paper or a book (or book chapter) then it is good practice to list all authors on the first use of the reference and from then on use the *et al.*:

Jones, Auton, Burton & Watkins (2008) have written a paper focusing on how service users have helped to develop stroke services.

Jones *et al.* (2008) outline their action research study through which they developed a stroke care pathway.

In a reference list

(Book) Gimenez, J. (2007) *Writing for Nursing and Midwifery Students*, Basingstoke: Palgrave Macmillan.

(Article) McSherry, R. & Proctor-Childs, (2001) Promoting evidence-based practice through an integrated model of care: patient case studies as a teaching method. *Nurse Education in Practice* 1 19–26.

If an author is cited in the text then it is essential that the full reference of that author and where it is cited is made clear. This is a **secondary source reference**:

Polit, D. F. & Beck, C. T. (2004) *Nursing Research: methods, appraisal and utilization*, (7th edn) Philadelphia: Lippincott Williams & Wilkins. Cited in Speziale, H. J. S. & Carpenter, D. R. (2007) *Qualitative Research in Nurs*ing, Advancing the Humanistic Perspective (*4th edn*). Philadelphia: Lipincott Williams & Wilkins.

If it is an actual chapter in a book that the actual reference you use comes from then it is important to reference it as such, as well as the page numbers for that chapter. This is still a **primary source reference**:

Tod, A. (2006) Interviewing. In: Gerrish, K. & Lacey, A. (eds) *The Research Process in Nursing* Oxford: Blackwell Publishing. Chapter 22: 337–352.

Vancouver system

In this system all references are cited in the reference list in the order in which they appear in the text. Some writers use the name of the author in the text but only attribute the information with a number.

An example in text: Holland (1) notes the different roles and functions of the nurse and illustrates her meaning with Savage's (2) four main functions of the nurse. She also cites Henderson's (3) definition of nursing.

In the reference list this would be written as:

1. Holland K. Nursing and the Context of Care **In:** Holland, K., Jenkins J., Solomon, J. & Whittam, S. (eds) *Applying the Roper-Logan–Tierney Model in Practice*, 2nd edn, Edinburgh: Churchill Livingstone (Elsevier), 2008: 22–43.

2. Savage, J. (ed) *Strengthening nursing and midwifery to support Health for All.* WHO Regional Publications, European Series, No. 48, World Health Organisation, Copenhagan, 1993 **cited in** Holland, K. Nursing and the Context of Care **In:** Holland, K., Jenkins J., Solomon J. & Whittam, S. (eds) *Applying the Roper-Logan–Tierney Model in Practice*, 2nd edn, Edinburgh: Churchill Livingstone (Elsevier), 2008: 22–43.

3. Henderson, V. *The nature of nursing*. Collier-Macmillan, New York, 1966 **cited in** Holland, K. Nursing and the Context of Care **In:** Holland, K., Jenkins, J., Solomon, J. & Whittam, S. (eds) *Applying the Roper-Logan–Tierney Model in Practice*, 2nd edn, Edinburgh: Churchill Livingstone (Elsevier) 2008: 22–43.

From these last two references the reader will be able to obtain not only the cited reference, but also the chapter where this was cited and the book in which the chapter had been written.

This accurate referencing is essential in order to be able to access the source of the supporting evidence and if necessary check its accuracy.

+ ....

EBP in action

Consider the following Harvard reference list and identify which are right and which are not and re-write these in the correct way.

Reference list exercise: identify the correct referencing format

Boote, J., Lewin, V., Beverley, C. & Bates, J. Psychosocial interventions for people with moderate to severe dementia: a systematic review. Clinical Effectiveness in Nursing, 2006, 951, 1–15.

Curran, & Brooker, (2007) Systematic review of interventions delivered by UK mental health nurses, *International Journal of Nursing Studies*.

Gerrish, K. & McMahon, A. (2006). In K. Gerrish & A. Lacey The Research process in nursing, Oxford: Blackwell Publishing, (2006), 1–15.

Haberman, M. & Uys, I. R. (2005) *The Nursing process: a global concept.*

Hockey, L. (1984) The nature and purpose of research. In Cormack, D.F.S. (ed) The Research Process in Nursing, (*1st edn*). London: Blackwell Science, 1–10.

Lauder, W., Roxburgh, M., Holland, K., Johnson, M., Watson, W., Porter, M., Topping, K. & Behr, A. Nursing and Midwifery in Scotland: Being Fit for Practice, University of Dundee, 2006.

All these references, written accurately, can be found in this book. You will find further exercises online.

....

Plagiarism and referencing in academic work

It is important to ensure that all material cited in quotes or paraphrased is referenced correctly. When material directly taken from a text is not referenced or attributed to the author from where it is taken and is used as if it were your own, then this is called plagiarism and is a very serious offence in academic terms. Sometimes a few words are changed or their order is changed but it is still plagiarism. If the student has not understood how to reference, especially if only just commencing academic study then they need to discuss it with their tutor as soon as possible. It is not acceptable to claim poor referencing if it is persistent throughout one assignment or a series of assignments, especially when one is claiming the work as their own. Students need to be aware that many universities have or are purchasing computer software which can detect plagiarism. All student assignments are then submitted electronically and are subjected to the software.

Students also need to be aware that lecturers marking their work for specific modules are also familiar with the texts or articles they have used as evidence, and can also identify areas of text where there is a clear difference in writing styles between that of the student and that of the original source of the evidence being used.

Consider the following paragraph:

Holland (2005: 1) stated that:

66 *A significant number of papers submitted to Nurse Education in Practice do not take into account a reader without prior knowledge and understanding of the context in which author's write. In addition there is a tendency to use terminology and language that is specific to individual cultural and organisational contexts within that individual's own country.* 99

Now consider this one:

A number of journals which authors send papers *to* do not *appear to* take *notice* of the reader *who does not have* prior knowledge and understanding of the context *they write about. There is also* a tendency to use terminology and language spe-cific *to the author's* own country.

Writing for publication does not sound like an easy job and it is really useful to be able to read papers in a journal which do not sound like gobbleedook and rubbish.

As you can see here, in the sections in green, we have many words that are similar to the full reference nor is it attributed to the original author. This is clear plagiarism. Sometimes there is also a complete change in writing style which alerts the reader to

---

Box 9.4 Examples of plagiarism

a. Handing in somebody else's work as your own.
b. Buying or borrowing somebody else's work.
c. Paying somebody to write for you.
d. Copying without citing.
e. Failing to use quotation marks.
f. Changing only a few words from the original.
g. Building upon somebody else's ideas without giving credit.
h. Changing the words in the original but keeping the essential ideas without citing.
i. Paraphrasing without citing.

Source: Gimenez (2007: 144)

a possible case of plagiarism, as can be seen in the second sentence in italics (this is exaggerated to make a point). Gimenez (2007) offers a very useful list of plagiarism examples in Box 9.4.

If you are found out to have plagiarized someone else's work consistently then you could be dismissed from your course of study. So getting to grips very early on with referencing is a must for all students. If you keep accurate records of references you use as you go along and ensure that you learn to develop good paraphrasing skills then this will stand you in good stead.

Using evidence in either practice or academic work is to be commended but only if the source is acknowledged so that others may have an opportunity to access it and widen their own knowledge base. We will be returning to this issue again in Chapter 10 when we consider writing for publication.

Summary

- Using evidence in assignments of any kind is both good practice and essential.

- Ensuring that this evidence is the best evidence to support your discussion or EBP is also a skill you need to learn.

- Referencing correctly both in text and in any list requires practice and is another essential skill to learn early in your programme of study.

- Using someone else's words, either from articles or other student's work is not acceptable. Neither is purchasing an essay from websites and passing them off as your own. Honesty is a fundamental value of nursing and being a nurse.

■ *Online resource centre*

 You may now like to visit the accompanying website for this book and explore the additional resources you will find there. **www.oxfordtextbooks.co.uk/orc/holland/**

■ References

Beverley, C., Edmunds-Otter, M. & Booth, A. (2006) Systematic reviews and secondary research. In: Gerrish, K. & Lacey, A. (eds) *The Research Process in Nursing*. Oxford: Blackwell Publishing, 316–334.

Bond, & Gerrish, K. (2006) Preparing a research proposal. In: Gerrish K. & Lacey, A. (eds) *The Research Process in Nursing*. Oxford: Blackwell Publishing, 123–137.

Chapman, G. E. (1983) Ritual and rational action in hospitals. *Journal of Advanced Nursing* 8 (1) 13–20.

Chevannes, M. (2002) Issues in educating health professionals to meet the diverse needs of patients and other service users from ethnic minority groups. *Journal of Advanced Nursing* 39 (3) 290–298.

Coates, V. (2004) Systematic reviews: best available evidence for clinical practice? *Journal of Diabetes Nursing*, March 2004. http://findarticles.com/p/articles/mi_m0MDR/is_3_8/ai_n6180340/

Cronin, P, Ryan, F. & Coughlan, M. (2008) Undertaking a literature review: a step by step approach. *British Journal of Nursing* 17 (1) 38–43.

Department of Health (2008a) *End of Life Care Strategy*. London: DH.

Department of Health (2008b) *Health Quality Care for All—NHS next stage review final report (Darzi report)*. London: DH.

Dingwall, L. (2008) Promoting effective continence care for older people: a literature review. *British Journal of Nursing* 17 (3) 166–172.

Doyle J. (2008) Improving sexual health education for young people with learning disabilities. *Paediatric Nursing* 20 (4) 26–28.

Field, P. & Morse, J. M. (1985) *Nursing Research: the application of qualitative approaches*. Kent: Croom Helm Ltd.

Gimenez, J. (2007) *Writing for Nursing and Midwifery Students*. Basingstoke: Palgrave Macmillan.

Hamilton, M. & Essat, Z. (2008) Minority ethnic users experiences and expectations of nursing care. *Journal of Research in Nursing,* 13, 102–110, http://jrn.sagepub.com/ at University of Salford on July 7th 2008.

Hannigan, B. & Burnard, P. (2001) Preparing and writing an undergraduate dissertation. *Nurse Education in Practice* 1 175–180.

Hatchett, R. (2006) A guide to academic essay writing. *British Journal of Cardiac Nursing* 1 (11) 546–549.

Holland, K. (1993) An ethnographic study of nursing culture as an exploration for determining the existence of a system of ritual. *Journal of Advanced Nursing* 18 (9) 1461–1470.

Holland, K. (1999) A journey to becoming: the student nurse in transition. *Journal of Advanced Nursing* 29 (1) 229–236.

Holland, K. (2005) Writing for an international readership. *Nurse Education in Practice* 5 1–2.

Holland, K. (2008) Health Quality Care for All—NHS next stage review final report. *Nurse Education in Practice* 8 (5) 299–301.

Leininger, M. (1978) Transcultural Nursing: Concepts, theories, and practices. New York: John Wiley & Sons cited in Chevannes, M. (2002) Issues in educating health professionals to meet the diverse needs of patients and other service users from ethnic minority groups. *Journal of Advanced Nursing* 39 (3) 290–298.

Nursing & Midwifery Council (2004) *Standards of Proficiency for Pre-registration Nursing Education*. London: NMC.

Nursing & Midwifery Council (2007) *The Code: standards of conduct, performance and ethics for nurses and midwives*. London: NMC.

Phipps, S. (2003) *The Impact of Poverty on Health—a scan of research literature*. Ottowa: Canadian Institute for Health Information. **http://psd.pwgsc.gc.ca/Collection/H118-11-2003-2E.pdf/**

Rawlings- Anderson, K. (2004) Assessing the cultural and religious needs of older people. *Nursing Older People* 16 (8) 29–33.

Salway, S., Platt, L., Chowbey, P., Harriss, K. & Bayliss, E. (2007) Long Term Ill Health, Poverty and Ethnicity. Bristol: Polity Press.

Spradley, J. P. (1979) *The Ethnographic Interview*. Orlando: Holt, Rheinhart & Winston In.

■ Further reading

Carnwell, R. & Daly, W. (2001) Strategies for the construction of a critical review of the literature. *Nurse Education in Practice* 1, 57–63.

Ely, C. & Scott, I. (2007) *Essential Study Skills for Nursing* Edinburgh: Mosby Elsevier.

Hart, S. (ed.) (2010) *Nursing: Study and Placement Skills.* Oxford: Oxford University Press.

■ Useful websites

LearnHigher—Centre for Excellence in Teaching and learning

http://www.learnhigher.ac.uk/learningareas/academicwriting/home.htm/
This site has a whole range of learning resources to support students and links to websites.

Dissemination of evidence
Writing for publication and presentation of learning activity

Karen Holland

The aims of this chapter are:

➤ To illustrate the importance of dissemination of research and evidence.

➤ To explore how students can get involved in dissemination activity such as conference presentations.

➤ To examine the requirements of a poster presentation.

➤ To develop the skills to undertake a book review.

➤ To examine what is required to write a short paper for publication in a journal.

➤ To explain the process of writing for publication generally.

Introduction

Nursing practice that has an evidence base is dependent as we have seen on accessing, evaluating and then utilizing that evidence. This assumes that the evidence has initially been disseminated in such a way that you are able to access it in the first place. Hence an invaluable form of evidence is that of a systematic literature review, where the 'quality' and form of the evidence on a topic has already been evaluated and the body of evidence summarized. Dissemination of research findings is an essential part of the research process and it can be said that the research is not complete until this has occurred (Newell & Burnard 2006).

As a student you may well be asked to undertake a review of the literature, but also required to demonstrate your own dissemination of learning through activities such as presenting the evidence you have found in literature reviews to your peers in either an oral presentation or a poster presentation. Some of you may also have already disseminated your own experience of practice through writing a reflective account in a journal such as the **Nursing Standard** or a written a book review or article in a peer-reviewed journal such as **Nurse Education in Practice**.

This chapter will help you to develop some of these dissemination skills and give you the confidence to be able to share your work or thoughts with others, either in the classroom, in clinical practice, or through writing in a publication which others can read. Firstly let us consider the wider implications of dissemination of research and evidence for nursing practice.

Dissemination of research and evidence

To be able to utilize research evidence in practice is dependent on being able to access it in the first instance (see Chapter 6), determine its quality and its value (see Chapter 7), and most importantly read what someone has already undertaken through its dissemination. To ensure that a complete picture of the research is obtained (see Chapter 3) the information must be in a form that is readily understood by those needing to use it. Mulhall & Le May (1999: 8) see evidence (i.e. the actual research evidence) as the first stage of a process, with dissemination (communication of information from the research) as the stage prior to acting on the evidence (implementation).

Dissemination of research and evidence is central to its being utilized in practice. It has been surprising during my own searching of the literature as background to the writing of this chapter that in fact the art of dissemination is not given a great deal of attention in books on research and evidence-based practice. Johnson (2007) however has written a complete chapter on the topic, but focusing very much on the 'ethics and aesthetics' of dissemination rather than a 'how to do it' approach. He stresses the importance however of dissemination in its value to society, or translated for this chapter, to nursing. He offers a number of ways in which to disseminate research outputs in particular, such as conference presentations, books, and journals, but as his book focuses on ethics of research he discusses mainly those issues such as plagiarism, authorship order, and constructive criticism. Johnson (2007: 204) states that:

> 66 *an explanation sometimes offered by those who fail to disseminate their work appropriately is the fear of criticism.* 99

and certainly from my personal perspective of being a journal editor this is often related to me by colleagues as one of the reasons why they do not wish to write articles. I am sure as a student you will also feel something similar when you have to disseminate your work to peers in the classroom, and presenting information to an audience can be daunting at any time without being assessed on your performance as well. We will return to this later when focusing on writing for publication.

Electronic initiatives

The importance of dissemination of research has led to a number of strategic and international initiatives through which nurses and other health and social care professionals can access current evidence. This has been undertaken through electronic access rather than by individual presentations of research to a local or international audience. These sites act as a repository for evidence to be disseminated. Here are some of the main examples:

1. The Joanna Briggs Institute (Adelaide: Australia) states that:

> 66 The Joanna Briggs Institute is an International not-for-profit Research and Development Organisation specializing in Evidence-Based resources for healthcare professionals in nursing, midwifery, medicine, and allied health. With over 54 Centres and groups, servicing over 90 countries, The Joanna Briggs Institute is a recognized global leader in Evidence-Based Healthcare 99
>
> (http://www.joannabriggs.edu.au/about/home.php/)

To be able to access some of the information on this site however requires registration and payment. You can register as a student member for a reduced rate to certain sections of the site.

2. The Cochrane Collaboration offers access to a vast database of systematic reviews and databases (http://www.cochrane.org/) and includes a UK based Cochrane Centre (http://www.cochrane.co.uk/en/index.html)

3. Centre for Reviews and Dissemination (York University, UK) is a part of the National Institute for Health Research (NIHR) and also offers a range of resources and publications in relation to evidence and systematic reviews. (http://www.york.ac.uk/inst/crd/projects/access_evidence.htm)

These sites are ideal if you are attempting to determine the body of evidence available on a specific topic.

Dissemination of evidence is undertaken not only through specific sites such as those above. Research studies and literature reviews, as well as papers explaining new ideas and theories are also disseminated via journals, books, and reports. Some research findings might also be disseminated through more popular type professional magazines or websites which inform readers in a less structured way, for example see this website http://www.communitycare.co.uk/ for summaries of (new) research on a range of topics such as Elder abuse: prevalence and prevention (O'Keefe *et al.* 2007) (http://www.communitycare.co.uk/Articles/2008/03/26/107725/learning-by-experience-elder-abuse-prevalence-and-prevention.html).

This kind of dissemination allows practitioners from health and social care to access a summary of the actual research study itself which would inform their practice without necessarily having to access the full report. It is important however to remember that if you wanted to use the research as part of a literature review, that you gain access to the full report or published article in order to ensure that you take account of the whole of its meaning rather than a brief summary. The research summary noted above however although referred to as a summary, does in fact report a great deal of detail about the actual research undertaken and the findings.

EBP in action

You have been asked to determine what evidence is available on one of the following topics:

1. Current interventions for venous leg ulcers
2. Self-care support networks for health and social care
3. Mental Health promotion
4. Childhood obesity
5. Elder abuse
6. Dental care and children
7. Nutrition and nursing care
8. Health promotion and alcohol use in adolescent

Choose *one* that relates to your practice and use the Centre for Reviews and Dissemination (NIHR) website (http://www.york.ac.uk/inst/crd/index.htm/) initially to determine what evidence is available. Following that, to access other forms of dissemination tools to add to the body of evidence you have collated.

You can use this as part of a planned session in university which may involve undertaking a similar exercise or be part of one. You can also consider the information as part of your practice learning. Make a list of all methods of dissemination accessed. How has the majority of research evidence on these topics been disseminated? Which one do you think was more effective in relation to helping you understand the evidence base available in order to recommend change in practice?

Disseminating evidence to change practice

Whichever method of dissemination you believed would be more effective in deciding how to recommend a change in practice, a key point to remember is that you have to be able to understand what the evidence is saying, and that there is clearly enough of it to suggest that the evidence is robust and valid to make a recommendation for change. It is also important to remember that changing practice requires more than simply knowing that some evidence would be very important to implement. A paper entitled '**Getting evidence into practice**', published by the NHS Centre for Reviews and Dissemination (1999) made this point very clear, and stressed that:

> ❝ Whilst knowledge of a practice guideline or a research based recommendation may be important, it is rarely by itself, sufficient to change practice. The literature on persuasive communication and advertising makes a distinction between communications that can increase awareness and those that actually bring about changes in behaviour. This distinction is helpful in understanding that dissemination and implementation may be considered as a spectrum of activity, where dissemination involves raising awareness of research messages and implementation involves getting the findings of research adopted into practice. ❞
>
> (NHS Centre for Reviews and Dissemination 1999: 2)

In their conclusion, following a discussion of a range of issues related to changing behaviour, models of change and changing practice, they make the point that is still valid 10 years later, in that 'dissemination activities by themselves are unlikely to lead to changes in behaviour' (NHS centre for Reviews and Dissemination 1993: 13) but that the awareness of 'the message still plays an important part in the process'. This is why it is important that, as a student nurse, you engage in activities which help to develop skills in all forms of dissemination activity, to enable you share with others evidence of either others research or your own research and evidence awareness.

Alongside the development of these skills, you will also be learning in your final year of study mainly how to engage others in changing practice, through such activities as developing leadership skills and working with others. All these skills are important in relation to meeting the outcomes of the NMC to become a qualified nurse. The NMC Standards of Proficiency for entry to the register (2004: 30) clearly includes dissemination as being necessary for qualifying as a nurse:

> ❝ *Care Delivery: .... identify relevant changes in practice or new information and disseminate it to colleagues* ❞
>
> (NMC 2004)

For a student nurse therefore dissemination involves sharing with others findings from other people's research or people's views on certain topics. One kind of nursing assessment that can identify learning about dissemination and how to disseminate is an assignment which asks you to present information to peers. This kind of activity is known as an oral presentation, which can also be undertaken outside of the classroom or practice area at a conference. The next section will look at this more closely.

Skills for disseminating evidence in presentations

Box 10.1 outlines a typical nursing assessment which asks you to present information to peers.

The NMC Standards of Proficiency for entry to the register states that as part of a student nurse's personal and professional development it is important to:

> 66 *Contribute to the learning experiences and development of others by facilitating the mutual sharing of knowledge and experience.* 99

> (NMC 2004: 34)

You may for example be asked to present your work to colleagues as part of a module, and to undertake this kind of activity requires similar skills to that of presenting to

---

Box 10.1 Dissemination of the evidence for care

Using an aspect of patient care from your recent clinical placement experience, you are required to present an evidence base rationale for this to your peers.

The presentation will take 15 minutes in total, allowing for at least 5 minutes of discussion and questions.

The focus for assessment will be on:

    a) The type of evidence for dissemination.

    b) Where you obtained this evidence.

    c) Your presentation of the evidence.

    d) The means you choose to disseminate your findings—as per guidelines.

Note: PowerPoint must be used.

people you may not know at an event such as an NHS Trust good practice day or at a conference. Brookes (2007: 32) found that qualified nurses did not disseminate their academic course work and that the main reasons were 'lack of confidence, lack of motivation and lack of awareness of the means to disseminate'. Kinn & Kenyon (2002) had shown however that if nurses had an opportunity to develop their skills in presentation that this would have a very positive outcome. They outlined their evaluation of a series of workshops for this purpose in Scotland and their findings clearly illustrated an increased number of nurses who did present their work at local events, nationally, and internationally.

You might be asked as part of the activity to reflect on how you disseminated to your peers and some key questions to use can be seen in Box 10.2.

Let us consider the presentation that you would undertake to disseminate your evidence-based findings as outlined in Box 10.1. Depending on the focus to your placement there are a number of possibilities. If you were on a surgical ward you may decide to focus on the need to ensure good practice in infection control. Your presentation will involve using PowerPoint and may include the following slides:

1. Title of the topic: Hand-washing and its importance in infection control and your name and student group, year, and placement name

2. Aims of the session:

   a. To outline the main reasons for why good practice in infection control procedures are important on a surgical ward.

   b. To explain why good practice in hand-washing is important in preventing infection.

   c. To provide evidence to support good practice in hand-washing by nurses.

3. Outline reasons for good practice in infection control procedures.

Box 10.2 Self-assessment questions: guide for reflection

1. What was the aim of the presentation?
2. Who were you presenting to?
3. How did you prepare for it and do you think you did this well?
4. What method of presentation did you use to present the evidence and do you still think that was the right one?
5. How did your peers respond to the presentation? Did they ask questions? Did they listen? How do you know this?
6. What do you think you did well and what you didn't? what would you do next time
7. What did you learn from the experience?

4. Explanation of hand-washing importance and good practice.

5. What the evidence is to support the need for effective hand-washing.

6. Conclusions in regards to the evidence.

7. Key references used in the supporting evidence.

For key points to remember regarding any slide presentation see Key Points box. Figure 10.1 illustrates the slides in the above presentation and the whole PowerPoint presentation can be accessed online.

EBP in action

Consider the presentation in Fig. 10.2 and determine if it fulfils the criteria in Box 10.1 (the content of the presentation relates to the issues to be considered by students in writing their research dissertation which is of relevance to Chapter 9)

Compare it to the one on hand washing in Fig. 10.1.

Remember both Powerpoint presentations can be accessed online.

This kind of presentation can be placed on the student Virtual Learning environment, such as BlackBoard to share your findings with colleagues. In other words you will be able to disseminate your own research-based evidence for the importance of hand-washing in infection control.

Some students may wish to share their reflection of the student experience with a wider audience, and may decide (often with support of their tutors or on occasion

---

! Key points

- Include in the first slide the title of your topic, name and group/course details, and where you study.

- All information should be understandable and use bullet points to make statements and then not too many per slide.

- Make sure that the presentation is in a colour which can easily be read by people and the same for the words.

- If including images make sure people will be able to see them clearly.

- Try not to overload your presentation with 'gimmicks' which detract the audience from the message you are trying to convey.

- Check for spelling and grammar errors.

- Use lower case type unless upper case appropriate.

- In your last slide include contact details should anyone wish to discuss the presentation further with you.

Hand washing and its importance in infection control

Student Nurse C Holland-Rees
September 2006
Ward B–Surgical Ward

1

Aims of the session

- To outline the main reasons for why good practice in infection control procedures are important on a surgical ward
- To explain why good practice in hand washing is important in preventing infection
- To provide evidence to support good practice in hand washing by nurses

2

The chain of infection

- Infectious agent
- Source of infection
- Portal of exit
- Modes of transmission
- Portal of entry
- Susceptible person
- Breaking the chain of infection

3

Reasons for good practice in infection control procedures on a surgical ward

- Prevent spread of infection from one patient to another or from nurse to patient when in hospital (hospital acquired infection)
- Meet the Department of Health requirements for reducing hospital acquired infection (DH 2007)
- Save patients' lives and reduce additional suffering and unnecessary pain and anxiety

4

Importance of hand washing in infection control

- Key to prevention and control of infection
- Choices of hand-decontamination: soap and water, alcohol based hand rubs or gel or antimicrobial hand wash
- Six-step hand wash technique (Endacott et al. 2009).
- Use of personal protective equipment: gloves, disposable aprons and eye and mouth protection
- Student nurses: importance of learning in clinical skills sessions

5

Evidence to support the need for effective hand-washing

- MRSA and Clostridium difficile rates of infection
- Dept of Health 2009
  http://www.dh.gov.uk/en/Publichealth/Healthprotection/Healthcareacquiredinfection/index.htm
- National Patient Safety
  http://www.npsa.nhs.uk/cleanyourhands/
- CQC survey shows patients think hand hygiene of doctors and nurses is improving (May 2009)

6

Key references and hand-washing

- Endacott R., Jevon, P. & Cooper, S. 2009
  Clinical Nursing Skills: Core and Advanced, Oxford University Press, Chapter 4: Essential Skills
- Delivering clean safe care
  http://www.clean-safe-care.nhs.uk/

7

Figure 10.1 Example of hand-washing presentation

Preparing for your dissertation

Karen Holland

Editor

Nursing evidence-based practice skills

1

Dissertation options

- Option A: a structured/comprehensive or systematized review of evidence on a particular topic/critical analysis of implications for practice
- Option B: a research proposal that includes a critical review of relevant research literature etc.

2

Developing the research design
Finding the topic

- Deciding on the research question
- Agreeing project aim and research objectives
- Identifying the methodology and methods
- Gathering evidence
- Analysing the evidence and determining the findings
- Writing up

3

Study question and aim(s)

- Refining the original idea (usually following reading and reviewing literature)
- Arriving at the research question
- Research aims: what is it that you need to know/determine?
- Research outcomes: what is it you want to have achieved at the end of the study?

4

Literature review—evidence base

- Searching the literature—systematically
- Critically appraising the research evidence
- Deciding on your position regarding the evidence, e.g. the political or social perspective
- Reference management: keeping details/ possible use of Endnote
- Being systematic about the evidence presentation

5

Methodology and method choice

- The research question (and or hypothesis) will determine the methodological approach to be taken
- What you need to find out will determine the research methods (data collection)

6

Ethical approval

- If you have chosen Option B assignment you will need to consider all aspects of gaining ethical approval from an Ethics Committee and issues around information to participants and/or informed consent
- If you have chosen Option A assignment you will need to consider the ethical considerations taken by researchers in the articles/reports you are reviewing

7

Writing and structuring the dissertation

- Be systematic from the beginning—it helps to outline the study structure into relevant chapters
- Ensure referencing in text matches reference lists/keep accurate reference material
- Liaise with supervisor on an ongoing basis
- Follow Project guidelines for presentation

8

Figure 10.2 Example of preparing for your dissertation presentation

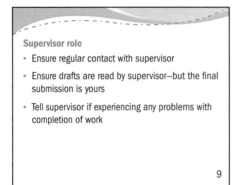

Supervisor role
- Ensure regular contact with supervisor
- Ensure drafts are read by supervisor—but the final submission is yours
- Tell supervisor if experiencing any problems with completion of work

9

Publishing from the assignment
- Once your assignment has been submitted and a successful outcome achieved you may wish to forget it ever existed!
- The brave among you might want to publish the work or have been told that it is worthy of publication
- Consider a number of issues if this is the case— including the type of paper you want to write, the journal and the writing involved (time)
- Most importantly take advice from someone with publishing experience as to whether or not this could be achieved

10

Figure 10.2 Example of preparing for your dissertation presentation (Continued)

with their tutors) that a conference presentation is an opportunity to do so. This is often spoken of as 'presenting a paper' but in reality you are making a presentation similar to the one in the classroom. The same skills are required for both but because the audience is different there will be some variation in how you undertake the presentation.

Unlike undertaking a presentation to peers in a classroom, however, presenting at a conference is normally preceded by having to submit an abstract of what you will be presenting. In addition for most conferences all the abstracts are considered for inclusion in the conference programme by a panel of reviewers. This means that if you want to have your abstract accepted for presentation that it will need to follow the conference guidelines for acceptance in the first place, but also offer something that will attract attention in ensuring successful acceptance. This next section will discuss writing an abstract for a conference.

Skills for writing an abstract

Firstly let us consider what an abstract is. In the context of a research study an abstract is very important. It is considered an essential part of summarizing the study for the final written report and as you will have seen from Chapter 6, an abstract (included in an article) then acts as a reference to determine whether the article which you have found through searching actually includes the information you might require. It needs (without resorting to the full article), in brief, to inform the reader:

- What the background context to the study was, i.e. what had led up to undertaking the study.

- What the focus to the study was, i.e. the actual research focus, which could also refer to some of the key literature.
- What methodology and methods were used in the study.
- How the research was undertaken—briefly mentioning data analysis.
- Main findings or results.
- Implications of the findings.

This kind of abstract in an article is usually required to be a certain word length, e.g. the *Journal of Clinical Nursing* (JCN) abstract is required to be 300 words in length and also structured according to specific headings. Each journal will have its own style in which to present an abstract. An example of an abstract from JCN can be seen in the Example Box below.

....

Example Death, empathy, and self preservation: the emotional labour of caring for families of the critically ill in adult intensive care

Abstract

Aim and objective. The purpose of this phenomenological study is to explore the emotional labour nurses face when caring for relatives of the critically ill in intensive care unit.

Background. The admission of a critically ill patient into adult intensive care is a crisis for both patients and their families. Family members of the critically ill may experience extreme levels of stress and emotional turmoil throughout the course of the relative's illness. A central tenet of providing holistic nursing care in the intensive care unit is to care for both patients and their families; however, the emotional involvement required places considerable demands on those delivering care. The support health care providers require is frequently overlooked in these challenging environments.

Design. Heideggerian phenomenological approach was adopted.

Methods. A purposive sample of 12 registered nurses working in an adult intensive care unit were interviewed. Interview transcripts were analysed using Colaizzi's framework. Data were collected in autumn 2005.

Results. Analysis of the participants' interview transcripts revealed the following themes: significance of death, establishing trust, information giving, empathy, intimacy and self preservation.

Conclusions. Emotional work forms an important part of the critical care nurses job. The significance of death, breaking bad news and interpersonal relationships are sources of emotional stress for the critical care nurse caring for the family of the critically ill. The impact of this stress on the nurse and the care they deliver requires further investigation.

»

> **Relevance to clinical practice.** Registered nurses caring for families who have relatives in adult intensive care units expend considerable emotional labour. Potentially, unless appropriately supported and managed, emotional labour may lead to occupational stress and ultimately burnout
>
> From Stayt, L. C. (2009) *Journal of Clinical Nursing* 18 (9) 1267–1275.

EBP in action

Identify three journals and consider the guidelines for the abstract. What were the main differences between them? Following this undertaking, and using the reviewing guidelines in Chapter 7 guidelines, determine if the abstract included the above points regarding content.

We will return to the above type of abstract when considering the steps required in writing an article for publication.

Writing an abstract for a conference presentation

Writing an abstract for a conference presentation has similarities to that for an article, in particular the importance of conveying the message of what your presentation will include. In terms of dissemination of evidence and research, presenting a paper at a conference is an important activity (Happell 2007), not only as a means of making others aware of what you want to share with them but also raising awareness of the topic itself. Most conference abstracts are also published in the conference proceedings or as happens at many conferences through being given a CD rom with all the abstracts and papers presented. Conferences also give possible presenters an option of either an oral (speaking) or poster presentation. We will consider both in this chapter.

In considering writing an abstract, which will be accepted by the conference review team or Scientific Committee, Coad and Devitt (2006: 113) state that one of the '*biggest hurdles is getting started*'. They recommend initially that you 'review the title and aims of the conference' as this will have an impact on how you both structure your abstract and most importantly what you intend to present in terms of content. For example, if a conference has a focus on nurse education and student learning, submitting an abstract which describes a clinical issue such as hand-washing technique will not be relevant. However if the topic you wished to present was how student nurses learn about hand washing and how this is then implemented in the reality of practice then the focus may well be feasible. Coad *et al.* (2007) have written a very useful paper on the issue of developing an abstract for conferences where they outline 'eight steps'. These eight steps are:

Step 1 Thinking about the purpose of your abstract

Step 2 Getting started

Step 3 Setting out your style

Step 4 Avoiding common pitfalls

Step 5 Getting the title to appeal

Step 6 Aims and outcomes

Step 7 Content

Step 8 References

Step 9 The submission process

Step 10 What happens next

These offer a very useful guide for anyone new to writing abstracts. Albarran (2007: 570) also writes about similar stages and why writing a conference abstract 'is a skilled activity requiring attention to detail and an ability to write clearly, fluently and informatively', but also offers examples of why abstracts are unsuccessful in being accepted. He offers the following reasons (Albarran 2007:570):

- Lacks stated aims and objectives.

- Is unstructured, fragmented and lacking rigour.

- Presents results in a vague and confusing manner.

- Fails to convey the implications for the profession simply and succinctly.

- Undersells—or oversells—the originality or uniqueness of the work.

Albarran (2007) also offers an example of a typical list of instructions for preparing a conference abstract, but advises checking the conference requirements to ensure these are met exactly as required (see Box 10.3).

Box 10.3 Typical list of instructions for preparing a conference abstract

1. List of authors, institutions, and contact details.

2. Contact details of corresponding author.

3. Preference for presentation mode (oral or poster).

4. Title (must be short, not more than 12 words).

5. Structure of presentation (e.g. research).

6. List of learning outcomes (if applicable).

7. Word limit (often 200-300 words maximum).

8. Font size (not larger than 12 point).

9. Specific type of font (e.g. Times, Arial).

10. Specified number of references (maximum of three).

11. Specified referencing system (Vancouver or Harvard).

12. List of key words (maximum of four).

13. Declaration of any conflict of interest.

14. Check whether tables/figures are permitted.

(From Albarran, J. (2007) Planning, developing and writing an effective conference abstract, *British Journal of Cardiac Nursing* 2 (11) 570–572.

Why do I need to know this?

Many of you may be thinking why should I know about submitting abstracts to a conference as it is unlikely that I will be considered for doing this? I attend a number of conferences where more and more students are now presenting their work, either in relation to their own studies or together with their tutors.

This kind of activity offers an excellent opportunity to undertake personal and professional development and also for meeting other students as well as authors whom they may have come across in writing assignments.

Attending conferences without doing a presentation is also an excellent opportunity for sharing ideas and being able to participate in discussions.

For example the NETNEP International Nurse Education Conferences have a student programme, **http://www.netnep-conference.elsevier.com/**, where not only are students able to submit a short paper for a competitive student scholarship to attend the conference itself, but also if they attend they have an opportunity to meet other students to share their student experiences as well as other social and academic activities.

There are other similar events where the student experience is considered an essential part of the conference experience. The Royal College of Nursing (UK) for example has a student community focus and there are a number of opportunities available to write, obtain support and submit short reports for their student paper and present poster presentations at the student day at their annual congress (see **http://www. rcn.org.uk/development/students/** for details). This is an excellent way to begin your dissemination activity and also promotes the development of your future professional practice.

Examples of conference abstract

An example of an abstract can be seen later on in the Example Box. This was chosen not just because it is one of the author's but also relates to the student experience of learning to be a nurse. It might be of interest to compare the findings with your own experiences.

+ ....

EBP in action

Although this was an abstract submitted to a conference in 1996 and involved evaluation of an experience that was a later Project 2000 curriculum where student nurses undertook a period of rostered practice (a pre-1996 curriculum) it still has merit as an abstract. There was an agreed word limit of 400 words without the author information and title. As an exercise, critique the abstract against the criteria identified by Albarran (Box 10.3) normally included in a conference abstract. Consider what is missing from the abstract and what you think, based on this, the author could have done to improve your understanding of what the aims of the presentation were.

....

Example of a conference abstract

Title 'A journey to becoming: The student nurse in transition

Authors Karen Holland MSc, BSc (Hon), RN, RNT

Lecturer Department of Nursing, University of Salford

This paper is based on a study undertaken to explore the nature of 'transition' as experienced by student nurses and through gaining an insight into their world sought to establish whether there was a clearly defined 'transition stage within their journey to becoming qualified nurses.

In keeping with the developing relationship between the disciplines of anthropology and nursing, the methodology of choice was ethnography. Thematic analysis of the data revealed a 'transition' for the student nurse which was not clearly defined and the lack of clarity was being perpetuated for many by their dual role as both 'student nurse' and 'worker'. This was also creating a potential role conflict and 'blurring' of the boundaries between 'professional' nursing and 'skilled' health care work. This was of concern on two counts:

1) the teaching of the auxiliary nursing skills that they equated with basic nursing skills essential for the first year student nurse to 'fit in' to the reality of practice

2) when they were acting in the auxiliary role, what were the boundaries between that and their status as student nurses?

The data also revealed that the rationale for 'learning to become a nurse' retains the idealized and vocational imagery of nursing as 'helping and caring' for 'sick' people. This is significant, in that despite the changes brought about by the

»

introduction of Project 2000 and the developing 'academic' nature of nursing, the majority of the student nurses continued to want to do so because of what one could only describe as an inner sense of vocation. The students also appeared to acknowledge that 'knowledgeable doer' and 'knowledgeable carer' were similar but in expanding this theme it became clear that 'knowledgeable doing' was viewed as being linked to actual task and job performance rather than the 'caring' qualities inherent within nursing. 'In limbo' states were discovered as well as the 'ritual' nature of their rostered practice experience.

It was considered imperative that further study be undertaken to determine the exact nature of the role and activities of student nurses within clinical practice and that in retrospect that they should be given full student status and in effect become 'students of nursing'. Central to this is the premise that in order to retain the caring ethos central to nursing's existence that they should also be referred to as 'knowledgeable caring doers'.

This abstract was submitted and accepted for the Nurse Education Tomorrow Conference 1996

Having an abstract accepted for presentation at a conference is not just about having a good quality abstract however. Unfortunately most conferences only have the capacity for an exact number of either oral or poster presentations, as well as having to balance out the number of presentations they have to include in their conference themes, and good abstracts may well not be accepted due to this reason and not because they did not meet the required standards. Most conference organizers will give feedback if this is the case.

Types of conference presentations

Some of you will have actually submitted the abstract for a poster presentation and some of you may also be offered the chance to present your work as a poster rather than an oral presentation and this should not be considered a lesser form of presentation at all. In fact poster presentations at many conferences offer a wider opportunity for dissemination, and indeed many conferences now allocate an equal amount of time for poster presentations as they do for oral presentations.

If you are offered this alternative by the conference organizers, firstly consider whether the content of what you would be presenting does in fact translate easily into a poster presentation, as certainly some kind of abstracts which communicate early findings of research study, for example, may not have enough detail to include in a poster presentation. The panel of abstract reviewers however (usually known as a scientific committee) will already have considered this prior to recommending the alternative to an oral presentation.

The main purpose for submitting the abstract may well have been to explore early ideas or literature. A student abstract may have presented experiences from practice supported by literature and evidence and could, with the right kind of re-focus, make an excellent poster.

If this happens to you then it would be advisable to discuss the possibilities, with either your personal tutor or one of the lecturers who you know has experience of presenting at a conference, before you make an final decision about accepting a poster presentation and not an oral one.

EBP in action

1. Find the details of submitting a conference abstract from three different conferences. These could be UK based or international. Compare them with each other and identify any differences from the points already made in this section. How many of them encouraged students to submit abstracts?

2. Using one of your own assignments write an abstract of 200 words, the content of which you would like to share with a group of students. Reflect on the challenges of doing this and what you also learnt about being concise when having to summarize your work of possibly 3000 words into a few paragraphs.

Once your abstract has been accepted you must then consider what you will need to do to actually undertake a presentation at the conference. Firstly we will consider presenting an oral presentation.

The oral conference presentation

First of all, if you have achieved success congratulate yourself for having your abstract accepted. Now you have to prepare the actual presentation and yourself. If the conference is in the UK or international there will also be travel and accommodation to organize and most importantly funding will need to be obtained for all of this plus the actual conference fees. Some conferences actually have reduced conference registration fees for students either wishing to attend the conference or if they are presenting. An example of this is the Nurse Education Tomorrow Conference (**http://www. jillrogersassociates.co.uk/conferences/netinternational.htm/**). Please check this on an annual basis. An excellent example of how students can participate in this kind of event is of a student where I work who won a student award during her clinical placement experience. She is using her award to attend an educational event which she believes will enhance her learning and also help her personal and professional development. It was a requirement of the award that she used the funds awarded for an educational purpose.

An example of a conference which had reduced student registration fees in 2009 was the National HIV Association (**http://www.nhivna.org/index.php/**) which had ten student concession awards for their 2009 annual conference.

Your abstract has been accepted, now you have to prepare yourself and your presentation. Some issues we have already covered in the early section on presenting to your peers but we will be looking at these again in this section with regards to conference presentation. The key points to a slide presentation using PowerPoint were covered in the previous key points box.

Remember this is about presenting evidence of one kind or another. It may be useful if you are presenting the results of an in-depth literature review on a topic to re-read the steps necessary for undertaking such a review (see Chapters 7 & 9). This will have given you clear areas for including in your presentation; areas such as background to the review, key questions being asked of the literature, your search strategy, key words used, how you chose the papers to include in the review, how did you categorize them, what was the evidence, how did you theme the literature and what were your findings and conclusion. An example can be seen in the presentation on Partnerships and Collaboration in Higher Education in Fig. 10.3.

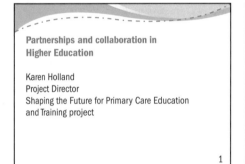

Figure 10.3 Example of a presentation on Partnerships and collaboration in Higher Education

Sub-projects 2

- A survey and questionnaire which can be utilized to determine workforce perspectives of education and training needs to deliver IHSC
- Focus groups and survey to determine local user/ carer perspectives of education and training needs to deliver IHSC
- Development and piloting of an Education and Training Needs Analysis Tool (ETNA) for identifying workforce needs to deliver IHSC   5

Collaboration

- Collaboration is open to many interpretations. Definition used in this project:
- Collaboration is defined as a dynamic transforming process of creating power sharing partnership for pervasive application in health care practice, education, research and organisational settings for the purposeful attention to needs and problems in order to achieve likely successful outcomes (Sullivan 1998)   6

Outcomes of project collaboration

- Proving to be instrumental in creating networks and stimulating dialogue acrossthe NW Region
- Acting as a catalyst for bringing people and organisations together
- Creating a community of learning in the Project team

7

Integrated Health and Social care: the inter-professional dimension

- Future workforce perspective: a student conference
- Key issue that arose from the day: need to understand each other's professional roles and responsibilities
- If we don't understand each other's roles how can we expect a patient to do so (Student comment)   8

Learning to work together

- Major theme throughout the student conference in particular the need to have the skills to work collaboratively within teams and the attitude of valuing others in those teams for the contribution they make to patient care
- Major theme throughout the project is working together across disciplines—not creating a new single multi skilled professional workforce Respect for uni-professional roles in care delivery   9

Key implications for health and social care services and education

- Systematic Review: six major themes which have been embedded throughout all the sub-projects. These are:
- Communication
- Team working
- Role awareness
- Personal and professional development
- Practice Development and leadership
- Partnership working   10

Example of role awareness implications

- Role awareness should become an essential element of all programmes relating to preparing the workforce to deliver integrated health and social care
- Shared learning initiatives between health and social care workforce students in practice should be encouraged to develop awareness and understanding of team roles
- Role awareness education for service users/carers should be considered essential to ensure effective communication and appropriate use of services   11

Conclusion

- Partnership and collaboration between education, health and social care is essential if future integrated services are to be delivered by an efficient, skilled and knowledgeable workforce
- It is our joint responsibility to ensure that the future workforce is given the educational experience to make this a reality
- Ref: Sullivan, T. J. (1998) Collaboration - A health care imperative, McGraw Hill, New York   12

Figure 10.3 Example of a presentation on Partnerships and collaboration in Higher Education (Continued)

EBP in action

Critically review the presentation in Fig. 10.3 and determine whether the presentation could be understood without any dialogue to go with it and in your view what could have been done differently. Remember the issues of key messages and time, plus the focus to the conference when reviewing this presentation. Undertake to devise your own presentation.

Preparing for your presentation

All presentations involve a level and type of communication. This also applies to presenting to your peers and tutors in the classroom. The material you will be preparing is one area; however, another important element of presenting in any context is that of how you use your voice, your body language, and most importantly your appearance. Hardicre, Coad and Devitt (2007) provide a useful ten steps approach to successful conference presentations see Box 10. 4.

Box 10.4 Ten steps to successful conference presentations

1. Step 1—Considerations: such as the audience, their level of knowledge, how many, time allowed.

2. Step 2—Preparing the content: such as not too much information, clarity of information.

3. Step 3—Visual aids: PowerPoint; data stick or disc.

4. Step 4—Handouts: helpful and appreciated; may be a website.

5. Step 5—Practice: timing must be right as must clarity.

6. Step 6—Preparing for the day: ensure you are there on time and too nervous (natural).

7. Step 7—Delivering your presentation: introduce yourself and topic; take your time and look at the audience.

8. Step 8—Tips to engage the audience: keep eye contact, ensure you speak to all audience by alternating this eye contact.

9. Step 9—Questions: Be confident and if they don't ask anything, you ask them.

10. Step 10—Networking: take some cards with you and if none available write contact details in a diary or notebook;make a point of talking to people.

From Hardicre, J. Coad, J. & Devitt, P. (2007) Ten steps to successful conference presentations. *British Journal of Nursing* 16 (7) 402–404.

Let us consider first the preparation required. It might be useful at this stage to re-visit the abstract you sent in. If we use the one in the last Example Box above as a guide, you will have noted in your critique that I reported on the actual research study carried out and not necessarily outlined in a very explicit way what I was going to present. You can determine however that I would be reporting on the research undertaken and my findings. You will also have noted that I would be presenting to a conference audience of nurse educators.

Based on this you need to consider:

- Why you are presenting the information in the first place.
- Who the audience that is going to listen to it and ask you questions.
- What you are going to be telling them, based on what they will already have read in the conference abstract book.
- How you are going to present the information.

Following this you need to consider:

- How long you have to present the information.
- What you want the audience to gain from listening to you.
- What the venue is like for doing the presentation.
- What time the presentation is taking place.
- Do you need to take a handout of the presentation with you or will there be other means to communicate with people who are interested in contacting you after your presentation.
- Making some notes of what you need to say, either with the slide handout or alternatively on some cards that you can refer to key points.

You will as a student be familiar with having to present to your peers in the classroom and know what it feels like before you do this. Most of you will have felt those 'butterflies' and be apprehensive beforehand. This is a normal reaction and even very experienced presenters still have these feelings, especially as you think they may not like what you have to say. However taking the time to practice beforehand will make a difference, either to colleagues or to yourself. This is also good practice in timing yourself to ensure that you do not have too much information to present or that you do not speak quickly or too slowly. You will also be very familiar as a student with how you feel in listening to a lecture straight after lunch for example—when a softly spoken lecturer and a topic that to you is not interesting makes you feel a bit sleepy! It is important to consider how the lecturer, or in this case the presenter, may be feeling as well—as it may be the first time they have given that lecture and they also have just had lunch!

If you know where you are going to be presenting, it is a good idea to check out the setting when you get to the conference venue, or if presenting to your peers in university, check out the classroom or lecture theatre you will be presenting in. Checking the size of the room, the seating arrangements and most importantly the technology available is essential. Most of you will be familiar with using either a pen drive (USB) or a CD, either for saving your assignments or notes. Ensure you don't forget to take them with you, or possibly the wrong one!

However, technology is not always reliable, as some of us know to our cost. I personally have been known to take at least two different pen drives with me plus a set of OHP slides in case of emergencies! I am aware of situations that students have found themselves in, when they have come to present their work in class to find that the computer will not allow them to use that particular model of pen-drive (USB).

It is always good to check these things before presenting whenever possible. Another option that I have found useful in such circumstances but again should not be necessary is to send the presentation to an email address which can be accessed via the internet (e.g. your own personal account). This latter option is for many an extreme one—but for those who are nervous of not having their presentation available to them, especially if first time presenters these issues are a possible option.

? Thinking about

Consider your own experience of listening to a presentation. What was the best one you experienced and what made it so? Consider the environment, the speaker, the topic, the length, and of course the opportunity for you to ask questions. You may also have chosen to present to other students as part of a learning outcome in a professional development module and know exactly what that presenter may have experienced.

Making the presentation

Now we come to the actual presentation itself. This is where you need to remind yourself that you know exactly what you want to disseminate to others. As a qualified nurse you will be expected to present information in a variety of ways and all the skills you learn from disseminating to your peers in class or in practice will all help you with this. Delivering the presentation may involve the following practical aspects:

- Make sure you have some way of timekeeping, e.g. watch or wall clock.

- You may need to make sure you have a drink available (normally provided at a conference) as your mouth can get dry if nervous—check with your university/school rules with regard to drinks in the classroom.

- At a conference you may well have someone introduce you to those listening—unlike the classroom where most of the students will know you.

- Start the presentation by explaining what the topic is and what you intend to do. (This may also be on a slide as aims.)

- Try and sound confident about what you are talking about.

- Try and focus on the audience as much as possible when talking and ensure that you look at both sides as well to the front so people will know you are talking to all of them not just those in front.

- Try not to speak too quickly and rush through the presentation, and particularly try not to mumble. This is very important if not everyone in the audience speaks English or may be hard of hearing. Speak clearly and at a right speed.

- Try not to stand in front of the screen.

- Try not to wander about the room—using an electronic pointer does help people who choose to do this but it can still be distracting.

- It may be possible for you if using PowerPoint presentation to use an electronic pointer—these can be very useful if you have a diagram on the screen which you need to explain and point to.

- Always remember to try and smile every now and again at the audience, although grinning or making jokes all the way through is not a good idea!

Questions

When your presentation is over, whether this is 10 minutes to your peers in classroom or 20 minutes at a conference, there is usually built in some time for the audience to ask you questions. This can be for about 5–10 minutes depending on time allocated. They have come to hear what you have to say and are interested in the topic you have spoken about. They are not there to try and trip you up on what you have said. In the classroom, how you answer questions might well be part of an assessment as well as how you disseminated the information. Learning the skills on answering as a student will stand you in good stead for doing the same at a conference. It is usual at a conference for there to be someone who keeps you to time and ensures that the session finishes when it is meant to. If no-one wants to ask a question, you could try and ask them one yourself; for example, as a student you could ask: has anyone experienced a similar situation or has anyone looked at a similar topic and did you find any evidence that I haven't?

When the session is ended there may well be an opportunity to talk to other people at a conference, this is what Hardicre *et al.* (2007) call networking. This is often an excellent opportunity to share experiences or interests and also for keeping in contact with others. It is also important to reflect on your experience of being at a conference itself and participating. An excellent example is by Tierney-Wigg (2009), a student from the University of Salford who won a scholarship to attend a conference and wrote about his experience in a journal. A section from his paper can be seen in Box 10.5.

Box 10.5 The student experience of conference attendance

Just looking at the list of lecturers, doctors, professors and experts in their respective field filled us with awe, tinged with apprehension. By the end of the 'Meet and Greet' on the first day this was swept aside as we were all made to feel welcome, and indeed valued for our unique perspective on the topics to be discussed. We were able to ask questions and give feedback in seminars as peers, and as the conference continued ideas were beginning to take shape as to the key elements I would take with me in my further training. Publishers were keen to have us on board with their own student programmes and our opinions were noted with genuine interest; something that we all felt added to the experience.

We really were service users in this environment, which gave us all something to reflect on with regards our individual career paths.

Extract from Tierney-Wigg S. (2009) The student experience of NETNEP 2008: A personal reflection. Nurse Education in Practice 9 (2) 84–85.

The main consideration with presenting either to your peers in classroom or to a conference audience is that you gain something from it personally and professionally and most importantly enjoy it.

Skills for disseminating evidence in posters

A popular form of assessment is that of presenting your work by preparing a poster. Regardless of whether you are a student presenting a poster for colleagues in clinical practice or at a conference, the basic principles of what you need to consider are the same. Halligan (2008) believes that the poster presentation is as valued a form as an oral presentation and many conferences now offer them both as very distinct opportunities for disseminating evidence. He does make a point however that in many instances conference organizers do not make any difference between judging abstracts for the different types of presentations and considers that the selection criteria for a poster should be different. He argues that 'poster presentations are visual tools; therefore the selection criteria should reflect this' (Halligan 2008: 44). He concludes that:

> 66 ...poster presentations offer a forum where educators, practitioners and researchers all convene to appraise knowledge illustrated in many creative ways. This can only assist in narrowing the research-practice gap and promote the concepts of evidence-based practice, reflective practice, excellence in research and scholarship, and to support continuous life-long learning among the nursing community. 99
>
> *(Halligan 2008: 45)*

You may be a student at a university where preparing and presenting a poster is part of either your formative or your summative learning experience. You may also have an opportunity to work within a group to develop a poster which illustrates some work you have been involved in within a seminar. Developing some skills in doing this will be invaluable to you, as not only will you gain practical experience but will also then be in a position to develop the skills in presenting information orally. Utecht & Tremayne (2008) explained how poster presentations were introduced into nursing education as a part of a module assessment that required students to complete a piece of written reflection on a poster presentation related to actual patient care. It was found that 'clinical practice staff said they felt they did not fully understand the module's requirements and students' anxieties about them', so they:

> 66 . . . decided that students would produce an informative piece of visual material in the form of a poster. The poster project, entitled 'patient-centred enablement in clinical practice' encourages students to think about concepts of enablement from the start of their clinical placement. The poster presentation should be part of the preliminary interview with mentors, covering aspects of care that could be addressed. 99
>
> (Utecht & Tremayne 2008: 26)

Utecht & Tremayne's (2008: 26–27) subsequent evaluation 'found that 735 of the students had displayed their poster at their clinical placement' and an example they describe was where 'one student had prepared a poster on dietary issues for renal patients and referred to this when educating a patient new to dialysis'. There were issues however that arose concerning the mentors and clinical practice staff's own skills and knowledge of what was involved in poster presentations and how to determine their effectiveness.

This study illustrates the value of posters in the dissemination of work by student nurses and in the evaluation of their work the students clearly agreed on the value for their own learning and skill development. Based on these examples and experiences what is then required to prepare and present a poster of a topic for dissemination? Hardicre et al. (2007) again offers a ten–step approach to successful poster presentation in Box 10.6, which is a useful guide for novice poster presenters.

The main consideration for a poster is that it is a visual presentation, albeit that the presenter will have a dialogue with people who come to look at the poster or ask questions about what is presented there. However being visual does not mean that the poster should be covered in pictures and graphs, there is a need for balance.

The second consideration is who the audience will be. If the focus to your presentation is on a topic you have worked on in the classroom and you are presenting to fellow students then the poster content will need to reflect their ability to understand. The RCN website for students wishing to present posters at Congress in April 2009 had the following tips for students if their poster abstract was accepted (see Box 10.7).

Box 10.6 Ten steps to successful poster presentation

Note: These steps are mainly focused on the presentation of a research study

1. Step 1—Planning your poster: need to be clear what you want to say; is it representing a research study or not.
2. Step 2—Things to consider before constructing your poster: limited space will direct amount of content for example. If a research study or systematic review of literature consider the Steps 3–7 in the layout of the poster.
3. Step 3—Developing the abstract and title.
4. Step 4—Introduction.
5. Step 5—Methods.
6. Step 6—Results.
7. Step 7—Discussion and acknowledgements.
8. Step 8—Putting it all together: dimensions are normally stated by conference or your tutors; computer programmes are available to help you; laminate it to avoid damage in carrying it.
9. Step 9—Seek advice: if not familiar for example with using technology; check spelling and grammar or other errors before finalizing.
10. Step 10—The day of presentation: check space to place it—often allocated day and a number.

From Hardicre, J. Devitt, P. & Coad, J. (2007) Ten steps to successful poster presentation, *British Journal of Nursing* 16 (7) 398–401.

Another useful site for examples of poster presentations is that of the Centre for Reviews and Dissemination: **http://www.york.ac.uk/inst/crd/posters_presentations.htm/**. However these are very detailed posters, focusing very much on systematic reviews on a number of topics.

Box 10.7 Some hints and tips for posters

- Make sure you know what you want to say and what the outcome or message of your work is and then try and be as creative as possible in presenting it.
- It helps to try and keep your poster visual by using charts or diagrams or pictures.
- You may not want to be with your poster all day to explain the content so ensure that it can be understood if you are not there.
- You may want to have handouts of your poster to give to people to take away.

From RCN website: **http://www.rcn.org.uk/development/students/**
accessed 14 April 2009

EBP in action

Access the site mentioned above (http://www.york.ac.uk/inst/crd/posters_presentations.htm/) and look at a number of the poster presentations. Consider in relation to Box 10.7 whether the posters viewed were presented in the best way for that information and determine who the audience was likely to be. Could you understand what the content of the posters were saying, i.e. the message and the topic for example? Finding this site will also help you develop the skills outlined in Chapter 6.

Practical considerations for posters

Returning to Hardicre *et al*. (2007) consider first the size that your poster has to be. Conference organizers are very clear in relation to the size required, for example if you have been told you have a space 3ft × 3ft to use you would not then prepare a poster that would be 5ft × 5ft!

Conversely if you had a 6ft × 6ft space and you designed a poster that was only 3ft × 3ft it may well appear 'lost' in this size of display area. All conferences will give you specific poster size requirements once your poster abstract has been accepted, and may also have guidance on their website prior to submission (see http://www. ukstrokeforum.org/ for example).

There are also a number of design issues to be considered in order to ensure people want to come and look at your poster, consider its message, and most importantly talk to you as the poster presenter! These are: colours used, size of fonts for different section headings and messages, use of pictures and graphics, ensuring the message is clear with contact details. One useful idea is to map out the poster sections on a piece of paper first, to get an idea of layout etc; of course using PowerPoint as a tool to do this can be a better idea (see this website for examples http://www.studentposters.co.uk/templates.html/).

EBP in action

Using the key points outlined in Hardicre *et al*. (2007) prepare your own poster for presentation to your student colleagues. The topic may be the one chosen for the first 'EBP in action box' in this chapter—the evidence on a key topic of your choice. The final presentation must measure 36 inches wide × 48 inches long, i.e. a portrait size poster. Check what guidelines may be available on your own university web-site for preparing and presenting a poster.

Once you have prepared the poster there is then the issue of ensuring that it is of the best quality for a conference presentation, in other words having it laminated by a professional company or university department. This ensures less damage to the poster in transporting it to a conference and it is also good practice to do this. Usually putting the poster in a poster tube is a good idea for transporting it, especially important if you have to travel long distances. This does have a cost implication, which is why it is critical that you have the content of your planned poster checked by someone, as you would an essay or a paper for publication, for grammar, typos, and other errors in the text. If it is for a student seminar it may be that a paper copy is sufficient, dependent of course on the size required to present your information. You will be given guidance on this by your programme or module leaders.

It is important to remember that all these of presentations we have discussed are about dissemination of evidence of different kinds, and that ultimately it is what ensures the success of that dissemination which is important. Essential to all of them is preparing yourself, as we know that presentations can be daunting even for the most experienced presenters.

If presenting a poster, as with the oral presentation, it is important to arrive on time, check the space where your poster has to be placed (most conferences allocate a set number, date and time for it to be set up), make sure you have different kinds of material to put the poster on a display board (again conferences will usually give guidance). Ensure you are then standing or sitting by your poster when required, and be ready to talk to people about it.

If you have an opportunity to share the poster with practice colleagues, you may even have an opportunity to display it in practice; it is always a very good idea to ensure that the content of the poster is given approval by your tutors beforehand. Your programme guidelines will advise on this.

Summary of issues regarding presentations

- Presenting any work is an essential part of disseminating all kinds of evidence, not just research studies but evidence of scholarship and academic or practice related course work.

- Presentations offer an opportunity for you to demonstrate a range of skills, including sharing knowledge about an important practice related topic, developing effective communication and information technology skills.

- Presentations also encourage the development of confidence as a developing professional who is expected to include dissemination of evidence as part of the evidence-based practice cycle.

Writing a book review

Writing a book review is another method of dissemination; however, this concerns your views about someone else's written work and there are certain protocols to be observed in doing this. It is also one of the ways in which individuals can engage in writing for publication.

As with any other form of writing, it requires a set of skills which enables readers to clearly understand what is written and also of value to others. We have already explored what is required of writing assignments in Chapter 8, it may be useful to re-cap at this stage on some of the main issues involved in writing generally. Whitehead (2002) undertook a study exploring the academic writing experiences of student nurses and considered it essential that they should receive support during their programme of study for this critical aspect of their academic, and indeed practice, experience. Gimenez (2007) provides us with a valuable resource on the particulars of writing, from how to structure sentences to how to write a research proposal.

Writing a book review encompasses many skills, not least of which is a balanced critique of a book in relation to its usefulness either for the reader themselves or for others. Johnson (1995) offers some excellent guidance on how to write a book review, although it is important to remember that it is now 14 years since its publication. There are however some very useful examples of book reviews in this article and some additional criteria to use in evaluating this book.

Johnson (1995) offers a statement by Cormack (1994) as to the value of book reviews, in that they are helpful to those wishing to borrow books as well as those purchasing books for libraries. In my view they are also of value in giving possible readers, i.e. students, an opportunity to have an insight into the content of a book and its value for the programme of study they are undertaking. Books are often recommended by course tutors for students, some may even be essential ones that they have to purchase in order to use as part of a module. It is important therefore that tutors have an opportunity to decide on which ones are the most appropriate for their students but also that students have an opportunity to review a book for themselves.

You can see examples of these on the Nurse Education in Practice website: http://www.elsevier.com/nepr/, where there are a number of published book reviews written by students, and also an opportunity for students to be included in a panel of book reviewers. This means that the Book Review editor will be able to send them a book (sent to them by publishers) to review and they can then review it and, more often than not, retain the book if they consider it of use to them. Personally I think it is essential that students review books which in effect have been written for their use, and am aware that many publishers now include student reviews of books as part of the author's book writing development.

In journals there are usually a set number of words for book reviews; check the journal websites for this information, and in the author guidelines or similar section. This can range from 200 to 400 words in the main.

What are the steps therefore when reviewing a book?

Johnson (1995) has some useful information which you can refer to. Here are my own criteria:

1. What does the title tell you about the book?

2. When you are reading it, does the title reflect accurately what the book includes? In other words does the book meet your expectations of what the title states.

3. Who are the authors?

4. Is the book focused on the UK nursing programmes or is it translated or 'adapted'? (See example book review)

5. Who is the readership of the book? I.e. is it aimed at foundation course students or post-graduate level students?

6. If you are a student for whom the book is aimed at in terms of content and level, is it understandable to you? Are you able to read it easily?

7. Does the book have additional supporting material that you can use? For example it could have a CD Rom included as part of the book, to which you can refer to at different chapters or may have direct links to online web-based resource (such as with this book) This is a developing trend with publishers, to provide supporting material for students.

8. Does the book follow a logical sequence in terms of chapters?

9. Is the content up to date with regards to supporting evidence or literature? Are these accessible should you wish to obtain them for reference?

10. If there are illustrations are these not too many to be distracting to you in relation to the content?

11. How much does it cost? Is this good value when it comes to what the content is?

12. Does the book have access to online material?

13. As a student would you recommend it to others?

As you can see from these points, there are similarities to critiquing an article (see Chapter 7) and it is important that a book review is undertaken with the same consideration. It needs to be a balanced view, and offer both positive and negative viewpoints.

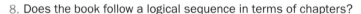

EBP in action

Consider the example book review in the example box below and, using the above questions as a guide, determine how many of the steps above the reviewer author had considered. Is the author for example a student or a lecturer? Using one of your own books undertake a similar review. If interested, and to encourage developing review skills, contact a book review editor on a journal and investigate what the requirements are to becoming a student member of a book review panel.

Example book review

Fundamentals of Nursing: Concepts, process and practice. Authors: Kozier, B, Erb G, Berman A, Snyder S, Lake R & Harvey S (2008) Pearson Education Limited.

This book is the European Edition of its US counterpart, yet the content in the main appears to focus on UK nursing. It is aimed at undergraduate level students nurses from only three branches: adult, mental health, and child (particularly those undertaking the Common Foundation Programme, page xi), omitting the learning disability branch. Given the importance of shared learning between the branches and the importance of caring for patients/clients of all ages, some who may have learning difficulties, this could be considered a significant omission.

On first reading the contents page (26 chapters) and the Guided Tour of the Book section, it looked to be a promising addition to my list of recommended reading for pre-registration nursing programmes. However there were some limitations to the book in translating to the UK market. Chapter 1 for example relied on many Royal College of Nursing (RCN) publications for its evidence, and when others were used these were very dated. It was disappointing also to see dated books when new editions were already in print, e.g. Hinchliff *et al.* (1993) and Parahoo (1997). References in most of the other chapters were in the main American, e.g. chapter on Health, Wellness and Illness and Chapter 11 on Infection Control, which may cause access issues for UK students, as well as not being able to link theory and evidence-based practice in these areas. Even the **Research Notes** mainly referenced US studies, e.g. 'Are nursing students mathematically prepared?' (Brown 2002: 521) when there are many significant European ones available. At the end of each chapter there was a Critical Reflection box linked to a case study at the beginning. It was difficult to see how this was a critical reflection, and it was left to the student to actually link theory and practice.

The chapter on Nursing Process was useful, but no evidence was provided to support the claim that 'diagnosing' was 'slowly developing in the UK' (p. 153). It was of some concern however in a **Clinical Alert**, the suggestion that a student could:

> *If possible, and with the patient's consent, take a digital or instant photograph of significant skin lesions for the patient record, include a measuring guide (ruler or tape) in the picture to demonstrate lesion size.*
>
> (p. 695)

In most NHS Trusts in the UK this is the role normally allocated to Medical Illustrations departments and the implication that a student nurse in the Common Foundation Programme could undertake this, even with the patient's consent, was in my view open to many kinds of interpretation.

On a positive note the diagrams, photographs, and practice notes were helpful, and the assessment interview questions in the practice focused chapters especially so.

(Holland, K. (2010) Unpublished Book Review.)

Writing an article for publication

As we have seen, writing a book review involves using a set of criteria on which to base your writing. Writing an article for publication uses a different set of criteria and steps but unlike a book review it is you that will be writing the article for others to review and critique (Devitt *et al.* 2007a). We have already seen in many of the other chapters the importance of being able to access well written and relevant articles which authors have written to disseminate various forms of evidence. This could be the outcomes of a research study or a systematic review of the literature, or in some cases a report of an education development and its usefulness for others.

There are a large number of journals available which are either country based e.g. **Nursing Standard** or international, e.g. **Journal of Clinical Nursing**. Each of these will have their own guidelines for authors as well as other specific information that will help authors to publish their work.

Some journals have specific sections where students can publish their reflections of practice, for example the **Nursing Standard** has a section entitled 'Student experiences in the real world of nursing'. Here students can submit a short description/reflection in no more than 500 words an example of an experience from practice (information for students on a number of issues can be found at: **http://nursingstandard.rcnpublishing. co.uk/resources/studentlife/**).

There are key steps to consider when writing an article for publication. In Box 10.8 you can see those I have identified as important. In particular please note the importance of reading the author guidelines. An example of those for the **Nursing Standard** can be found at: **http://nursingstandard.rcnpublishing.co.uk/resources/articles/author.asp/** and

---

Box 10.8 Writing an article for publication: some key points

1. Decide on what you want to write about.

2. Decide on your target readership.

3. Choose the most appropriate journal.

4. Read the author guidelines.

5. Read some articles from the journal.

6. Decide on the type of article presentation which best suits your topic.

7. Plan your writing time-scale and evidence gathering.

8. Write the paper.

9. Ensure that you check the author guidelines again and that the article follows the right structure (e.g. research papers).

10. Check abstract covers the content of the paper.

11. Have the paper peer reviewed by a colleague for readability, clarity of content, grammar & typos.

12. Ensure all acknowledgements made to either funding body or someone who has helped you with developing /reading the paper.

13. Check the submission process—is it online for example?

14. Submit to the journal.

for **Nurse Education** in *Practice* at: http://www.elsevier.com/wps/find/journaldescription.cws_home/623062/authorinstructions/.

Heyman & Cronin (2005) and Devitt *et al.* (2007b) offer some guidance on how students can convert their academic assignments into a journal article.

An important issue that is highlighted in these and other papers is that of ensuring that the same paper is not submitted for publication elsewhere and also that if writing with someone else that all authors have agreed the order of authorship. It is also important to acknowledge the contribution that anyone who has not written any of the article but may involved in aspects of the work, such as reading it and offering comments or possibly involved in collecting data. It is not acceptable to submit the same paper to different journals at the same time, but if a paper is rejected by one journal it could then be reviewed and, using the new author guidelines, be revised for another journal.

Some of you may well have had feedback on your assignments and comments from tutors to say: 'this is an excellent piece of work—you should consider getting it published'(Sbaih 1999). It is important to remember that written work for an assignment is not what is required of a journal article, and that you will be required to make considerable adjustments to it, using the journal author guidelines, to prepare it for submission for publication. If you wish to pursue this consider discussing it with someone who has had experience of writing articles which have been published or if possible the editor of a journal.

EBP in action

Using one of your own assignments, especially one where you may have had feedback as above, consider what you would need to do to turn it into a publishable piece of work? If it is a reflective piece of work involving an experience in clinical practice, could part of it be used to submit to a journal such as the **Nursing Standard**? (See student experience section of 500 words.) Consider discussing your interest in publishing either an article or book review with a tutor who has experience of doing this.

The peer review process

Once you have submitted a paper however there is another process that you need to be familiar with, and that is the actual publishing side of publication, which also includes what is called the peer review process. Some journals do not have this for certain types of articles, such as short reports or reflective accounts. Being a peer-reviewed journal is of critical importance in terms of ensuring quality of the publication as well as enabling the journal editor to make a judgement of whether to accept a paper or not. This review process can be either an open review where the authors know who the author is or a blind peer-review (normally two reviewers) who will not know who they are. Most review-ers undertake the work in their 'free time' and do not receive payment for doing so. There is a time commitment involved but for most journals this is not onerous. Those who undertake this role are committed to developing the scholarship of their discipline and are usually experienced authors themselves. It is expected that a journal reviewer has some knowledge of the specialist field, e.g. orthopaedic nursing—if reviewing for the **Journal of Orthopaedic Nursing,** or have some other related skills and knowledge such as expertise in a specific research methodology.

There is an expectation that they offer constructive comments to authors, be willing to help them develop their papers for publication, and generally keep up to date with what is happening in the context of their discipline or specialist field. They also have to keep to deadlines for return of reviewed papers. If they are reviewers for an international journal they need to take account of the fact that for some authors English is not their first language and that any article they review needs to be understood by readers in different countries.

Generally feedback by the reviewers to editors requires a decision to be made as to the article's strengths and weaknesses and also its overall value to the body of knowledge of that discipline. Decisions made range from advising rejection to requesting major revi-sion, and it is very unusual for an article to be accepted without any revision at all.

Some examples of reviewer comments are.

- This is very difficult to read—the language very complicated.
- The structure needs further work—this could in fact be an assignment.
- It has exceeded the word limit.
- International readers will not be able to understand all the abbreviations and no explanations of the context of the paper offered (see Holland 2005).

So given all these issues why is writing for publication a good thing for student nurses to learn about and actually undertake themselves? Timmons & Park (2008) undertook a study to establish what the factors were that influenced whether stu-dents published their dissertations. Although there were sound reasons why gradu-ates did not publish, the main one being it was not a priority at the end of their degree programme, there was an overall feeling that there were benefits to it. These included personal gain in terms of enhancing their *curriculum vitae* (CV) and their careers but also supported a co-authorship role for the supervisor once the disser-tation had been completed. They considered a number of measures to ensure that submission for publication became a consideration of the programme: making it part of the assessed part of the course was one possibility and also including being made aware of the possibilities of writing for publication as part of the course timetable.

The students in the study had chosen topics where they wanted to know what the evidence base was and 'to evaluate a new practice such as nurses doing thrombolysis' (Timmons & Park 2008: 746).

Dissemination of research findings is the final stage in the research cycle and it could also lead to the beginning of new research questions. Dissemination and sharing of new knowledge from literature reviews can also lead to new developments and often illustrate the gap in evidence supporting nursing practice. This was highlighted in Professor Dame Jill Macleod Clark's presentation to the RCN Research Conference in 2009 (http://www.rcn.org.uk/development/researchanddevelopment/rs/research2009/keynotes/), and her key message focused on the need for more research into the outcomes and impact of nursing interventions, such as managing and preventing skin breakdown, the outcomes of which affect the quality of life for a patient.

Summary

This chapter has highlighted the importance of dissemination of evidence of all kinds and stressed the importance of student nurses both learning the actual skills involved in dissemination activities and also having the opportunity to actually participate and engage in various ways of doing so.

- Learning to present the outcomes of your studies as a student and also learning to write for publication will enable you to establish the foundation skills that are essential for dissemination in your professional career as a qualified nurse.

- Learning about the importance of dissemination will clearly help in understanding the importance of utilization of evidence in your practice, for without dissemination in its various forms there would not be the up-to-date evidence available to assure that your nursing interventions are evidence based.

■ *Online resource centre*

Remember that you can access the PowerPoint slides for Figs 10.1, 10.2 and 10.3 online as well as other online resources **www.oxfordtextbooks.co.uk/orc/holland/**

■ References

Albarran, J. (2007) Planning, developing and writing an effective conference abstract. *British Journal of Cardiac Nursing* 2 (11) 570–572.

Brookes, D. (2007) Why nurses do not disseminate academic coursework. *Nursing Times* 103 (12) 32–33. (**www.nursingtimes.net**)

Coad, J. & Devitt, P. (2007) Research dissemination: the art of writing an abstract for conferences, *Nurse Education in Practice* 6 112–116.

Coad, J., Devitt, P. & Hardicre, J. (2007) Ten steps to developing an abstract for conferences. *British Journal of Nursing* 16 (7) 396–397.

Cormack, D.F.S. (1994) *Writing for Health Care Professionals*. Oxford: Blackwell.

Devitt, P., Hardicre, J. & Coad, J. (2007a) Ten steps to getting your paper published in a professional journal. *British Journal of Nursing* 16 (5) 290–291.

Devitt, P., Coad, J. & Hardicre, J. (2007b) Ten steps to convert your assignment into a journal article. *British Journal of Nursing* 16 (5) 290–291.

Giminez, J. (2007) *Writing for Nursing and Midwifery Students*. Basingstoke: Palgrave Macmillan.

Halligan, P. (2008) Poster presentations: valuing all forms of evidence. *Nurse Education in Practice* 8 41–45.

Happell, B. (2007) Hitting the target! A no tears approach to writing an abstract for a conference presentation. *International Journal of Mental Health Nursing* 16 447–452.

Hardicre, J., Coad, J. & Devitt, P. (2007) Ten steps to successful poster presentation. *British Journal of Nursing* 16 (7) 398–401.

Hardicre, J., Coad, J. & Devitt, P. (2007) Ten steps to successful conference presentations. *British Journal of Nursing*, 16 (7) 402–404.

Heyman, B. & Cronin, P. (2005) Writing for publication: adapting academic work into articles. *British Journal of Nursing* 14 (7) 400–403.

Holland, K. (2005) Writing for an international readership *Nurse Education in Practice* 5 1–2.

Johnson, M. (1995) Writing a book review: towards a more critical approach. *Nurse Education Today* 15 228–231.

Johnson, M. (2007) Dissemination: ethics and aesthetics. In: Long, T. & Johnson, M. (eds) *Research Ethics in the Real World*. Edinburgh: Churchill Livingstone/Elsevier, 193–206.

Kinn, S. & Kenyon, M. (2002) Presentation skills workshops for nurses. *Nurse Education Today* 22 144–151.

Mulhall, A. & Le May, A. (1999) *Nursing Research: dissemination and implementation*. Edinburgh: Churchill Livingstone.

Newell, R. & Burnard, P. (2006) *Research for Evidence-Based Practice*. Oxford:Blackwell Publishing.

NHS Centre for Reviews and Dissemination (1999) *Getting Evidence into Practice: effective health care. University of York: NHS Centre for Reviews and Dissemination* 5 (1) 1–16.

Nursing and Midwifery Council (2004) Standards of proficiency for pre-registration nursing education. London: NMC.

O'Keeffe, M., Hills, A., Doyle, M., McCreadie, C. *et al.* (2007) *UK Study of Abuse and Neglect of Older People*. Prevalence survey report. London: National Centre for Social Research.

Sbaih, L. (1999) Helping student convert assignments into articles: tips for teachers. *Accident & Emergency Nursing* 7 112–113.

Tierney-Wigg, S. (2009) The student experience of NETNEP 2008: a personal reflection. *Nurse Education in Practice* 9 (2) 84–85.

Timmons, S. & Park, J. (2008) A qualitative study of the factors influencing the submissions for publication of research undertaken by students. *Nurse Education Today* 28 744–750.

Utecht, C. & Tremayne, P. (2008) Using poster presentations in nursing education. *Nursing Times* 104 26–7 (www.nursingtimes.net/).

Whithead, D. (2002) The academic writing experiences of a group of student nurses: a phenomenological study. *Journal of Advanced Nursing* 38 (5) 498–506.

Further reading

Oermann, M. H. (2002) *Writing for Publication in Nursing*. Philadelphia: Lippincott Williams & Wilkins.

Newell, R. (2000) Writing academic papers: the clinicale effectiveness in nursing experience. *Clinical Effectiveness in Nursing* 4 93–98.

Useful websites

Centre for Reviews and dissemination:

http://www.york.ac.uk/inst/crd/projects/getting_evidence_into_practice.htm/

Writing for Publication workshop:

http://www.science.ulster.ac.uk/inr/groups/wwop/pdf/Kader_Parahoo.pdf/

Glossary of terms

A

Anonymity Principle in research ethics that individuals should not be identifiable by name or sufficient personal details to reveal their identity.

Audit A process of gathering data on performance or output that can be used to compare with a standard or previous audit measure. It is used to provide local information and cannot be generalized to other situations. It does not increase our understanding of a concept or topic and so is not research. Although, because of some of the tools used, e.g. patient questionnaires or observation check-lists, it can look similar.

B

Backward chaining Method of searching the literature where the references section of one article is used to find possible relevant articles that have been used by the author. In this way the search goes back through the literature from one article to another.

Bias This relates to any part of a study that creates a distortion in the results or the interpretation of the results. It is usually associated with the sample, but can be found in most of the parts of the research process.

Blinding In an experimental design, an attempt to conceal from those involved, who is in the experimental group and who is in the control group. This is also called 'masking'.

C

Case study Method of research that attempts to answer a question by studying the details of one individual or setting that is analysed in depth.

Clinical guidelines Principles of treatment covering certain diagnoses or health pro-

blems that are based on the best available evidence and therefore help practitioners make evidence-based decisions.

Confidentiality Principle in research ethics that ensures that personal details are not shared with others and that all data are kept securely to protect those in the sample.

Confounding variable In an experimental design, a variable present in the situation that can interfere with the assumed relationship between the independent and dependent variable due to its influence on the dependent variable.

Control group *See also* experimental group Participants in an experimental design who are compared to the experimental group on the same outcome measure to establish the success of an intervention or procedure.

Correlation A statistical relationship between variables that illustrates a pattern or association. The size and nature of the relationship is illustrated by the correlation coefficient.

Clinical effectiveness Involves the measurement, monitoring, and improvement of care and determines whether an intervention is effective or not.

Critique/critiquing (as in an article) A critical review. Making a judgement about the value or quality of a written piece of work against a set of criteria.

Cross-sectional studies Descriptive study design, such as a survey, that involves collecting data from several sub-groups at one point in time rather than following a single group over time, e.g. nursing students in different academic years.

D

Data collection Part of the research process where the researcher applies the research tool to gather data.

Dependent variable   This is the variable that forms the outcome measure of a study. This usually forms the focus of a study, such as level of pain.

Descriptive research   A category of research where the purpose is to paint a picture of a situation in numbers or words, allowing a clear and accurate representation to emerge.

Descriptive statistics   Statistical processes that allow the findings of a study to be summarized and described in easily assimilated and useful ways, such as giving the mean (average) of a variable for the group.

Dissertation   A piece of written work which describes a researcher's actual study or a piece of work which follows a similar process, undertaken at the end of a degree programme. This is sometimes known as 'desk top' research where material is gathered from a range of published resources and the structure follows that of a 'research study'.

Dross   Information, often in a qualitative study, that is not relevant to the main focus and outcome of the research.

Emic   The insider's view (such as a research participant) and a discription of a situation.

Empirical/empirical evidence   Information gathered in the everyday world using measurements assessed through the senses.

Ethics   The code of practice followed by researchers to ensure the protection of individuals involved in studies. This relates to such principles as doing good and avoiding harm; protecting the human rights of the individual, including the decisions about taking part in a study under informed consent; treating everyone fairly; protecting the identity of those involved in studies and gaining approval from an ethics committee (LREC) set up to protect the individual's human rights and safety, and control the actions of researchers.

Ethics committees   Committees which consider the ethical considerations of a research study, such as safety of the participants and

researcher, protection of vulnerable participants and obtaining informed consent

Etic   This is the opposite of the 'emic' view and is that of the outsider (such as the researcher).

Evidence   Information that provides a confirmation or support for sound (clinical) judgements.

Experimental design   Quantitative method of research used to identify the existence of cause and effect relationships between variables. Usually consists of an experimental group and a control group.

Experimental group   *See also* **control group** Participants in an experimental design who receive the independent variable, usually in the form of a treatment or intervention. The outcome measure or dependent variable is then compared to the outcomes from a control group.

Ethnography   A study which describes a culture, where the researcher or ethnographer normally 'lives with' or participates in activities related to that cultural group. They record their observations and communications with the group in various ways, such as field notes (notes whilst observing) tape recorders or sometimes video diaries.

Forward chaining   Similar to backward chaining but instead of using the references section of an article and going back in time, databases are used to find 'similar articles' or 'cited by' to take the search forward to possibly relevant articles that have appeared on the same topic since a particular article was published.

Focus group   A small group who volunteer to be asked questions about a particular topic in qualitative research—representative of the community/group being studied.

Generalizability   The ability to apply the findings from one study and be reasonably confident they will apply to other similar situations.

Hierarchy of evidence   A rank order of evidence listing what are considered to be more trustworthy forms of evidence at the top and less accurate ones towards the bottom. This is a controversial view and not everyone agrees with its application.

Historical research   Research which involves analysis of past events, records or accounts and draws conclusions from these and also considers relevance to present day.

Hypothesis   Researcher's prediction or expectation concerning the relationship between variables in a study.

Inferential statistics   Statistical techniques that allow 'inferences' or assumptions to be made about the larger population of interest based on the findings of the sample in a current study. This does require the way the sample was selected to follow some strict rules to ensure that they are closely representative.

Interactionism   Approach from sociology that is based on a way of looking at the world and how people interact using symbols in order to communicate with one another and establish meaning. Sometimes known as symbolic interactionism.

Inter-observer (rater) reliability   The extent to which different observers agree when observing the same event or variable. Inter-rater reliability is a term used to describe the same situation.

Interpretative research   A qualitative approach that attempts to understand phenomena through attempting to understand the meanings those involved in a study assign to them—e.g. how they make sense of their lives and their world.

Interviews   A type of conversation between the researcher and participant (interviewee) using a series of set questions or in what is known as an open-ended interview, possibly one very broad question or statement which then allows the participant to present their 'story'.

Likert scales   Developed by the American psychologist Rensis Likert, this is a scale designed to measure attitude or opinion through a respondent's level of agreement with statements in a questionnaire. Options usually ranging along five alternatives from 'strongly agree' to 'strongly disagree'.

Literature review   See review of the literature.

Masking   See Blinding.

Mean, median, mode   These are all used in descriptive statistics to provide a measure of what is 'typical' in the group. In everyday use we talk about the 'average' which follows a similar idea.

Narrative   Data in the form of a long written description or story provided by someone.

Non-participant observation   Direct observation by the researcher who does not interact with those being observed.

Observation   Systematic method of data collection, watching, and recording behaviour or events. Can be used in both quantitative and qualitative studies, although the form of observation will be different.

Operational definition   Description of the way a concept is being measured in a study, e.g. pain using a 10 point pain scale.

Paradigm   This is the view of research held by the researcher and can be divided broadly into a quantitative view: where the main purpose is to concentrate on accurate measurement and relationships between variables, and a qualitative view: where the purpose is to present the view of the world through the eyes of those involved in an interpretative way. A paradigm refers to a world view that affects the way people see things, e.g. nursing paradigm refers to a shared understanding of what is meant by nursing—it is a 'taken for granted' view that we all share the same understanding of what nursing is; however we may use a nursing theory to help us understand what nursing is from a specific perspective.

Participant   An individual taking part in a study. A more polite term than 'subject'.

Participant observer   Researcher who gathers data while being a member of the group being observed.

Peer-reviewed journals   Journals that try to set a standard on the quality of the articles published by having these scrutinized by experts in the field before they are published.

Phenomenon   Element or focus that forms the subject of the research. In qualitative research it replaces the word 'variable' used in quantitative studies.

PICO   An acronym that stands for Patient Intervention Comparison group, and Outcome measure. It was developed to make it easier to develop reviews of the literature that would take into account all the essential elements that are needed to determine best practice.

Pilot study   This is a mini version of a study used to check the accuracy of the tool of data collection and to ensure that any practical problems with data collection are identified before the main study begins.

Plagiarism   Taking or copying someone else's work or words and presenting it as your own.

Positivist approach or paradigm   Positivism is a belief about the nature of research that emphasizes the objective nature of the information gathered through the human senses that is 'factual', and helps to establish laws or principles that apply generally rather than depending on human interpretation and limited to the research setting where they took place. It concentrates on measurement

and relationships between variables, often referred to as the 'scientific' approach to research.

Power calculation   A method of calculating the sample size needed in a study to ensure that statistical analyses are accurate and will detect real differences or relationships between the variables or outcome measures.

Primary reference   An original source of work that has been directly accessed. *See also* Secondary reference.

Primary source of evidence   The original study written by the researcher(s) responsible for collecting the data, as opposed to secondary sources, which are reports by others of primary studies, for example, a review of the literature or summary of someone's research that may have 'filtered' the research to some extent.

Prospective study   Research design where data are collected from a particular time and date onwards. The data collection period is in the future, as opposed to the past as in a retrospective study.

Purposive sampling   A method of selecting a sample by 'hand-picking' those who represent a typical cross-section of the group of interest to the researcher. This is based on the researcher's knowledge of what is typical in such a group.

Quantitative research approach   A way of designing research where the emphasis is on measurement and the search for relationships between variables in order to answer a hypothesis or describe what is known through this measurement.

Qualitative research approach   A way of collecting in-depth 'rich' data following the rules and principles of this approach. There is an emphasis on preserving the views of individuals and using flexible methods of data collection to ensure the results match the original situation as closely as possible. The aim is to gather insights and understandings of a phenomenon.

Quasi-experimental design Design where the researcher introduces an intervention and makes a comparison with a group that does not receive the intervention, but there is no randomization of the sample. This limits the interpretation of the result. No cause and effect relationship can be demonstrated as there may be factors already existing in the two groups responsible for variations in the outcomes.

R

Random allocation or assignment A systematic method of allocating those in an experimental study to either the experimental or control group where everyone has an equal chance of being in either group. This is to reduce bias between the groups.

Randomized Control Trial (RCT) Method of conducting research involving, usually, an experimental group and a control group. It is regarded as a 'scientific' method as it allows conclusions to be made concerning the existence of 'cause and effect' relationships.

Reactive effect The way individuals in a study may change their behaviour in a positive way because of their inclusion in a study rather than as a consequence of the intervention.

Refereed articles/peer-reviewed articles These are articles that have been judged by experts as worthy of publication for a particular journal. They often include the wording 'this article has been subject to double-blind review, to indicate this.

Reliability This relates to the accuracy or consistency of the tool of data collection and is an important criterion for the collection of sound and accurate data.

Research aim The statement(s) of intent which stresses the outcome of the research and derived from the research question or hypothesis (see Hypothesis).

Research approach or research strategy See qualitative research approach and quantitative research approach.

Research design The research design is the category or type of research plan followed by the researcher such as 'survey' or 'experimental' design. Each follows certain principles and serves a specific research purpose.

Research governance This is a broad set of criteria or standards that are there to ensure that research continually achieves and improves its quality.

Research method This is the method of collecting research data in a study. It describes the tool(s) of data collection used. Examples include questionnaires, interviews, or observation.

Research problem An area of practice which requires further examination in order to provide an evidence base.

Research process The stages of a research study broken down into the major steps the researcher follows in carrying it out. Can be referred to as the Research design.

Research proposal The (written) outline of a study constructed in the planning stage by the researcher. It is used to seek permission and ethical approval for the study. Each of the key stages of the study are outlined to allow judgements to be made on the justification for the study and the decisions made for the approach that will be taken throughout the study.

Research question This is the question which directs the researcher in their study and which also directs the research approach to be followed.

Retrospective study A study where the data already exist at the start of the study and the researcher gathers the data from the past through experiences, or records.

Review of the literature See also Systematic review This is a careful conducted examination of published work that can help answer a specific question. The review should be based on good quality information and should include the writer's views on the information.

Rigour The extent to which the researcher has attempted to produce high quality research. This is achieved by demonstrating they were aware of possible problem areas in the study and have tried to reduce them as far as was possible. NB Rigour is spelt here in its UK form and care should be taken to avoid the US spelling of 'rigor' in UK based work.

Role modelling   Basing personal and/or professional behaviour on what others do, in the context of a student nurse this would be considered to be based on the good practice of a qualified nurse.

Sample   A proportion of those in the total group in whom the researcher is interested.

Sample inclusion and exclusion criteria   To ensure that a sample matches (represents) the main study population as closely as possible: the researcher should identify, inclusion criteria; that is those desirable characteristics that would make the sample resemble the study population, and exclusion criteria; that is those characteristics that are undesirable and unrepresentative, or that might be a danger to those taking part in a study.

Sampling frame   A list of those to be included in a study where each 'unit' is given a number. The list is used in conjunction with a table of random numbers or computer generated numbers to select those included in a study or allocated to a particular group. The method demonstrates an absence of researcher bias.

Sampling strategy   The method used by the researcher to select individuals (things or events) to be included in a study.

Search engines   An information retrieval system in the form of a website that will search for articles or information from a variety of sources on the web.

Secondary reference   Work by one author that is mentioned or cited in the work of another author but that is not directly accessed.

Secondary source of evidence   See primary source of evidence.

Selection bias   In sampling where those included in a study do not represent those in the larger group because of the way they were selected or criteria used to search for eligible individuals.

Seminal work   These are studies from which other studies have grown. They are the ones usually referred to in studies as the classic work that still has relevance, e.g. Ervin Goffman's work on asylums.

Semi-structured interview   An interview which uses a set of questions which can be added to in a flexible way at each interview, but the main set of questions are set for all participants to ensure some degree of consistency across all the participants in relation to the required information.

Social desirability   Element in data collection where individuals may give an inaccurate response to questions based on their desire to be seen in a positive light by the researchers. Answers will tend to be influenced by socially approved values or standards, e.g. sensible drinking limits.

Source   Used as a verb 'to source' and describe the process of locating, obtaining or tracking down a supply of information. This is usually published literature, such as articles, statistical information, or policy documents. All of these need to be 'sourced' from a reliable location.

Statistical analysis   Systematic method of analysing data from quantitative studies to describe or interpret numeric outcomes.

Study population   Those people, things, or events the researcher wants to say something about or explore.

Survey   Research approach designed to collect information from a large sample to give a general picture of a situation. Usually involves questionnaires or interviews.

Systematic review of the literature   A form of review of the literature utilizing a specific method of searching and retrieving evidence which is then critically analysed and used to ensure that decisions are then based on the best available evidence, e.g. clinical guidelines.

Timeframe   The period of time covered by a review of literature.

Triangulation   The use of more than one tool of data collection or research approach, etc.

It is used to answer a research question from different aspects to try to increase the accuracy of the results.

Transcribing   Process of transferring audio recordings of interviews into a written format as accurately as possible.

Trustworthiness   In qualitative research, a general term to indicate how much confidence we can have in the accuracy of the findings. This uses a variety of ways to ensure for instance, that findings are believable, can be confirmed and may relate to other settings.

Validity   The extent to which the information collected in as study has measured what it was intended to collect, for instance the extent to which the frequency that someone washes their hands has actually been measured rather than the guesses made by individuals of the frequency.

Variable   This is the focus of the researcher's interest and is the concept that varies, such as pain level, or experience of chronic pain. In experimental studies variables can be divided into *dependent variables*, and *independent variables*.

Vignettes   This is a short 'story' or scenario which may derive from an actual experience or event from practice which is then used as way of obtaining views and perceptions of participants about what is taking place or what they would do if faced with a similar situation. They can also be used to determine people's beliefs on sensitive topics.

INDEX